Aging Skin

CLINICAL DERMATOLOGY

Series Editor

ALAN R. SHALITA, M.D.

Professor and Chairman
Department of Dermatology
State University of New York
Health Science Center at Brooklyn
Brooklyn, New York

1. Cutaneous Investigation in Health and Disease: Noninvasive Methods and Instrumentation, *edited by Jean-Luc Lévêque*
2. Irritant Contact Dermatitis, *edited by Edward M. Jackson and Ronald Goldner*
3. Fundamentals of Dermatology: A Study Guide, *Franklin S. Glickman and Alan R. Shalita*
4. Aging Skin: Properties and Functional Changes, *edited by Jean-Luc Lévêque and Pierre G. Agache*
5. Retinoids: Progress in Research and Clinical Applications, *edited by Maria A. Livrea and Lester Packer*

ADDITIONAL VOLUMES IN PREPARATION

Clinical Photomedicine, *edited by Henry W. Lim and Nicholas A. Soter*

Oxidative Stress in Dermatology, *edited by Jürgen Fuchs and Lester Packer*

Cutaneous Antifungal Agents: Selected Compounds in Clinical Practice and Development, *edited by John W. Rippon and Robert A. Fromtling*

Aging Skin

Properties and Functional Changes

edited by

Jean-Luc Lévêque

L'Oréal
Aulnay-sous-Bois, France

Pierre G. Agache

University Hospital
Besançon, France

Marcel Dekker, Inc.   **New York • Basel • Hong Kong**

Library of Congress Cataloging-in-Publication Data

Aging skin : properties and functional changes / edited by Jean-Luc
    Lévêque, Pierre Agache.
        p.   cm.—(Clinical dermatology ; 4)
    Includes bibliographical references and index.
    ISBN 0-8247-8791-9 (alk. paper)
    1. Skin—Aging.   I. Lévêque, Jean-Luc.   II. Agache, Pierre.
III. Series.
    [DNLM: 1. Skin Aging—physiology.   W1 CL69L v.4 / WR 102 A267]
QP88.5A375   1993
612.7'9—dc20
DNLM/DLC
for Library of Congress   92-48688
                                                                             CIP

This book is printed on acid-free paper.

MARCEL DEKKER, INC.
270 Madison Avenue, New York, New York 10016

Current printing (last digit):
10 9 8 7 6 5 4 3 2 1

PRINTED IN THE UNITED STATES OF AMERICA

Series Introduction

During the past decade there has been a vast explosion in new information relating to the art and science of dermatology as well as fundamental cutaneous biology. Furthermore, this information is no longer of interest only to the small but growing specialty of dermatology. Scientists from a wide variety of disciplines have come to recognize both the importance of skin in fundamental biological processes and the broad implications of understanding the pathogenesis of skin disease. As a result there is now a multidisciplinary and world-wide interest in the progress of dermatology.

With these factors in mind, we have undertaken a new series of books specifically oriented to dermatology. The series will be purposely broad in focus and will range from pure basic science to practical, applied clinical dermatology. Thus, while there will be something for everyone, all editions in the series should ultimately prove to be valuable additions to the dermatologist's library.

The latest addition to the series, by Jean-Luc Lévêque and Pierre Agache, is a worthwhile and excellent addition. Other volumes, including a comprehensive clinical review of acne, an introductory dermatology text, and a review of clinical application of the retinoids, are planned and will appear in the near future.

I sincerely hope that you will enjoy reading these books as much as I have enjoyed planning them with the authors and editors of this series.

Alan R. Shalita
SUNY Downstate Medical Center
Brooklyn, New York

Foreword

The past decade has brought an enormously increased awareness of skin aging as a legitimate but neglected area of research and therapeutics. More than a half-dozen texts are now devoted to the subject, and virtually all new editions of the leading textbooks in dermatology and geriatrics have added chapters on this previously invisible subspeciality. Skin-aging symposia are now regularly organized around the world, with intended audiences ranging up to several thousand health professions and/or researchers. Public and private research funding for cutaneous gerontology has grown to many millions of dollars annually, and development of agents that prevent, reverse, or symptomatically improve age-associated skin changes has acquired a high priority at many forward-looking pharmaceutical and cosmetics firms.

In the rapidly approaching twenty-first century, it is estimated that fully 20% of the population in the developed nations of the world will be aged 65 years or older. Those aged 85 years and older are already the fastest growing segment of these societies. Skin changes, both physiologic and pathologic, figure prominently among the medical and psychosocial problems to be faced. There is thus an urgent need to define these problems and to develop quantitative measures of their severity.

The present volume comprises 21 chapters by acknowledged world authorities on the assessment of aging skin by noninvasive techniques. These authors provide comprehensive in-depth and up-to-date reviews of topics ranging from the mechanical properties of aged and photoaged skin, cutaneous vasculature and vasoreactivity, and physical and biochemical surface characteristics, to permeability and barrier function. There is a strong and appropriate focus on methodology, with most chapters providing definitions of terms often misunderstood by the nonexpert and including when appropriate their mathematical derivations. A particular strength is the thorough discussion of the limitations of available methodologies and acknowledgment of controversies. Data interpretation, particularly as related to cutaneous physiology, is better accomplished in some areas than others, but overall the interested reader receives far more assistance in this regard than from other available references.

In brief, this concise text provides an optimistic but rigorous assessment of the noninvasive techniques now available to assess skin aging. It is also an excellent single-source summary of recent data. One cannot help being impressed by the progress that has been made in the past 10 years and by the additional advances undoubtedly awaiting us in the coming decade. Dr. Lévêque and Professor Agache are to be congratulated not only on their own original contributions to the field, well reviewed in this text, but on creating a masterful overview of this complex area.

Barbara A. Gilchrest
Professor and Chairman
Department of Dermatology
Boston University School of Medicine
Boston, Massachusetts

Preface

At first glance skin aging looks like a morphological phenomenon, a change in outer aspect. That is true mostly for exposed body areas but also for covered areas. Accordingly, any analysis of skin aging should start with a morphological, eventually semiquantitative description, which would permit a certain classification to be made.

However, a major part of the visible alterations associated with skin aging reflects functional changes, that is, modifications in the behavior of various tissue components within the skin. For example, the emergence of deeper furrowing and wrinkling is related to a mechanical failure as shown by loss of tension and elasticity. The complexion is altered in relation to changes in skin vasculature. The reduction in the water-holding capacity of stratum corneum and its subsequent dryness also influence the general aspect of the skin. These phenomena and others that do not appear visually, such as changes in sweating capacity or sebaceous secretion, also contribute to the behavior and/ or pathology of skin aging.

Our goal in planning this book was to present some of the modifications of the skin linked to aging, quantitatively assessed by noninvasive methods in vivo.

In the 1970s, visual descriptions of skin changes were strikingly precise, whereas evaluations of functional alterations were somewhat vague since the terminology used was imprecise. Toward the end of the 1970s techniques enabling the characteristics of the human skin to be assessed directly became available. In addition, because they were noninvasive, quantitative, and suitable for routine use, they permitted necessary statistical methods to be applied to the results. The first studies of skin aging based on these methods began to be published during the same period, and we believe that an overview of the data obtained is now justified.

This book could not have been written without the collaboration of a large number of specialists, most of whom were pioneers in the use of noninvasive methods; some are friends, but we express our gratitude to all those who participated in any way.

Population aging in the developed countries is not simply a socioeconomic problem. There is also the question of the social status of the elderly, which depends on cultural criteria, themselves affected by the excessive individualism of an increasingly materialistic society.

Self-esteem is strongly conditioned by the way others see us, and this is all the more important in the relationship between individuals of different generations. As a result, dermatology and cosmetology have special roles to play. This is the major driving force behind research into skin aging—an ongoing effort in which this book is only one step.

Jean-Luc Lévêque
Pierre Agache

Contents

Contents

Contributors

H. Adhoute, Ph.D. Director, Laboratoire d'Explorations Fonctionnelles Cutanées, Clinique Dermatologique, Hopital Hôtel Dieu, Marseille, France

Aude Agache, M.D. Department of Functional Dermatology, University Hospital, Besançon, France

Pierre G. Agache, M.D. Professor, Department of Dermatology and Venerology, and Head, Department of Functional Dermatology, University Hospital, Besançon, France

Roland Bazin Chef de Service, Department of Biophysics, L'Oréal, Chevilly-Larue, France

Enzo Berardesca, M.D. Associate Professor, Department of Dermatology, University of Pavia, Pavia, Italy

P. Berbis, M.D. Assistant, Department of Dermatology, Hopital Hôtel Dieu, Marseille, France

Andreas J. Bircher, M.D.   Department of Dermatology, University of Basel, Basel, Switzerland

Pierre Corcuff   Research Engineer, Department of Biophysics, L'Oréal, Aulnay-sous-Bois, France

Olivier de Lacharrière, M.D.   Department of Biophysics, L'Oréal, Aulnay-sous-Bois, France

Jean de Rigal, Ph.D.   Department of Biophysics, L'Oréal, Aulnay-sous-Bois, France

Brigitte Faivre, M.D.   Dermatologist, Department of Functional Dermatology, University Hospital, Besançon, France

Gary L. Grove, Ph.D.   Vice President of Research and Development, K.G.L.'s Skin Study Center, Broomall, Pennsylvania

Richard H. Guy, Ph.D.   Professor, Department of Pharmacy and Pharmaceutical Chemistry, School of Medicine, University of California—San Francisco, School of Medicine, San Francisco, California

Albert M. Kligman, M.D., Ph.D.   Professor, Department of Dermatology, University of Pennsylvania, Philadelphia, Pennsylvania

Jean-Luc Lévêque, Ph.D.   Director, Department of Biophysics, L'Oréal, Aulnay-sous-Bois, France

Alain Lucas, M.D., Ph.D.   Department of Functional Dermatology, University Hospital, Besançon, France

Howard I. Maibach, M.D.   Professor, Department of Dermatology, University of California—San Francisco, School of Medicine, San Francisco, California

R. Marks, M.D., Ph.D.   Professor, Department of Dermatology, University of Wales College of Medicine, Cardiff, Wales

Jean Mignot, Ph.D.   Professor, Laboratoire de Métrologie des Interfaces Techniques, Institut Universitaire de Technologie, Besançon, France

G. E. Piérard, M.D., Ph.D.   Department of Dermatopathology, University of Liège, Liège, Belgium

Y. Privat, M.D.   Director, Department of Dermatology, Hopital Hôtel Dieu, Marseille, France

Kathleen V. Roskos, Ph.D.   Research Chemist, Controlled Release and Biochemical Polymers Department, SRI International, Menlo Park, California

Terence John Ryan, M.D., F.R.C.P.   Department of Dermatology, Churchill Hospital, Oxford, England

D. Saint-Léger   Research Engineer, Department of Applied Biology, L'Oréal, Clichy, France

Jørgen Serup, M.D., Ph.D.   Assistant Professor, Bioengineering and Skin Research Laboratory, Bispebjerg Hospital, University of Copenhagen, Copenhagen, Denmark

Klaus P. Wilhelm, M.D.   Departments of Dermatology, Medical University of Lübeck, Lübeck, Germany, and University of California—San Francisco, School of Medicine, San Francisco, California

Yang Xie, Ph.D.   Laboratoire de Biophysique Cutanée, Faculté de Médicine, Besançon, France

Aging Skin

1

Aged Skin: Clinical Signs and Methodologic Aspects

PIERRE G. AGACHE and BRIGITTE FAIVRE

University Hospital
Besançon, France

I. INTRODUCTION

For ages, humankind has attempted to retard the deleterious effect of years on the skin: "retarder des ans l'irréparable outrage," wrote the French dramatist Racine in *Athalie* (Act II, Scene 5, Verse 496). That the damage could not be fully repaired was evident; That it could be partly amended was a belief that over the centuries steadily encouraged the use of cosmetics. Cosmetic use is an understandable expression of the importance of skin beauty in many societies (1,2).

It was no small surprise recently when it was discovered that retinoic acid can reverse the signs of aging previously thought to be ineluctable, and moreover that ointments used as placebos can have a similar although less intense effect (3), supporting the belief that cosmetics are beneficial in delaying skin aging. The recent discoveries were possible only because clinical data were assessed scientifically, using statistics. These statistical techniques were originally developed mostly by psychologists for rating human behavior (4) and later by clinicians for assessing drug efficacy and such subjective symptoms as pain or conditions like acne or psoriasis.

When trying to use these techniques to assess the skin alterations associated with aging, we are first faced with the following question: are these

1

attempts of value when we have at our disposal an increasing array of objective biochemical and physical parameters that rely upon changes in skin structure and function rather than appearance only and accordingly give in-depth information and precise and reliable chemical or physical data? The following chapters discuss salient examples of such possibilities. Notwithstanding, how brilliant they may be, these physical techniques describe and measure only one aspect of skin aging that is not found in every person and often does not follow the same course as the skin overall, which is the end point of therapeutic or scientific research. Objective assessments cannot describe the diversity of skin aging. Furthermore, to be validated as reliable skin aging parameters, they must be comparable to an overall skin aging assessment.

If we assess skin by visual and tactile methods, we must realize that we are experiencing a psychosensorial phenomenon. First, exposed body areas are almost the sole concern of therapeutic research because of their psychological impact. These are the only areas seen by other people and even by the individual in front of a mirror. This is why skin aging is often synonymous with photodamage. Nevertheless, the study of covered areas is of utmost interest not only in fundamental research but also in helping to understand the complicated patterns of photodamage. Extracutaneous factors can influence judgment about an individual's age. Fatigue causes shadows around the eyes and increases skin laxity. Unusual worrying may increase the permanent contraction of facial muscles and make wrinkles more visible. Sweating, a good meal, smart clothing, or a ''young'' hairstyle can alter the apparent age of the face. An investigator trying to assess skin photodamage should be aware of such possible biases.

The main difficulty, however, is in the multiplicity of signs that together constitute aged skin. These are presented in Tables 1 through 4. Obviously senescence does not alter the skin similarly in all body regions. The damage depends on many factors, including the frequency and angle of solar exposure, the density of skin vasculature, and gross or subtle peculiarities in structure. Subareas can be isolated within the face, such as cheeks, forehead, temple, chin, and nose, that often age differently or at different rates (Fig. 1). Not all the signs of photodamage are seen in every area. Moreover, some lesions correspond to certain specific areas. The clinical parameters of aging should be selected according to the area to be studied.

The next difficulty to surmount is avoiding a misunderstanding of the phenomenon in question. The lists presented in Tables 1 through 4 are unclear for some categories that have not yet been analyzed and described by dermatologists because they have been considered ''normal.'' For example, ''yellow discoloration'' is quite imprecise and probably merges with Milian's *peau citréine* (lemonlike skin), which associates a *peau d'orange* phenomenon with

Table 1 Skin Alterations of the Face Associated with Aging

1. DIFFUSE LESIONS
   Coarse wrinkling (expression wrinkles)
   Fine wrinkling
   Yellow discoloration
   Peau d'orange
   Mottled hyperpigmentation
   Cutis rhomboidalis (leathery skin)
   Roughness and dryness (upon palpation)
   Laxity
   Thinness (atrophy)
   Diffuse elastoma
   Favre-Racouchot syndrome
   Telangiectasias
2. CIRCUMSCRIBED LESIONS
   Actinic keratoses
   Senile sebaceous adenoma
   Seborrheic warts
   Actinic lentigines
   Eyelid hidradenomas

Table 2 Skin Alterations of the Neck and Nape Associated with Aging

1. DIFFUSE LESIONS
   Coarse wrinkling
   Fine wrinkling
   Cutis punctata linearis colli (atrophy)
   Laxity
   Cutis rhomboidalis
   Diffuse elatoma (Dubreuilh)
   Favre-Racouchot syndrome
   Roughness and dryness (upon palpation)
   Erythrosis interfollicularis colli
   Mottled hyperpigmentation
   Telangiectasias
2. CIRCUMSCRIBED LESIONS
   Actinic keratoses
   Seborrheic warts
   Acrochordon (skin tags)
   Actinic lentigines

Table 3 Skin Alterations of Dorsum of Hands and Forearms Associated with Aging

1. DIFFUSE LESIONS
    Fine wrinkling
    Mottled hyperpigmentation
    Roughness and dryness (upon palpation)
    Laxity (through skin folding)
    Thinness (atrophy)
2. CIRCUMSCRIBED LESIONS
    Actinic keratoses
    Actinic lentigines
    Bateman's purpura
    Stellate spontaneous scars
    Guttate hypomelanosis

a yellow discoloration. The latter is also observed, however, in cutis rhomboidalis, diffuse elastoma, and Favre-Racouchot syndrome (5) and accordingly this term requires a more accurate description. Coarse wrinkling can apply to the wrinkles of expression that occur on the forehead, above the base of the nose, at the outer corners of the eyes (crow's-feet), and vertically on either side of the mouth. Not all of these wrinkles have the same depth or cosmetic importance, or even the same anatomic background. Accordingly the location of the wrinkles being investigated should be indicated. Fine wrinkling was described by Weiss et al. (6) as either "coarse, pebbly topog-

Table 4 Skin Alterations of Covered Body Areas Associated with Aging

1. DIFFUSE LESIONS
    Fine wrinkling
    Laxity (through skin folding)
    Thinness (atrophy)
    Roughness and dryness (upon palpation)
2. CIRCUMSCRIBED LESIONS
    Cherry angiomas
    Seborrheic keratoses (trunk)
    Mollusca pendula (groin and axilla)

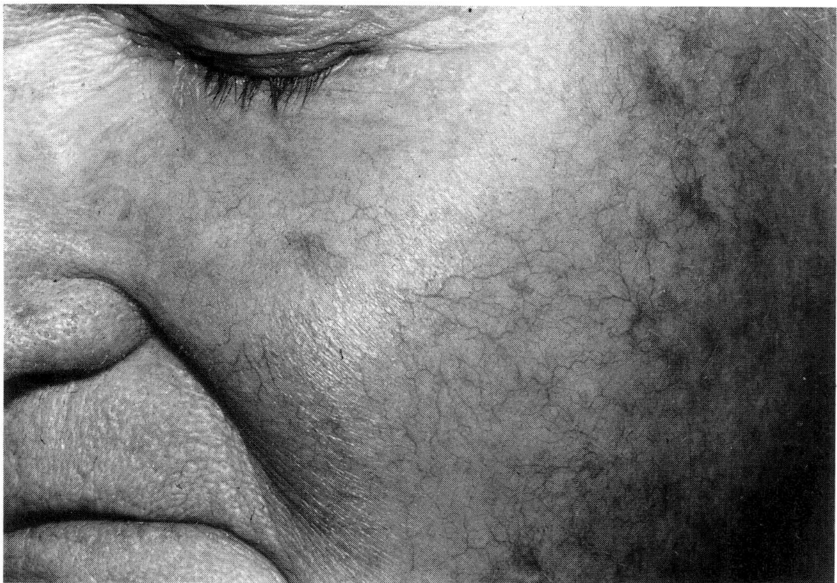

Figure 1 Female 66 years old. Different types of aging are seen on the upper lip (thick peau citréine skin) and cheek (thin atrophic skin with telangiectasias).

raphy'' or a ''shallow meshwork of indentations'' and was illustrated by photographs. There are other types of fine wrinkling, however, for example those associated with skin atrophy (7). In a fine description of ''smoker's face,'' Model referred to ''a subtle gauntness of the facial features with prominence of the underlying bony contours,'' giving ''a slight sinking of the cheeks'' and/or ''a plethoric slightly orange, purple, and red complexion'' (8). Clearly these descriptions, although detailed, merge with sun-induced alterations and need explanatory photographs at least to be used by other investigators.

Some clarification could be afforded by indicating the way the parameter is assessed (Fig. 2). For example, *laxity* (loss of tension or recoil) can be reliably assessed on the dorsum of the hands by lifting a fold of full-thickness skin about 1 cm above the surface for 1–2 s and then allowing the skin to recoil. The laxity is indicated by the duration of the fold.

In conclusion, apart from such typical lesions as telangiectasias and circumscribed alterations well known to dermatologists, there is a need for new and more precise analysis of most of the clinical parameters of aging skin so that a consensus might be reached on definitions and designations.

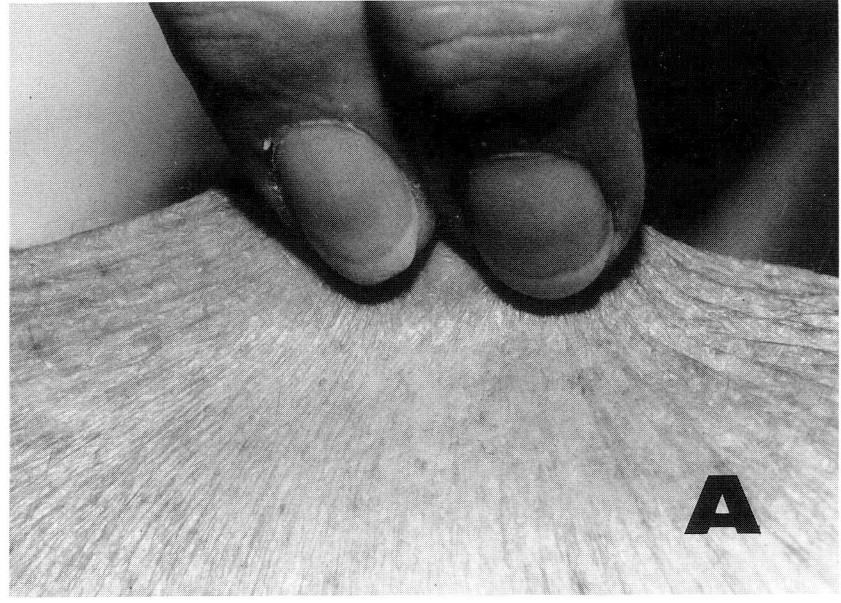

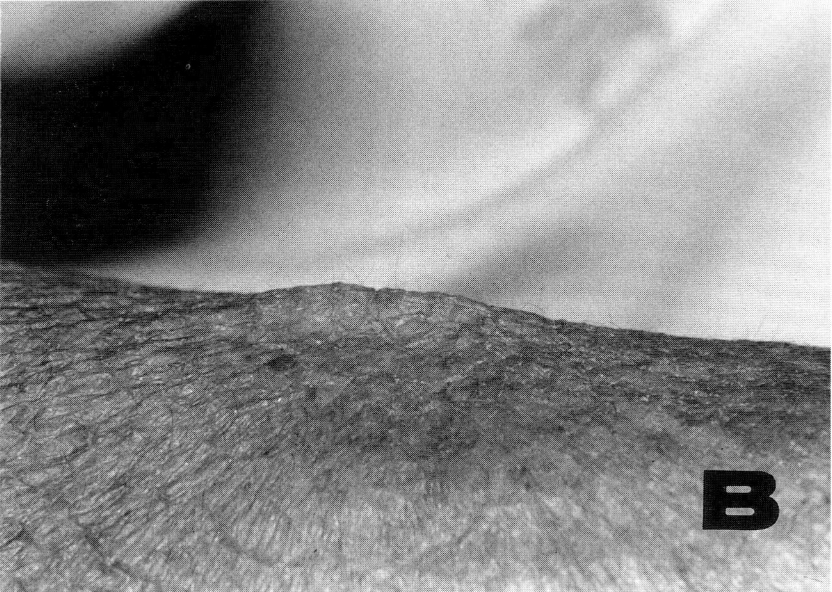

Figure 2 Clinical assessment of skin laxity: (A) lifting a skinfold; (B) delay in skin recoil.

II. ANALYTIC QUANTIFICATION OF SKIN AGING

Quantification of discrete or circumscribed lesions is by simple counting. Using this method, Misiewicz et al. (9) demonstrated the efficacy of retinoic acid derivatives on actinic keratoses. When lesions are numerous and small, however, it is often necessary to decide below what size a lesion should be ignored.

Alterations that cannot be counted because they are either too numerous or too diffuse should be evaluated semiquantitatively. Three types of scoring systems are available, which apply to specific situations and require different statistical procedures. These are usually referred to by statisticians as the nominal, ordinal, and interval scales (4).

Nominal scoring is the only way to assess data that are different in nature and consequently cannot be lumped together in a single scale. It uses words instead of figures. For example, the overall response of actinic keratoses to treatment is rated as worsening, no response, partial response, and complete response (9). The χ^2 test is the most common way of processing such samples.

Using words in a classification does not mean that the items are different in nature. For example, the side effects of topical tretinoin therapy can be recorded as none, mild, moderate, and severe (10). The words might have been replaced by 0, 1, 2, and 3, respectively, because it is the intensity of the same phenomenon that was assessed. Here we are dealing with an ordinal scale.

Such scales typically rank data that are of the same nature but of different intensity or degree and are used when the intervals between degrees are presumably different or the variation is obviously nonuniform. Leyden et al. (11) used a four-grade scale to rank the degree of improvement in overall skin aging following topical tretinoin treatment: much improvement, moderate improvement, slight improvement, and the same. An ordinal scale was also used by Misiewicz et al. for assessing erythema and scaling as a whole: none, minimal, moderate, and severe. Obviously the difference in intensity of the sign(s) between none and minimal is not the same as that between moderate and severe. Accordingly, only ranking was possible and no intermediate values could be allocated to the data. The statistical processing of ordinal scales uses non-parametric tests, such as the Mann-Whitney or Wilcoxon signed-rank test. These tests work with numbers or percentages of individuals, not with parameter values.

When assessing a clinical component of skin aging, one often has the feeling that the variation in a phenomenon—crow's feet, tactile roughness, and yellow discoloration, for example—among the general population or over a period of follow-up is continuous. Not only a ranking but a true, although subjective measurement can be attempted in such a situation using a continuous scale in which the possibilities of rating within the limits are infinite. Digital continuous scales are made up of a horizontal line graduated in equal intervals that represent an arbitrary unit of measurement and facilitate the assessment. On the other hand, statisticians stress the point that such scales favor the accumulation of data around the bars, which disrupts the random distribution of the data and invalidates the scale for further parametric statistics. Recently the analog continuous scale has been used. This is simply a horizontal line, usually 10 cm long, without graduation, on which the investigator places a mark corresponding to the estimated value of the parameter. The distance to the minimum end is then taken as the measurement.

Using an analog scale, Grove et al. (12) were able to compare visual and profilometric assessments of crow's-feet in 22 subjects aged 24–64 years. Some discrepancies were found for low wrinkle grades for which the authors believed the visual assessment was better. Lever et al. (10) successfully assessed the individual signs of photoaging on a 0–10 visual analog scale in 20 subjects treated on one side by tretinoin, the other side serving as control. By week 12 the difference between the two sides was highly significant. In 1988, we conducted a similar experiment in 12 subjects aged 41–91 years. Although the sample was very small, we obtained significant results (Table 5) (13).

Weinstein et al., in assessing the components of skin aging, collected data through an ordinal scale and then processed them as if the scale were continuous. This was because there is no clear-cut demarcation between the two types of scales. Strictly speaking, a scale on which only grade (or half-grade) values are given to individual data is discontinuous and consequently should

Table 5 Results of Tretinoin Treatment of Fine Wrinkles of Face[a]

Day	Tretinoin	Vehicle	Difference
0	733	735	−2
30	692	712	−20[b]
60	700	729	−29[b]
90	710	747	−37[b]
120	717	768	−51[b]
150	694	749	−55[b]
180	745	769	−24[b]

[a]Fine wrinkles on the face in 12 subjects treated on one side by tretinoin and on the other side by vehicle only, at random. Mean scores (0–10 visual analog scale) × 100.
[b]$p < 0.05$.

be considered a ranking, not a real measurement. In fact, Weinstein et al., when breaking this rule, were probably right because the variation they observed was continuous in nature and the sample sizes were more than 30. In their work, each of eight components of aging was separately classified into 10 grades (0–9), and only grade values were given. Each sample mean score was calculated, and the differences with time and between samples were evaluated by parametric statistics.

When using a discontinuous scale, the number of grades should be related to the maximum sensitivity of the investigator's judgment; otherwise, intermediate values are thought necessary. Also, when the number of grades increases within the same range, the scale approaches a continuous scale insofar as the length of the interval between grades is reduced to the limit of sensitivity of a continuous scale. In this case, the two scales are somewhat similar in precision although they are mathematically different. This is shown in the Grove et al. study on crow's-feet. These authors found a high correlation ($r = 0.94$) between a five-grade discontinuous scale and an analog scale. The only discrepancy arose with subjects over 60 years who were either overrated (assigned grade 5 instead of 4) by the discontinuous scale or underrated by the analog scale. The latter seemingly gave a crisper evaluation but a greater coefficient of variation (55% compared to 46% as recalculated from the data). When the two scorings were compared with the mean depth of wrinkles (R_z) as measured by optical profilometry of replicas, the correlation coefficient with R_z was better for the results by digital scale ($r = 0.85$ instead of 0.79, as recalculated from data). No conclusion can be drawn owing to the small size of the sample (22 subjects), but this work and the remarkable epidemiologic studies done on crow's-feet among smokers (14,15) show the precision of well-used and well-designed discontinuous scales.

In summary, the first step in selecting the appropriate scale is to examine the nature of the data. Are they categorical and not convertible into figures? A nominal scale should be used. If they are of the same nature and vary in degree but the variation is not uniform and it is not possible to find equally distanced grades, a ranking should be used, that is, an ordinal scale. When data are identical in nature and vary in intensity and the variation appears continuous and uniform—that is, amenable to equally distanced milestones over the range of the variation—then measurement is possible using a continuous (interval) scale.

Whatever the type of scale, the second step is to raise the power of the assessment, that is, to achieve the maximum chance to differentiate the present set of data from another set if such a difference exists. This includes using (preferably) continuous scales rather than ordinal scales and ordinal scales rather than nominal scales to take advantage of all available information and avoid spoiling the data. Selection often requires thorough discussion because the limits of each scale type are somewhat blurred.

Another fundamental step is to increase the power of separation within the range of measurement by increasing the number of ranks in ordinal scales or decreasing the size of intervals in digital continuous scales as much as possible. The limits of such an attempt are the sensitivity and the reproducibility of the assessment. Both are increased if the ends of the scales and also grades are clearly defined by photographs and explanations, as seen in Weinstein et al. and Grove et al. The human eye is remarkably efficient in perceiving and scoring differences between two pictures observed simultaneously. Accordingly, for assessing a topical treatment, it is advisable whenever possible to treat one side of the body, the other side serving as control. Studies done in this way achieved results with smaller samples (10, 13).

Results recorded by trained observers are always crisper and less variable. The variability is also reduced when two or more observers' ratings are averaged, if they are not statistically different (16).

Finally, the accuracy of the measurements depends on the data themselves. A clinical sign, such as wrinkling or yellowness, is always heterogeneous: it is the result of several phenomena weighed differently among individuals. Reducing the heterogeneity facilitates the rating and increases its sensitivity. Hence a single body area or subarea should preferably be examined in a single scale. Observing one sign also gives more precise and reliable results. This poses the problem of global aging assessment.

III. QUANTIFICATION OF GLOBAL SKIN AGING

Skin aging as well as overall photodamage cannot be reduced to the sum of the individual components because of their different weights not only in senile or sun-damaged skin but also among normal subjects. For example, a 50% increase in the amount of telangiectasia does not have the same influence on the visual appearance of the skin as a 50% increase in fine wrinkling. Also, phenomena other than sun damage may influence the apparent age, for example the loss of adipose tissue that is the primary cause of cheek sagging. Preservation of the cheek fatty pad in contrast helps keep a younger face over decades by maintaining the skin taut and minimizing wrinkling. Accordingly, skin aging overall has its own value and should be evaluated as the end point of any cosmetic or therapeutic endeavor.

Why, then, is knowledge of age not sufficient? This is because several factors other than time (e.g., solar exposure) have a major influence on skin aging. Furthermore, we do not know whether the function aging $= f(\text{time})$ is linear and uniform.

What type of scale is best? Skin aging is a continuous process and does not change over the life span. Along this continuous line, is it possible to determine intervals of equal length that allow measurement and consequently use of a continuous scale? This is possible for individual signs, such as wrinkling, because grade 4 can correspond to twice the number of wrinkles as grade 2 and grade 2 twice as many as grade 1. Can we set up a scale of global skin aging in which the lesions at grade 3 are three times greater than at grade 1? Not for the time being. We can distinguish aging grades, but without knowing the distance between them; accordingly, we should use ordinal scales.

The power of the scale depends on the number of grades. When a four-point scale of photodamage was used (none, slight, moderate, and severe), it was apparently not processed statistically (6, 17) before and after treatment but aimed solely at defining the sample better than by age only. We used a five-grade rating (none, slight, moderate, severe, and very severe) in assessing photodamage in 12 subjects aged 45–91 years treated at random on one side by 0.01% tretinoin and on the other side by vehicle alone (13). Nonparametric variance analysis allowed us to demonstrate a significant difference from control from month 4 (Table 6), and the average rate displayed the changes versus time in the two cohorts. Weinstein et al. subdivided a four-point photodamage scale (none, mild, moderate, and severe) into 10 grades (none; 1–3, mild; 4–6, moderate; and 7–9, severe), each illustrated by reference color photographs. A sample of 251 subjects aged 29–50 years was assigned grades 1–6 and further treated by 0.05% tretinoin, 0.01% tretinoin, or vehicle alone. By week 24, the overall severity of photoaging was significantly reversed in the three cohorts but more in the 0.05% tretinoin-treated

Table 6 Results of Tretinoin Treatment of Global Photodamage to the Face[a]

Day	Tretinoin	Vehicle	Difference
0	317	317	0
30	308	317	−9
60	308	308	0
90	292	308	−16
120	267	308	−41[b]
150	258	300	−42[b]
180	292	317	−25[b]

[a]Global photodamage to the face in 12 subjects treated on one side by tretinoin and on the other side by vehicle only, at random. Mean scores (0–4 points visual rank scale) × 100.
[b]$p < 0.05$.

group. The changes in cohort mean grade versus time could also be clearly displayed. This study confirms the usefulness of sharply delineated scales.

Increasing the discriminating power is limited by the inter-individual variation at each stage, which arises from the diversity of aging pattern according to the type of skin and the prevalence of external or endogenous factors. Inter-individual variations would be much reduced if such patterns were selected and accurately described, so that aging variations could be assessed along homogeneous lines, similar to those that allow us to say of someone that he looks over or under his age. It would also permit us to set up standard milestones over the entire course of aging.

For this, we need thorough studies of both skin photodamage and chronologic aging, to describe fully the still unclear clinical signs of "normal" aging, sorting out those that tend to be associated or, in contrast to preclude each other (e.g., telangiectasia is rarely associated, if ever, with leathery skin). Obviously, subareas not only of the face but also of other body regions deserve in-depth analytic and morphologic studies.

IV. PROBLEMS POSED BY PHOTOGRAPHY

Photodamage evaluation can be made in real time, for example when treatment is applied on one side and placebo on the other side. In general, however, photographs are of utmost value.

Standard photographs help to set up the boundaries of scales of whatever type and render the grading more precise and reliable. When placed in a scale as reference to a step, photographs play the same role and divide the scale into smaller increments. In Weinstein's experiment, for example, the overall 10-step scale was divided into nine 1-step scales by reference photographs.

Photographs of all subjects in a study are needed for global evaluation at the start and end of treatment. They also permit a rating by two or several experts, which is of value in reducing the risk of individual variation. Finally, they allow image analysis, which is an attractive technique but awaits publication of validated results.

All those who use color photographs in skin photodamage assessment have experienced the difficulty of obtaining reproducible pictures. The many unsuspected pitfalls include (1) variations in film sensitivity to color components, according to manufacturer or even to batch; (2) differences in film processing techniques (in automatic processing the total range of luminance is usually reduced so that darker colors may be minimized; accordingly, manual film processing is preferable using the same batch); (3) changes in focusing distance and centering; (4) difficulty in maintaining the lighting over a period of time, that is, direction, composition, and intensity of the light; and

(5) variability in facial expression even after rest and when sitting with closed eyes. Also, hairstyling and a younger or older way of dressing may unconsciously influence experts when they rate skin aging on photographs.

Polaroid film may be used because the photograph is available immediately and can be checked for accuracy. However, it often lacks crispness. A close-up camera loaded with Polaroid film may give useful enlarged pictures of a limited skin area under invariable light.

V. CONCLUSION

The visual and tactile morphologic analysis of skin is a valuable tool that enables a scientifically acceptable assessment of both global aging and its various clinical components. For the present, there is no way to replace it by noninvasive objective assessment, although such techniques are already useful and promising.

The reliability and preciseness of such psychosensorial assessments are related to the use of appropriate scales and the use of good-quality color photographs as both standards and records. For this last purpose, however, the reproducibility of photographs is still difficult to obtain.

The near future will bring many studies on the effect of various cosmetics, drugs, and techniques on age-associated skin lesions. It will provide opportunities of improving the methodology, mostly in setting up appropriate standards of aging or photodamage, selecting the more suitable type of scale, and finding clues for easier and more rapid, reliable photography.

Should analog continuous scales be preferred to digital scales? Theoretically they have the advantage of infinite sensitivity and of avoiding the clustering of data around milestones. However, digital continuous or even discontinuous scales, when provided with reference photographs at each point, seem to improve the reliability of rating. Further methodologic studies are needed to answer the question.

Such investigations will be of value not only for therapeutic or cosmetic purposes, but also for fundamental research on the chronology of skin aging and its still poorly understood relations to aging of other tissues.

REFERENCES

1. Graham JA, Jouhar AJ. The importance of cosmetics in the psychology of appearance. Int J Dermatol 1983; 22:153–6.
2. Kligman AM, Graham JA. The psychology of cutaneous aging. In: Balin AK, Kligman AM, eds. Aging and the skin. New York: Raven Press, 1989; 347–55.
3. Weinstein GD, Nigra TP, Pochi PE, et al., Topical tretinoin for treatment of photodamaged skin: a multi-center study. Arch Dermatol 1991; 127:659–65.

4. Siegel S. Non parametric statistics for the behavioral sciences. International student edition. London: McGraw-Hill, 1956.

5. Burton JL, Ebling FJG. Disorders of connective tissue. In: Rook A, Wilkinson DS, Ebling FJG, Champion RH, Burton JL, eds. Textbook of dermatology, 4th ed. Oxford: Blackwell, 1986; 1787–857.

6. Weiss JS, Ellis CN, Headington JT, Tincoff T, Hamilton TA, Voorhees JJ. Topical tretinoin improves photoaged skin: a double-blind vehicle-controlled study. JAMA 1988; 259:527–32.

7. Tsuji T, Yorifugi T, Hayashi Y, Hamada T. Light and scanning electron microscopic studies on wrinkles in aged persons' skin. Br J Dermatol 1986; 114: 329–35.

8. Model D. Smoker's face: an underrated clinical sign? Br Med J 1985; 291: 1760–2.

9. Misiewicz J, Sendagorta E, Golebiowska A, Lorenc B, Czarnetzki BM, Jablonska S. Topical treatment of multiple actinic keratoses of the face with arotinoid methyl sulfone (Ro 14-9706) cream versus tretinoin cream: a double-blind, comparative study. J Am Acad Dermatol 1991; 24:448–51.

10. Lever L, Kumar P, Marks R. Topical retinoic acid for treatment of solar damage. Br J Dermatol 1990; 122:91–8.

11. Leyden JJ, Grove GL, Grove MJ, Thorne EG, Lufrano L. Treatment of photodamage facial skin with topical tretinoin. J Am Acad Dermatol 1989; 21: 638–44.

12. Grove GL, Grove MJ, Leyden JJ. Optical profilometry: an objective method for quantification of facial wrinkles. J Am Acad Dermatol 1989; 21:631–7.

13. Faivre B, Rochefort A, Agache P. 1988 Unpublished data.

14. Daniel HW. Smoker's wrinkles: a study in the epidemiology of "crow-feet" Ann Intern Med 1971; 75:873–80.

15. Kanduce DP, Burr R, Gress R, Kanner R, Lyon JL, Zone JJ. Cigarette smoking: risk factor for premature facial wrinkling. Ann Intern Med 1991; 114:840–4.

16. Walter SD. Measuring the reliability of clinical data: the case for using three observers. Rev Epidemiol Sante Publique 1984; 323: 206–11.

17. Caputo R, Monti M, Motta S, et al. The treatment of visible signs of senescence: the Italian experience. Br J Dermatol 1990; 122(suppl. 35): 97–103.

2

Influence of Aging on the Mechanical Properties of Skin

JEAN de RIGAL and JEAN-LUC LÉVÊQUE

L'Oréal
Aulnay-sous-Bois, France

I. INTRODUCTION

The study of changes in skin structure with age is becoming all the more important with the increase in life expectancy, the resulting increase in the number of elderly individuals, and the desire to preserve a youthful and attractive appearance. Changes in the skin with age involve mainly the emergence of lines and wrinkles, together with a loss of tonicity partly due to atrophy. These modifications are principally attributable to the constraints to which this barrier organ are subjected (solar radiation and mechanical solicitation, for example) and to genetically programmed aging. The atrophy that occurs during aging is accompanied by more profound changes, with a loss of organization within the elastic collagen network and alterations of the basal elements.

The mechanical properties of the skin reflect the behavior of these various elements, as well as their structural organization. As a result, biomechanical measurements should permit a simple, rapid, and noninvasive characterization of the changes that occur during aging of the skin at the level of the different components. Methods used in vivo allow repeated measurements, thus providing a means of evaluating the efficacy of numerous preparations proposed either to slow the effects of aging on young skin or to reestablish firmness and elasticity in aged skin.

Numerous methods have been advanced over the last 20 years. Schematically these can be divided into two classes:

1. Those in which the deformation is applied perpendicular to the plane of the skin (indentation, levarometry, ballistometry, and suction). These methods are dealt with in the following three chapters.
2. Those in which the constraint is applied parallel to the skin surface (uniaxial extensibility, torsion, and elongation vibration).

The latter methods have the advantage of permitting the results to be interpreted independently of attachments and the influence of the subcutaneous tissues, at least when the area of skin subjected to the constraint is not too large (1). In addition, measurements of torsion are only partially dependent on anisotropy and the orientation of the skin's natural lines of tension.

Section II is a review of the various studies performed using such torsion methods, with a comparison of the different results obtained. Factors capable of modifying the biomechanical properties of skin are also mentioned. Section III reviews the other methods available for characterizing the properties of skin along its plane, together with the main results obtained.

II. TORSION METHODS

A. Principle

Torsion torque is applied to the plane of the skin by means of a disk glued to the surface (double-sided adhesive film or cyanoacrylate glue); an angular displacement sensor measures the resulting deformation. The response of the skin takes the form shown in Figure 1. Various parameters corresponding to the different phases of the response are generally used:

$$U_E = \text{immediate extensibility}$$
$$U_R = \text{immediate recovery}$$
$$U_V = \text{viscoelastic deformation}$$
$$U_F = \text{final deformation}$$

To characterize the response of the skin, most authors adopt a mathematical model of the type

$$U = U_E + U_V(1 - e^{-t/T}) + At^m$$

This equation can also be used to calculate recovery.

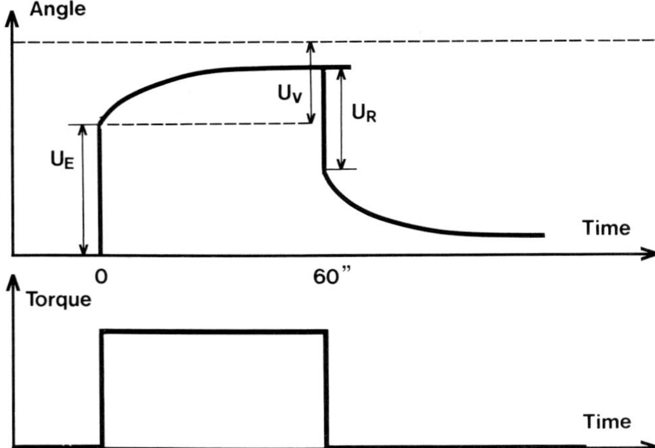

Figure 1 Time representation of the measurement, showing the main parameters used: (U_E; immediate extensibility; U_V; viscoelastic deformation; and U_R; immediate recovery).

The value of m varies according to different teams, although Sanders (2), Wjin (2), Finlay (4), Lévêque et al (5), and Escoffier et al. (6) agree on a value of 1. More recently, Pichon et al. (7) advanced a value of $m = 1/3$, which is closer to the real situation and based on a study of the phenomena involved in the behavior of the skin. The measurements obtained with most equipment are of the creep type (2–6); only one author has measured relaxation in terms of torque for a given angle of deformation (8).

As early as 1971, Finlay showed the advantage of limiting the zone of measurement by using a guard ring around the mobile disk (4); under these conditions the influence of the subcutaneous tissues is limited.

For well-defined geometries, a certain number of hypotheses and approximations are used to obtain working equations. These consist of considering the skin as a homogeneous and isotropic material (which is clearly not the case). Two such attempts have been made and the results obtained are similar, leading to an identical interpretation of the phenomena observed (3,9). Both authors obtained the equation

$$E = \frac{M}{4\pi e 0.4 R_1 R_2 \theta}$$

which relates Young's modulus to the torque M, skin thickness e, characteristics of the zone of measurement (R_1 and R_2), and the angle of rotation θ; 0.4 is derived from the approximation $E = 0.4\mu$, where μ is Lame's coefficient.

A rheologic interpretation of the response curves of the skin has also been proposed; it is based on a simple model that predicts its behavior. The two versions of this model correspond to two types of creep, one of which is linearly dependent on time (3):

$$U = U_E + U_V(1 - e^{-t/T}) + At$$

and the other involves a far slower creep (7):

$$U = U_E + U_V(1 - e^{-t/T}) + At^{1/3}$$

More recently (10), the use of a weak torque (90×10^{-4} N·m) and a guard ring defining a very thin layer of skin has favored measurement of the superficial layers (stratum corneum and epidermis).

B. METHODS WITHOUT A GUARD RING

The various methods can be used either with or without immobilization of the skin at a given distance from the disk (by the use of a guard ring). Wlasblom (1) and Sanders (2) used methods with no guard ring.

Using a very low torsion torque (8.3×10^{-4} N·m), Sanders obtained a virtually linear increase in the angle of rotation with age for a certain number of parameters, with 2.3° per decade for immediate extensibility and 3.6° for final extensibility. These results reflect a decrease in the elastic modulus with age. Using the equation calculated by Wlasblom (1), Sanders evaluated the skin modulus ranging from 2×10^4 to 10^5 N/m^{-2}, the higher value being for the youngest skin. There was no apparent change in the relaxation constant with age. However, it should be remembered that these results were obtained over an age range of 6–61 years and concerned a limited number of subjects. In addition, they reflect the overall behavior of the skin, including its natural state of tension, more than intrinsic rheologic properties.

C. METHODS WITH A GUARD RING

Finlay (4) was the first to limit the zone submitted to a constraint, measuring relaxation phenomena. The results showed that the relaxation constant is independent of age. In contrast, there was an age-related decrease in the immediate deformation induced by a torque of 2×10^{-3} N·m. Furthermore, none of the parameters characteristic of a relaxation curve were found to vary significantly with age. The changes observed were not modified when prestress was applied.

Chronologic aging has long been studied on the ventral surface of the forearm (6). Measurement of skin thickness within the same zones provides information on the intrinsic properties of the tissue studied. Indeed, the equation relating thickness, extensibility, and Young's modulus used by most authors (3,5,6,9) shows that the product of thickness and extensibility is inversely proportional to the modulus. Results (6) obtained with a force of 2.3–10.4 × 10^{-3} N·m show that the intrinsic elastic properties of the skin (U_E^*) do not vary before the seventh decade of life (Fig. 2), whereas recovery (U_R) (Fig. 3) and the relaxation constant T (fig. 4) diminish significantly with age at the highest torque used. The parameter best reflecting aging is elasticity (U_R/U_E Fig. 5). These results provide qualitative confirmation of those previously observed on another area (dorsal forearm) (5,9) and using a different apparatus at a torque of 9–28.6 × 10^{-3} N·m. Only the sex-related differences were not confirmed, as was the case for Wijn (3). It should be noted that the zones of measurement were different and that the dimensions of the

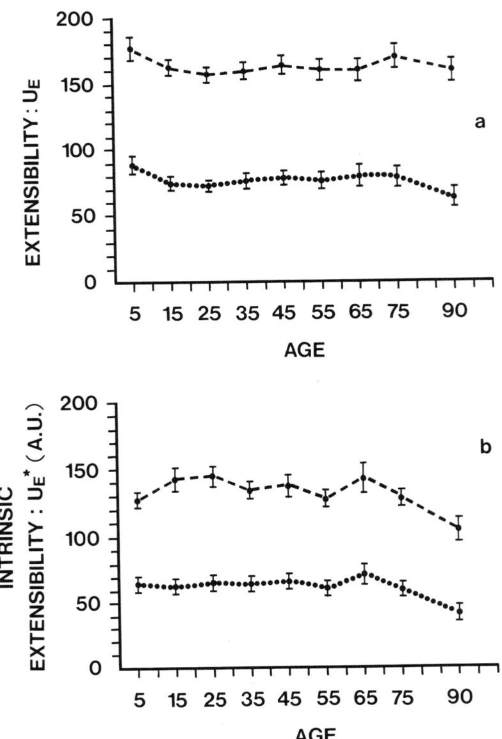

Figure 2 Immediate skin extensibility U_E (a) and intrinsic skin extensibility U_E^* (U_E * Skin Thickness) (b) as a function of age for high torque (dashed line) and low torque (dotted line).

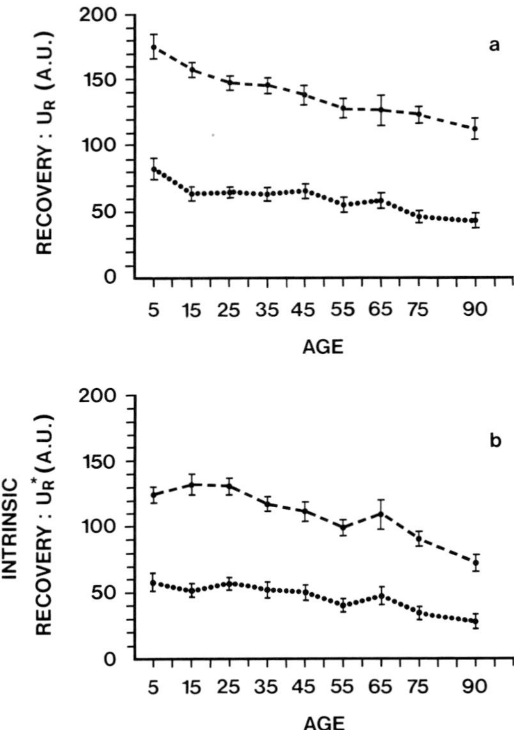

Figure 3 Immediate skin recovery U_R (a) and intrinsic skin extensibility U_R^* (U_R * Skin Thickness) (b) as a function of age for high torque (dashed line) and low torque (dotted line).

ring of skin submitted to the constraint were far larger. The decrease in elasticity with age was observed regardless of color or ethnicity (blacks, Hispanics, and whites) or the area studied (dorsal and ventral forearm) (11).

A description of aging phenomena using the characteristic parameters in Burger's model was first given by Wijn (3), who showed that the coefficient of elasticity diminished with age (by about 15% between the ages of 20 and 65 years); the other parameters showed no apparent variation or could not be determined. The results were fragmentary and concerned a small number of subjects ($n = 45$) with a limited age range (20–65 years). Furthermore, the author normalized the results for a standard skin thickness of 1.3 mm, regardless of age, which may have masked variations in thickness with the aging process (5,6).

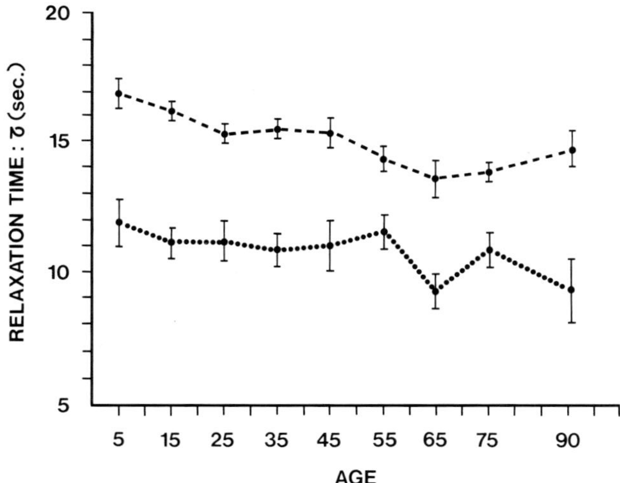

Figure 4   Relaxation time as a function of age for high torque (dashed line) and low torque (dotted line).

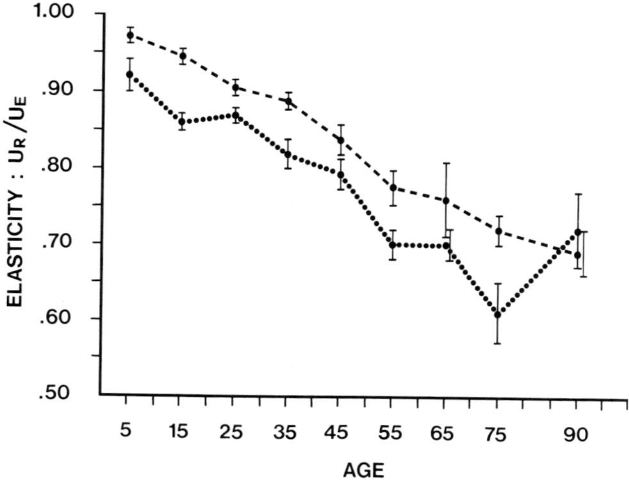

Figure 5   Skin elasticity or recovery-extensibility ration (U_R/U_E) as a function of age for high torque (dashed line) and low torque (dotted line).

D. DISCUSSION OF THE MAIN RESULTS

The most important results obtained by the various authors are reported in Table 1. The experimental conditions were widely different with regard to both the torque applied and the geometric characteristics of the area of skin subjected to the stress. However, two age-dependent trends emerge clearly:

1. A decrease in the stiffness modulus associated with low values (below 10^5 N/m^2) when the zone studied was not limited
2. An increase in the stiffness modulus at higher values (above 10^5 N/m^2) when the study zone was limited

These two observations suggest that in the first case measurements reflect the natural state of tension and the subcutaneous tissue and the variations observed reflect the increase in flaccidity of the skin with age. In the second case the observed variations reflect alterations induced by the effect of aging on the main structures of the skin.

Elastic fibers are chiefly responsible for the mechanical properties of the skin, at least when the deformation is relatively minor, and their degradation leads to a loss of elasticity (12). This would explain why, regardless of the methods used in vivo (6,13), the various authors all found a decrease whether the constraints were applied perpendicular or parallel to the skin surface. The morphometric changes in the dermal elastic network with age have been clearly described for an area of unexposed skin (14); they explain the loss of elasticity and recovering capacity. Oxlund et al. (12) showed the important role of elastic fibers in viscous deformation, with the elimination of elastin leading to a decrease in the relaxation constant. This illustrates the modulatory role of elastic fibers in the interactions between collagen and glycosaminoglycans. More recently, Fleishmajer et al. observed a decrease in the glycosaminoglycan content of the skin with age (15). The role of this fundamental substance was first suggested by Daly and Odland (16).

In summary, elastin is involved at two levels: in maintaining the collagen network and in controlling the movements of this network within the ground substance.

III. OTHER METHODS INVOLVING MEASUREMENTS PARALLEL TO THE SKIN SURFACE

Such methods can be divided into two classes: dynamic methods (shear wave propagation) (1,18) and static or quasi-static methods (extensometry) (3,19).

TABLE 1 Main Results Obtained by Torsional Measurements and Variation with Age of Computed Parameters

Torque (N·m)	Area	R_1/R_2 (mm)	Skin thickness	Results				Reference
				Extensibility	Relaxation	Recovery	Modulus (N/m^2)	
		8.7^a			$\sim$30		$7\text{--}20 \times 10^4$	Wlasblom (1)
8.3×10^{-4}	Dorsal forearm	8.7^a	Not measured	Increased	15 No variation		Decreased $10^4\text{--}10^5$	Sanders (2)
20×10^{-4}	Dorsal forearm	15/23		Decreased	Increased			Finlay (4)
90×10^{-4}	Dorsal forearm	25/35	Yes	Decreased		Decreased	Increased	Agache
286×10^{-4}							$4 \times 10^5/8 \times 10^5$	and Lévêque (5,9)
40×10^{-4}	Calf	5/12.5		Increased	$\sim$3.5		$\simeq 10^5$	Wjin (3)
23×10^{-4}	Ventral	18/24	Yes	No variation, then decrease after 70	No variation	Decreased	No variation then increase	Escoffier et al. (6)
104×10^{-4}	forearm		Yes	No variation, then decrease after 70	Decreased	Decreased	$\sim 11 \times 10^5$	

^{a}Without guard ring.

A. SHEAR WAVE PROPAGATION

The principle of this method is described in detail in Reference 18. A fine probe is placed perpendicular to the skin surface and vibrates; two sensors perpendicular to the excitation axis measure the speed at which the wave is propagated. The speed of propagation V_p is studied as a function of the frequency, ranging from 8 to 1016 Hz. The amplitude variations recorded by the two sensors are used to calculate a damping distance D, which is inversely related to the damping coefficient. The changes in these two parameters according to the frequency present a minimum for a value f_{min}. The degree of skin dehydration influences the value of f_{min}, which is about 400 Hz for well-hydrated skin compared to 700 Hz for dry skin.

The three parameters defined previously change with age, as follows:

1. A quasi-linear increase in f_{min} with age is evident, for both the damping distance and the speed of propagation.
2. The speed of propagation increases with age, particularly at low frequencies.
3. The damping distance varies with age, with a decrease at high frequencies and an increase at low frequencies.

These results are interpreted in terms of water content of the superficial layers of the skin. The two parameters are related either to viscosity or to the shearing modulus (20). The differences are most marked at low frequencies, at which the skin of the elderly has a higher coefficient of viscosity (approximately 50%) than that of younger subjects. As these authors have shown, the changes due to age are opposite to those produced by hydration; however, only the stratum corneum can be strongly modified. This study concerned a small number of subjects ($n = 16$) with a limited age range (24–63 years), but the authors concluded that the variations observed were solely related to the water content of the stratum corneum and that the largest variations are detected at low frequencies.

B. QUASI-STATIC MEASUREMENTS OF EXTENSIBILITY

Two patches of well-defined shapes are glued to the skin with double-sided adhesive film (as in the torsion method) at a distance that varies according to the area of skin to be submitted to the uniaxial constraint (3,21).

The force is generated either by an electromagnet (3) or by a motor associated with an endless screw (22), and the measurements can be of two types: relaxation or creep. Contrary to the measurement of torsion, it is necessary to define the constraint axis to take into account the natural tension of the cutaneous tissue (Langer's lines); some authors have defined parameters of anisotropy from the initial elasticity and from the coefficient of viscosity (3).

There are few published results concerning skin aging. Wijn studied a relatively small number of subjects with a limited age range and observed a large reduction (50%) in recovery; anistotropy was not affected. The coefficients of retarded elasticity (viscous deformation) also diminished with age (3). The author interpreted the results as underlining the importance of the elastic fibers in the mechanical properties of the skin, the coefficient of elasticity directly reflecting the number of elastic fibers.

C. MEASUREMENTS BASED ON SONIC VELOCITY

The speed at which pulses of acoustically white noise are propagated is measured in the plane of the skin by means of two piezoelectric sensors (23). The ultrasound waves are propagated along the axis of the emitter receiver, with no detectable transverse movement. The velocity of propagation is measured along a distance of 7 mm, the optimal distance for the back of the hand and the forearm. The authors found that the acoustic waves were mainly propagated within the superficial layers of the stratum corneum. They interpreted the variations in terms of differences in density due mainly to the degree of hydration. Although the authors reported an increase in the elastic modulus with age at a value of approximately 10^7 N/m^2, they gave no details of their results.

Two remarks can be made concerning these observations. First, the use of minor deformations (shear wave propagation) or ultrasound waves to study the aging of cutaneous tissues leads one to interpret the results in terms of modifications of superficial structures and variations in the water content of the stratum corneum (20,23). In contrast, methods based on uniaxial extensibility can be interpreted in terms of deeper modifications, particularly alterations of elastic fibers.

IV. CONCLUSION

Among the numerous methods developed to assess the in vivo biomechanical properties of the skin, torsional measurements are used more commonly. These methods give a clear definition of the evolution of skin properties during the aging process. When the skin area (quantity or surface) under study is well defined, the decrease in its extensibility induced by the aging process is very weak. In contrast, when this area is not demarcated, for a given torque the deformation is larger for old than for young people. This could be explained by the increasing mobility of skin and by propagation of the deformation over long distances.

The most striking result is the loss of elasticity—about 3% per decade—observed over the entire life span, whatever the method used. This decrease in elasticity is the measurement perceived by clinicians in aged skin as they pinch it.

Other methods should be used more intensively to obtain clearer conclusions about the evolution of the aging process using all the parameters they provide. For instance, uniaxial methods are of great interest because they yield information about the mechanical anistropy of skin. It is well known that this anisotropy is due to the reorganization of collagen bundles under the action of repeated stresses.

Overall, the most valid results concern the properties of the dermis and the role of the elastic fibers, even though methods exist for studying epidermal aging, based on torsion (10) or displacements of very low amplitude (18,20,23).

Finally, the few published results of dynamic methods seem promising, but interpretation of the phenomena is being discussed. Dynamic methods represent a large field of investigation for the future; by the choice of frequency, amplitude, and orientation of deformations they should allow investigations of the different layers of the skin.

REFERENCES

1. Wlasblom DC. Skin elasticity. Ph.D. thesis, University of Utrech, The Netherlands, 1967.
2. Sanders R. Torsional elasticity of human skin in vivo. Pflugers Arch 1973; 342:255–60.
3. Wjin P. The alinear viscoelastic properties of the human skin in vivo for small deformations. Ph.D. thesis, Catholic University of Nijmegen, The Netherlands, June 1980.
4. Finlay B. The torsional characteristics of the skin in vivo. Biol Med Eng 1971; 5:567–73.
5. Leveque JL, de Rigal J, Agache P, Monneur C. Influence of aging on the extensibility of human skin at low stress. Arch Dermatol Res (1980); 269:172–37.
6. Escoffier C, de Rigal J, Rochefort A, Vasselet R, Leveque JL, Agache P. Age-related mechanical properties of human skin. An in vivo study. J Invest Dermatol (1989); 93:353–7.
7. Pichon E, de Rigal J, Leveque JL. In vivo rheological study of the torsional characteristics of the skin. Congress of bioengineering and the skin, Stresa, Italy, 1990.
8. Finlay B. Dynamic mechanical testing of human skin in vivo. J Biomech (1970); 3:557–68.
9. Agache P, Monneur C, Leveque JL, de Rigal J. Mechanical properties and Young's modulus of the skin in vivo. Arch Dermatol Res (1980); 269:221–32.

10. De Rigal J, Leveque JL. In vivo measurement of the stratum corneum elasticity. Bioeng Skin (1985); 1:13–23.

11. Berardesca E, de Rigal J, Leveque JL, Maibach HI. In vivo biophysical characterization of skin physiological differences in races. Dermatologica (1991); 182:89–93.

12. Oxlund H, Manschot J, Vidik A. The role of elastin in the mechanical properties of skin. J Biomech (1988); 21:213–8.

13. Robert C. Effet des conditions socio-professionelles sur le vieillissement de la peau. J Med Esthet Chir Dermatol (1988); 15:235–8.

14. Lavker RM, Zheng P, Dong G. Aged skin a study by light, transmission electron, and scanning electron microscopy. J Invest Dermatol (1988); 73:235–8.

15. Fleishmajer R, Perlish JS, Bashey RL. Human dermal glycosaminoglycans and aging. Biochim Biophys Acta (1972); 279:265–75.

16. Daly CH, Odland GF. Age-related changes in the mechanical properties of human skin. J Invest Dermatol (1979); 73:84–7.

17. Potts RO, Buras EM, Chrisman DA. Changes with age in the moisture content of human skin. J Invest Dermatol (1984); 82(1):97–100.

18. Potts RO, Chrisman DA, Buras EM. The dynamic mechanical properties of human skin in vivo. J. Biomech (1980); 16:365–72.

19. Wijn PFF, Brakkee AJM, Kuiper JM, Vendrik AJH. The alinear viscoelastic properties of the human skin in vivo related to sex and age. In: Marks R, Payne PA, eds. Bioengineering and the skin. Cardiff: MTP Press, (1980); 135–45.

20. Potts RO, Buras EM. In vivo changes in the dynamic viscosity of human stratum corneum as a function of age and ambient moisture. J Soc Cosmet Chem (1985); 36:169–76.

21. Gigbon T, Stark T, Evans JH. Directional variation in extensibility of human skin in vivo. J Biomech (1969); 2:201–4.

22. Burlin TE, Hutten WC, Ranau HS. A method of in vivo measurement of elastic properties of skin in radiotherapy patients. J Invest Dermatol (1977); 69:321–3.

3

Mechanical Properties and Photoaging

ENZO BERARDESCA

University of Pavia
Pavia, Italy

HOWARD I. MAIBACH

University of California—San Francisco, School of Medicine
San Francisco, California

I. AGING VERSUS PHOTOAGING: CLINICAL AND ANATOMIC CONSIDERATIONS

Photoaging defines a clinical condition characterized by cutaneous aging exacerbated by exposure to ultraviolet light. This condition has been recognized since the nineteenth century, when an increased degree of aging was described in individuals chronically exposed to sun (sailors and farmers) compared to indoor workers.

Photoaged skin shows increased wrinkling, thickness, and laxity; its color acquires a yellow hue with areas of brown pigmentation. The epidermis is usually acanthotic, and keratinocytes may be atypic and show polarity loss. Sebaceous gland hyperplasia may be seen, and premalignant and malignant lesions may appear. In "intrinsic aging" the skin thickness is decreased (1) and there is a progressive flattening of the dermo-epidermal junction (2); senile angiomas are the only lesions that usually grow in protected areas.

Photoaging has a different pathogenic impact on skin structures than intrinsic aging, and the dermal alterations in photoaged areas of the face and hands are different from those of protected skin of aged individuals (3). Severely photodamaged skin presents numerous degenerated elastic fibers that finally become an amorphous mass (4). Ultrastructurally these changes begin with the granular appearance of the elastic matrix and the formation of several electron-lucent areas (5). Thus, dermal changes in photoaged skin are mainly related to the hyperplasia of elastic tissue that ends in fiber disintegration. In contrast, in intrinsic aging the hyperplasia and thickness of elastic material are only modest (6) and fibers show mild degeneration (4).

The effect of excessive sun exposure on the amount of collagen that appears decreased differs according to the type of collagen; soluble collagen decreases; and insoluble collagen increases (7); type III collagen increases in proportion (8,9). This effect seems to be the result of a repair process. In photoaged skin, type I collagen is degraded by the products of chronic inflammation released after ultraviolet (UV) damage, whereas in intrinsic aging mature collagen becomes more resistant to enzymatic degradation (10). Other changes differentiating photoaging from intrinsic aging are related to the ground substance, which is apparently increased in chronically sun-exposed areas (11).

We know less about the effects of chronic solar exposure on fibroblasts and elastic fibers. After UVA or UVB radiation, fibroblasts in the dermis appear numerous and larger, with a high metabolic activity (12). Besides these morphologic changes, it remains to be demonstrated whether there are qualitative biochemical changes in fibroblasts, ground substance, or elastic fibers.

Blood vessels in the upper dermis show a thickening of the wall due to the deposition of basement membrane like material and have a dilated and tortuous clinical appearance; protected aged skin may show these changes, even if to a lesser extent. Moreover, thin vessel walls have been reported in very old subjects (13).

II. EFFECTS OF UV RAYS ON SKIN STRUCTURES

Both UVA and UVB can produce epidermal cell alterations. The higher energy produced by UVB made them responsible for all the damage induced in the course of photoaging. Low UVB doses are required to produce photodamage of tissue: severe elastosis in experimental animals could be induced after exposure of 6 minimal effective doses (MED) a week for 30 weeks (14); after UVB exposure of 30–50 MED hyperplasia of elastic fibers may be seen in mice (15).

UVA penetrates the skin more deeply, inducing more damage to dermal structures. Because of its relative low energy, higher UVA doses are required to produce the same effects on tissue. Nevertheless, it is reported that single high UVA doses can damage blood vessels (16). Kligman et al. (14) compared the effects of exposure to UVB and UVA in hairless mice: animals exposed to ~3000 J/cm^2 of UVA developed a significant degree of elastosis. The degree of damage was less severe than in animals irradiated with UVB, but it extended deeper to the dermis. On the other hand, UVA had no histologic effect on collagen. Ground substance is reported to increase after both UVA and UVB radiation (14); as a result of the penetration patterns of the different wavelengths, the increase in ground substance is located mainly in the upper dermis after UVB, whereas UVA produces an homogeneous increase in the entire dermis.

III. SKIN MECHANICAL PROPERTIES, AGING, AND PHOTOAGING

Age-related changes in the mechanical properties of skin have been studied in vivo using different noninvasive techniques (17) and methods (18–20). Most of the work has been done in the attempt to understand and quantify so-called intrinsic aging. Uniaxial and biaxial tensile tests are straightforward methods (21) and show a marked age dependence because the magnitude of the initial elastic deformation decreases with age according to the degenerative changes induced in the dermal elastic network (22); compression tests give similar results, with a progressive loss of elastic recovery of the skin and thus a progressive increase in the time required for viscoelastic recovery after deformation due to changes in the ground substance (17). Torsional extensibility has been investigated with twistometers to measure skin deformation after the application of a torque parallel to the skin surface (23–26). This technique reduces differences induced by anisotropic forces and allows the quantification of several biomechanical parameters, such as immediate extensibility and recovery, viscoelastic deformation, elastic recovery, and creep relaxation time.

Skin biomechanics are related to the site investigated and to skin thickness: an inverse relationship exists between skin extensibility and skin thickness, the latter varying during the aging process (27,28). Skin thickness slowly decreases with age; the trend is higher in men. Using a twistometer during intrinsic aging, the skin maintains its extensibility until the seventh decade, whereas its elasticity or elastic recovery decreases from the early decades (26). Similar findings have been reported with an indentometric technique (29,30). No significant differences besides skin thickness are detected between men and women (26,30), and quantification of skin elasticity or elastic recovery appears the more sensitive parameter to evaluate the biomechanics of the intrinsic aging process. The viscous part of the deformation is constant through life and the creep relaxation time decreases linearly, suggesting a progressive fluidization of the medium (31). The viscous part of the cutaneous deformation is due to the displacement of interstitial fluid in the fibrous network (17); the viscosity of this fluid changes with age according to the presence of glycosaminoglycans (32).

Leveque et al. (33) first described the effects of chronic sun exposure on the mechanical properties of skin. They investigated the arms 1 cm below and above the sleeve mark in 35 cyclists participating in the Tour de France. The unprotected area was chronically sun exposed and deeply tanned. They measured skin thickness with pulsed ultrasound and skin extensibility and recovery using a torsional device and the size of desquamating corneocytes. The study reported striking differences in all the parameters investigated between chronically exposed and protected areas. These differences were not detectable in a control group of matched age. Long-term solar irradiation led to a decrease in skin extensibility and elastic recovery. The skin appears thicker, more rigid, and less susceptible to deformation. The authors suggest that changes in skin extensibility could be related to the increase in epidermal thickness (34). At the same time, the size of corneocytes decreased 13.5%, consistent with an increased epidermal turnover.

We investigated the immediate effects of low UV doses on mechanical parameters of the skin in vivo to elucidate possible differences between the mechanical behavior of the skin during intrinsic aging and photoaging (35) and to assess the efficacy of topical sunscreens in preserving skin mechanical efficacy. A group of 20 healthy volunteers of both sexes belonging to two age groups (10 young, age range 25–35, and 10 old, age range 45–55) were investigated. Subjects were exposed on the volar forearm every third day to increasing doses of UVB + UVA rays generated by a Waldmann UV 180 lamp. UV exposure increased from 1.5 to 6.5 minutes during 3 weeks of treatment. These low doses were administered to mimic normal daily solar exposure. Two control groups matched for age underwent the same treatment after topical sun protection with a cream containing 2% octyl methoxycinnamate and 0.5% butyl methoxydibenzoylmethane (Sun protection factor, SPF = 2). For each measurement a load of $3.8 \times 10^4 \, \mathrm{N/m^{-2}}$ was applied to the skin surface five times consecutively for 5 s using a suction device. To avoid the influence of possible hydration induced by the sunscreen, recordings were done before and after the 3 weeks of UV exposure on the same marked site 72 h after the last UV dose. The following mechanical parameters were measured: extensibility, elasticity, and hysteresis. Data were normalized for skin thickness measured with pulsed ultrasound. In both young and older subjects treated with the sun-protective cream no significant differences were recorded, whereas a significant decrease in skin elasticity was demonstrated in the untreated groups after UV irradiation (Table 1). In 3 of 20 untreated subjects slight erythema followed by tanning was present in the

Table 1 Skin Elasticity After Acute UV Irradiation[a]

| | Skin elasticity | | | |
| | Treated | | Untreated | |
Group	Before UV	After UV	Before UV	After UV
Young	50.2 ± 10.8	49.0 ± 7.1	54.7 ± 6.6	45.6 ± 11.3[b]
Old	44.2 ± 5.6	43.5 ± 8.3	49.7 ± 7.6	41.6 ± 4.4[b]

[a]A significant decrease is evident in both groups investigated
[b]P < 0.01 versus untreated value before UV.
Source: From Reference 33.

first days of exposure. No other signs were detectable in the other subjects (treated or untreated).

Our data show that skin mechanical function impairment may occur after a few weeks of moderate UV exposure and that low UV doses may cause changes in skin elasticity. Kligman et al. demonstrated that short-term UVB exposure may produce severe elastosis (14), and fibroblasts in animal skin appear hyperactive and more numerous. The dermis is thickened, with increased deposition of newly formed collagen. Higher UVA doses are required to produce this effect; nevertheless, single UVA doses produce erythema (36), and UVA is present in sunlight all day long in all seasons in greater doses than UVB; furthermore UVA, as mentioned earlier, is more penetrating, making connective tissue and fibroblast accessible targets. Erythema or subliminal erythema generated after low UVA + UVB exposure in skin not protected from sun may result in some degree of skin inflammation and edema, causing changes in skin resilient distension and thus affecting skin elasticity. This effect has been recorded in young and elderly subjects, allowing us to assume that photoaging progresses throughout life and its prevention is necessary even in adult life.

Impairment of skin elasticity after low UVA + UVB exposure is related to the acute effects of UV rays on skin, such as erythema and edema, whereas elastosis occurs after long-term exposure. Moreover, both conditions affect skin resilient distension, which results in skin elasticity changes. Skin elasticity in this case seems to be a reliable parameter to quantify and measure not only intrinsic aging but also photoaging and may be useful to detect early changes in skin biomechanics after UV exposure.

The reliability of elasticity as a parameter in monitoring photoaging was further confirmed in a study evaluating the efficacy of an antiaging treatment with topical tretinoin (37). The study, performed using the same technology described earlier, compared the effects of a cream containing 0.05% tretinoin versus a placebo applied daily on the volar forearm for 4 months. The 18 white subjects (age 39 ± 8) were treated daily for 4 months on the left forearm with topical 0.05% tretinoin. The right forearm was treated daily with a placebo-base cream. Using a load of $3.8 \times 10^4 \, \text{N/m}^{-2}$ (Table 2), a significant increase in skin elasticity was detected (P < 0.01). Values recorded were 58.9 in the placebo-treated site and 66.0 in the tretinoin-treated site (Table 2), (95% confidence intervals of the difference between 2.55 and 11.6). On the other hand, extensibility was unchanged and hysteresis was slightly increased from 0.26 to 0.32 in the tretinoin-treated site (confidence intervals between −0.14 and 0.16 and −0.01 and 0.1, respectively).

The study reveals that topical treatment with tretinoin influences skin elasticity but not other mechanical parameters of the skin, such as extensibility and hysteresis. Data were obtained using forces that involve collagen fibers in the response: collagen synthesis has been reported to increase after topical tretinoin treatment (38); no effect was detectable on elastic fibers. Indeed, in the same experiment, using lower forces ($1.2 \times 10^4 \, \text{N/m}^{-2}$) in the attempt to measure mainly the elastic fiber responses, no changes were recorded.

Interestingly, hysteresis, a parameter reflecting viscoelasticity, is not affected by the treatment, although an increased content of dermal glycosaminoglycans is reported after tretinoin treatment (39).

A different model of UV-induced damage is represented by oral methoxsalen photochemotherapy (PUVA). The combined treatment of UVA light with peak emission at 365 nm plus systemic 8-methoxypsoralen is used in the treatment of several resistant dermatoses, such as eczema and psoriasis. Recently we investigated the effects of this particular model of photoaging to correlate, from a biophysical point of view, the morphologic and biochemical changes in aging, photoaging, and PUVA photodamaging processes (40,41). The model was represented by the selective PUVA-induced damage of unexposed areas compared with chronically sun-exposed and occasionally sun-exposed sites. The 44 subjects (divided into four age groups) with psoriasis treated with PUVA and the 38 control subjects in the same age groups were treated. In both groups elasticity, hysteresis, and tensile distensibility were

Table 2 Biomechanical Parameters After 4 Months of Tretinoin (Average ± SD)[a]

	Treated	Placebo	P
Extensibility	2.06 ± 0.35	2.05 ± 0.5	NS
Elasticity	66.0 ± 12	58.9 ± 13	< 0.01
Hysteresis	0.32 ± 0.12	0.26 ± 0.08	NS

[a]A significant increase in skin elasticity is detected after tretinoin treatment using loads involving collagen fibers.

Table 3 Variations in Biomechanical Properties of Skin (Buttocks)[a]

	Tensile distensibility	Elasticity
PUVA-treated patients	2.10 ± 0.383[b]	58.06 ± 17.138
Control subjects	2.78 ± 0.447	63.82 ± 13.738

[a]Long-term PUVA-treated psoriatic patients (> 1000 J/cm^2) compared with a control group.
[b]$p < 0.001$.
Source: From Reference 38.

investigated on chronically sun-exposed (cheek), occasionally sun-exposed (volar forearm), and unexposed sites (buttocks). Elasticity was confirmed to decrease during intrinsic aging and photoaging, and significant changes in tensile distensibility were detected during PUVA treatment. This is significantly lower (Table 3) on the buttocks of PUVA-treated subjects (a site where the effects of photoaging are not detectable); no changes in this parameter were related to age. These data may be correlated to the photosclerosis (i.e., the increase in newly formed collagen in the papillary dermis) induced by the methoxsalen combined with UVA. The papillary dermis after PUVA treatment shows collapse of the venous capillaries, since long-UV rays have an effect on blood vessels (42,43); furthermore, a homogeneous, eosinophilic material is present at the dermoepidermal junction, devoid of elastic fibers that do not have amyloid or colloid characteristics. The collagen fibers are oriented parallel to the skin surface. The nature of the dermal remodeling after PUVA differs markedly from changes induced by other wavelengths (44). These morphologic changes justify the alterations in mechanical parameters just described. These studies, obviously performed on pathologic skin, need further investigation to confirm in depth the functional and histopathologic correlations.

IV. COMMENT

Different patterns of mechanical reactions of the skin can be elicited during the different processes of aging. Great importance in the acquisition of the data is determined by the force used; differentiation of forces can help in involving different structures of the skin, measuring the efficacy and the integrity of different compartments. Photoaged skin results in a decrease in skin extensibility not specifically different from intrinsic aging, but some aspects of its treatment can be better investigated using selective loads directed to the compartment targeted by the molecule used in the treatment (37). The choice of parameters to investigate is important, too. Specific models of photoaging (such as photoaging induced by PUVA therapy), giving particular histopathologic patterns, can be better monitored by assessing skin extensibility rather than elasticity. The combination of the intensity of the load applied to the skin and the dimension of the measured area can focus with more specificity on a particular layer or structure of the skin. Indeed, the size of the probe applied to the skin surface is an important factor influencing the experimental result. Small probes measure superficial layers of the skin, whereas larger probes involve the responses of deep dermal and subcutaneous structures. Investigation of the mechanical properties of skin can lead to a better understanding of skin function and skin responses to light, improving related therapeutic approaches in terms of prevention or treatment of skin aging and photoaging.

REFERENCES

1. Tan CY, Statham B, Marks R, Payne PA: Skin thickness measured by ultrasound: its reproducibility, validation, variability. Br J Dermatol 1982; 106: 657–67.
2. Montagna W, Carlisle K. Structural changes in aging human skin. J Invest Dermatol 1979; 73:47–53.
3. Kligman LH, Kligman AM. Photoaging. In: Fitzpatrick TB, Eisen AZ, Wolff K, Freedberg IM, Austen KF, eds. Dermatology in general medicine, Vol. 1, 3rd ed. New York: McGraw-Hill, 1987; 1470–5.
4. Kligman AM. Early destructive effects of sunlight on human skin. JAMA 1969; 210:2377–80.
5. Bravermann IM, Fonferko E. Studies in cutaneous aging. I. The elastic fiber network. J Invest Dermatol 1982; 78:434–43.
6. Lavker RM. Structural alterations in exposed and unexposed aged skin. J Invest Dermatol 1979, 73:59–66.
7. Smith JG, Davidson EA, Sams WM, Clark RD. Alterations in human connective tissue with age and chronic sun damage. J Invest Dermatol 1962; 39: 347–50.
8. Lowell CR, Plastow SR, Russell-Jones R, Thomas J: Collagen and elastin in actinic elastosis. J Invest Dermatol 1984; 82:566a.
9. Plastow SR, Lowell CR, Young AR. UV-B induced collagen changes in hairless mouse skin. Br J Dermatol 1984; 111:702–3.
10. Bentley JB. Aging of collagen. J Invest Dermatol 1973; 73:80–3.
11. Smith JG, Davidson EA, Sams WM, Clark RD. Alterations in human dermal connective tissue with age and chronic sun damage. J Invest Dermatol 1962; 39:347–50.
12. Kligman LH. Skin changes in photoaging: Characteristics, prevention and repair. In Balin HK, Kligman AM, eds. Aging and the skin. New York: Raven Press, 1989; 331–46.

13. Bravermann IM, Fonferko E. Studies in cutaneous aging. I. The microvasculature. J Invest Dermatol 1982; 78:444–8.
14. Kligman LH, Akin FJ, Kligman AM. The contribution of UVA and UVB to connective tissue damage in hairless mice. J Invest Dermatol 1985; 84:272–6.
15. Sams WM, Smith JG, Burk PG. The experimental production of elastosis with ultraviolet light. J Invest Dermatol 1964; 43:467–71.
16. Gilchrest B, Soter NA, Hawk JLM, et al. Histologic changes associated with ultraviolet A induced erythema in normal human skin. J Am Acad Dermatol 1983; 9:213–19.
17. Daly CH, Odland G. Age related changes in the mechanical properties of human skin. J Invest Dermatol 1979; 73:84–7.
18. Christensen MS, Hargens CW, Nacht S, Gans EH. Viscoelastic properties of intact human skin, instrumentation, hydration, effect and the contribution of the straum corneum. J Invest Dermatol 1977; 69:282.
19. Kijdd WL, Daly CH, Nansen PD. Variation in the response to mechanical stress of human soft tissues in the elderly and the young. J Prosthet Dent 1974; 32:493–500.
20. Brody GS, Landel RF, Peng TJ. Nondestructive rheologic analysis of normal and abnormal human skin. Bioeng Skin Newls 1979; 2–1:10.
21. Wan Abas WAB, Barbenel JC. Uniaxial tension test of human skin in vivo. J Biomed Eng 1982; 4:65.
22. Bravermann IM, Fonferko E. Studies in cutaneous aging: the elastic fiber network. J Invest Dermatol 1982; 78:434–43.
23. Agache PG, Monneur C, Leveque JL, deRigal J. Mechanical properties and Young's modulus of the skin in vivo. Arch Dermatol Res 1980; 269:221–32.
24. Wijn P. The alinear viscoelastic properties of human skin in vivo for small deformations. Thesis, University of Nijmegen, The Netherlands, 1980; 34.
25. Alexander H, Cook T. Variations with age in the mechanical properties of human skin in vivo. In: Kenedi RM, ed. Bedsore biomechanics. London: Macmillan, 1976; 109.
26. Leveque JL, deRigal J, Agache P, Monneur C. Influence of aging on the in vivo extensibility of human skin at low stress. Arch Dermatol Res 1980; 269:127.
27. Pierard GE, Lapiere CM. Physiopathological variations in the mechanical properties of skin. Arch Dermatol Res 1977; 260:231–9.
28. Pierard GE. A critical approach to in vivo mechanical testing of the skin. In: Leveque JL, ed. Cutaneous investigation in health and disease, New York: Marcel Dekker, 1989; 215–40.
29. Dikstein S. In vivo mechanical properties of the skin measured by indentometry and levarometry. Bioeng Skin Newsl 1979; 2(1):23.
30. Pierard GE. Evaluation des proprietes mechanique de la peau par les methodes d'indentation et de compression. Dermatologica 1984; 168:61.
31. Escoffier C, deRigal J, Rochefort A, Vasselet R, Leveque JL, Agache P. Age-related mechanical properties of human skin. An in vivo study. J Invest Dermatol 1989; 93:353–7.

32. Fleischmajer R, Perlish JS, Bashey RL. Human dermal glycoaminoglycans and aging. Biochim Biophys Acta 1972; 279:265–75.

33. Leveque JL, Porte G, deRigal J, Corcuff P, Francois AM, Saint Leger D. Influence of chronic sun exposure on some biophysical parameters of human skin: an in vivo study. J Cutan Aging Cosmet Dermatol 1988/89 1:123–7.

34. deRigal J, Leveque JL. In vivo measurements of the stratum corneum elasticity. Bioeng Skin 1985; 1:13.

35. Berardesca E, Vignoli GP, Borroni G, Rigano L, Gasparri F. Acute effects of UV rays on mechanical properties of the skin in vivo. In: Proceedings of the 16th IFSCC: cosmetic science in the 1990s and beyond. New York, October 1990.

36. Kaidbey KH, Kligman AM. The acute effects of long wave ultraviolet radiation on human skin. J Invest Dermatol 1979; 72:253–6.

37. Berardesca E, Gabba P, Farinelli N, Borroni G, Rabbiosi G. In vivo tretinoin-induced changes in skin mechanical properties. Br J Dermatol 1990; 122:525–9.

38. Nelson DL, Balean G. The effects of retinoic acid on collagen synthesis by human dermal fibroblasts. Collagen 1984; 4:119–28.

39. Schiltz JR, Lanigan J, Naibial W, et al. Retinoic acid induces cyclic changes in epidermal thickness and dermal collagen and glycosaminoglycan biosynthesis rates. J Invest Dermatol 1986; 87:663–7.

40. Borroni G, Zaccone C, Vignati G, et al. Assessment of biomechanical changes induced by long-term PUVA treatment ($> 1,000$ J/sqcm) in psoriatic patients. Abstract, VIII international symposium on bioengineering and the skin, Stresa, June 13–16, 1990; 59.

41. Borroni G, Vignati G, Vignoli GP, et al. PUVA-induced viscoelastic changes in the skin of psoriatic patients. Med Biol Environ 1989; 17:663–71.

42. Ramsey CA, Challoner AVJ. Vascular changes in human skin after ultraviolet irradiation. Br J Dermatol 1976; 94:487–93.

43. Willis I, Cylus L. UVA erythema in skin: is it a sunburn? J Invest Dermatol 1977; 68:128–9.

44. Pierard GE, Ackermann B. Histopathology of remodelling induced by PUVA in the superficial dermis. Br J Dermatol 1979; 100:251–6.

4

Ballistometric Properties of Aged Skin

H. ADHOUTE, P. BERBIS, and Y. PRIVAT

Clinique Dermatologique
Hopital Hôtel Dieu
Marseille, France

I INTRODUCTION

Chronologic or actinic skin aging is accompanied by important changes in the physical properties of the stratum corneum, epidermis, and dermis. These changes are due to a disorganization of elastic fibers and deterioration of conjunctival tissue. In combination with dysplasia of the dermoepidermal junction, these modifications lead to decreased elasticity and increased extensibility and constitute one of the main functional signs of skin aging.

Until recently, skin aging was assessed mainly through clinical examination. However, with the great advances in technology and computer science, a variety of new methods have been developed that allow noninvasive, in vivo measurement of the physical properties of skin. Although these techniques have been used mainly to evaluate the efficacy of pharmaceutical and cosmetic products, they also allow functional study of the effects of aging as well as physiopathologic variations caused by diseases affecting conjunctival tissue.

Ballistometry is a biomechanical technique in which cutaneous tone is evaluated by measuring the rebound of a light weight from a surface. The method was originally developed for evaluating the density of metallic surfaces. The first to apply it in dermatology were Tosti et al. in 1977 (1), who used ballistometry to evaluate the "plasticoelastic" consequences of such diseases as psoriasis, dermal sclerosis, and aging. The purpose of this chapter is to describe the measurement technique and then give our findings related to skin aging.

II. MATERIALS AND METHODS

A. Materials

The main characteristics of the ballistometer are summarized in Figure 1. It consists of a 4.7 g hammer and a counterweight attached to either end of a 20 cm long shaft. This assembly pivots in seesaw fashion on an axis perpendicular to the shaft.

Measurements are made by dropping the hammer on the target area. The hammer is placed in contact with an electromagnet at a 35° angle of deviation from the horizontal plane. To avoid manual handling, release is controlled by a microcomputer. After impact the hammer rebounds several times before coming to a stop. These rebounds are measured by an inductive linear potentiometer (ILP; Precilec 25H3, 9 V, 1600 Hz) that delivers an analog signal

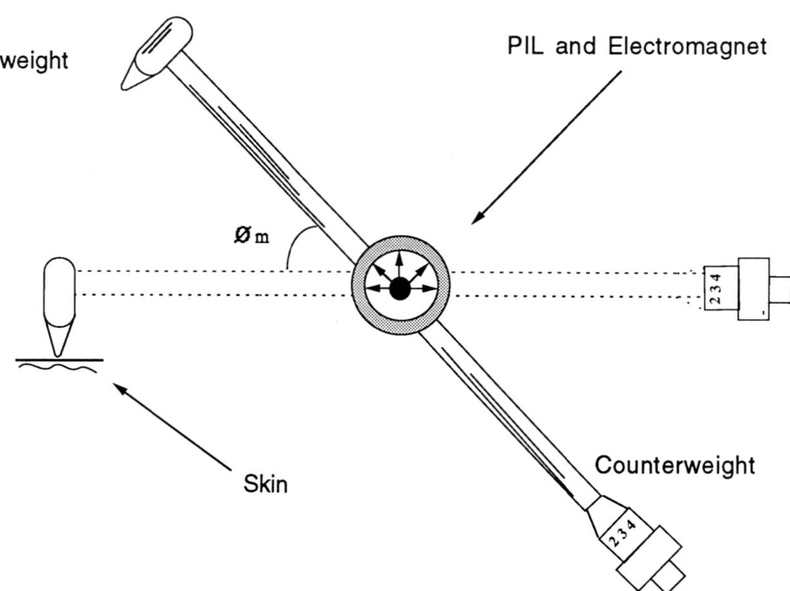

Figure 1 Fundamental principle of the ballistometer.

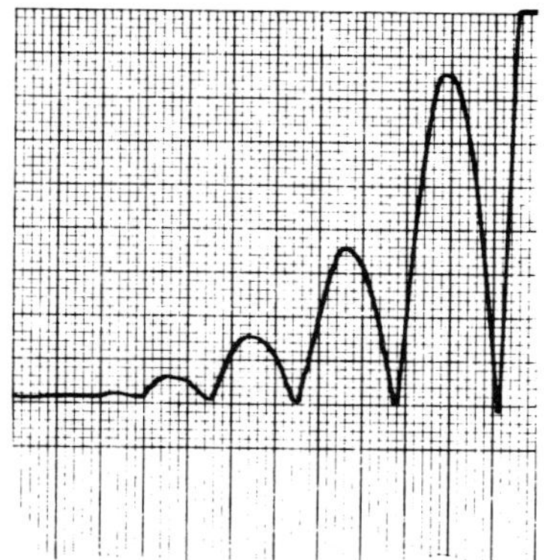
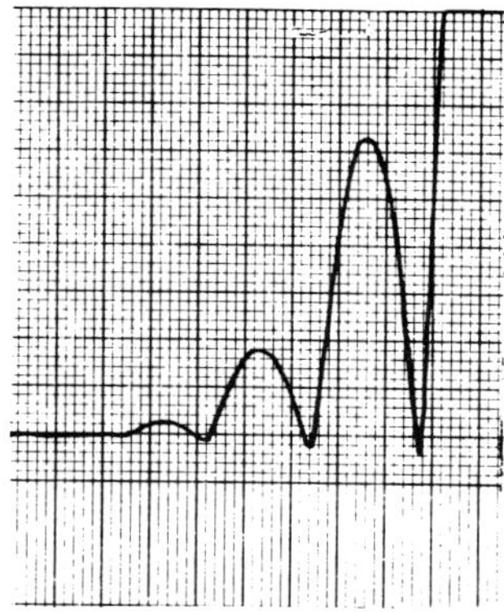

Figure 2 Ballistometric tracings of young and aged skin.

directly proportional to the degree of rotation of the axis. This analog signal is converted to a digital signal, thus enabling monitoring and processing by a microcomputer (PC XT).

Adjustment of the ballistometer is achieved by two controls. One is used to reset the ILP, and the other allows adjustment of the angle of deviation from the horizontal plane, which determines the amount of kinetic energy applied to the skin at the moment of impact. The microcomputer is programmed to calculate the amount of kinetic energy absorbed by the skin at the moment of impact and the cutaneous absorption coefficient. The rebounds are also visualized on a plotter. Figure 2 shows typical graphs.

B. Method of Calculation

The first parameter designed to assess changes in skin firmness during aging was called the coefficient of restitution e. This parameter, which was proposed by Tosti et al., is obtained by measuring and calculating the ratio between two peaks (1). We have developed another method of calculation based on the quantity of energy absorbed by the skin at each rebound. We use this calculated value to select a parameter derived directly from tracings recorded during measurement.

Figure 3 shows the different physical parameters used to construct the mechanical model:

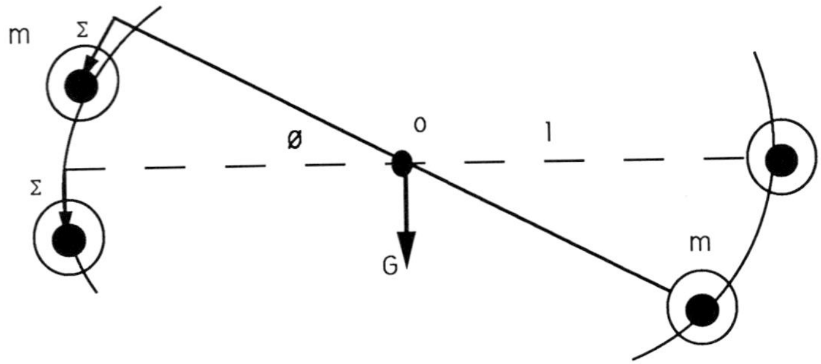

Figure 3   Mechanical model of the ballistometer.

$$m_1 = \text{weight of hammer}$$
$$m_2 = \text{weight of shaft}$$
$$G = \text{center of gravity of the system}$$
$$J = \text{moment of inertia of the system}$$
$$L = \text{length of shaft}$$
$$\theta = \text{angle of deviation}$$
$$g = \text{gravity constant}$$

Let J be the moment of inertia of the system with a center of rotation O. Taking into account the mass of the weight, counterweight, and shaft concentrated on the center of gravity G of the system, we obtain the equation

$$J = \frac{1}{3}m_2 l^2 + m_1(2l^2 + \epsilon^2)$$

If ϕ is the angle of deviation between the shaft and the horizontal plane, the potential energy of the system can be expressed as

$$E_p = -mg\epsilon \, cos \, \theta$$

and the law of energy conservation can be written

$$E_n = \frac{1}{2}J\theta^2 - mg\epsilon \, cos \, \theta \tag{1}$$

E_n between two successive impacts.

Since the kinetic energy at the peak of each rebound is zero ($\frac{1}{2}J\theta^2 = 0$), the energy absorbed at each rebound $n + 1$ can be expressed as

$$\Delta E = E_n - E_{n+1} = mgl[cos \, \theta_m(cos \, \theta_n - cos \, \theta_{n+1})] \tag{2}$$

Let X represent the coefficient of restitution (the ratio of restituted energy to incident energy). Assuming that absorbed energy is proportional to incident energy and based on equations (1) and (2), we can write

$$1 - X = \frac{mg\epsilon(\cos \theta_{n+1} - \cos \theta_n)}{-mg\epsilon(\cos \theta_n - 1)} = \frac{\cos \theta_{n+1} - \cos \theta_n}{1 - \cos \theta_n}$$

When θ_n is small, this equation can be simplified to

$$\theta_n = 1 - \frac{\theta_n^2}{2} \qquad \text{and} \qquad \delta\theta_n = \theta_n - \theta_{n+1}$$

whence

$$X = \left(1 - \frac{\delta\theta_{n+1}}{\theta_n}\right)^2$$

The second step in the constructed model consists of selecting an experimental parameter from the rebound tracings. The equation of the profile of the tracing representing the decreasing amplitude of the shaft's movement on the skin surface is

$$Y = Y_0 e^{-kt}$$

where Y_0 is the initial position of the shaft and K represents the form of the curve (Fig. 4). This parameter depends on the amplitude and number of rebounds. Y can be used as the experimental parameter to evaluate the capacity of the skin to absorb mechanical energy and to characterize its "firmness." This parameter is the cutaneous absorption coefficient (CAC).

C. Correlation Between the Theoretical Model and Experimental Calculation

The CAC is selected from experimental tracings. This choice is checked by measuring the correlation between this coefficient and the coefficient of restitution obtained from the theoretical model. We calculated the correlation between the CAC and coefficient of restitution x in a sample of 50 subjects. Figure 5 shows the different values attributed to the correlation coefficients between CAC and X calculated for the different rebounds.

Statistical analysis showed that values obtained by combining the second, third, and fourth rebounds were most characteristic of the reaction of the skin at impact. This is understandable since the first rebound is proportional to the initial energy, which is the greatest amount of energy applied to the surface during testing. It may be assumed that the first rebound depends on structures below the cutaneous layers, that is, on subcutaneous tissue. Given

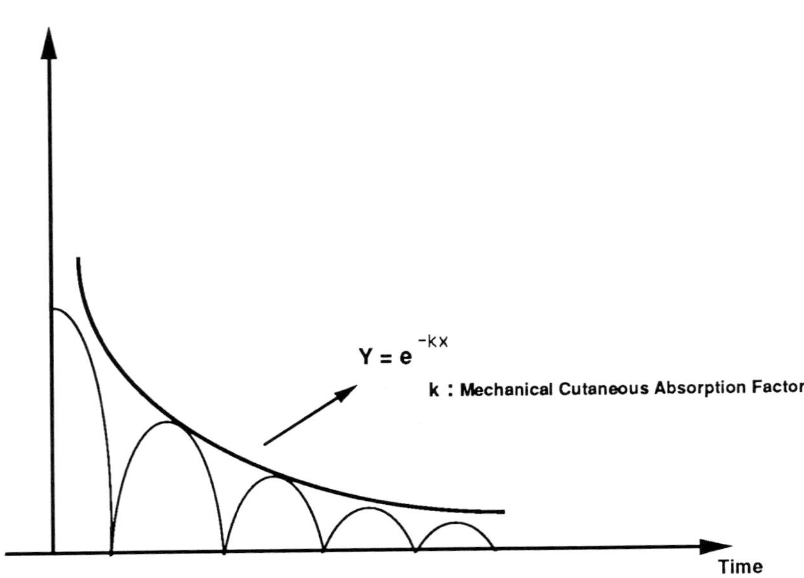

Figure 4 Rebound measurement showing the parameter used.

N° of rebounds	Correlation coefficients between CAC and X
1st - 2nd	R = 0.071 (P = 0.080)
1st - 3rd	R = 0.564 (P = 0.029)
2nd - 3rd	R = 0.654 (P = 0.008)
2nd - 4th	R = 0.664 (P ≤ 0.007)

Figure 5 Correlation of the CAC calculated by the mechanical model with the coefficient of restitution defined by Tosti and colleagues (1).

the relatively large amount of energy involved, the first rebound is virtually the same in all cases. This was proven by experimental measurement of first rebounds.

Kinetic energy values (ergs) were not used in the theoretical calculation. This is because the amount of kinetic energy applied to the skin during testing is always the same. Only the amount of kinetic energy absorbed at each rebound varies. The variable is represented by both the CAC and the coefficient of restitution.

D. Terminology

Before discussing our results, a comment on terminology should be made. In the various studies of the mechanical properties of skin, such terms as plastoelasticity, viscoelasticity, mechanical absorption, tone, and firmness have been used. The physical property studied by ballistometry is mechanical absorption, which characterizes the capacity of the skin to absorb low-level kinetic energy. This property can be evaluated by measurement of the CAC as already defined.

III. RESULTS

A. Ballistometric Skin Measurements

Very few studies have been published concerning the evaluation of viscoelastic characteristics by ballistometry. We present the results of two studies. The first was by Tosti et al. (1). In this publication, the authors presented ballistometric data from 46 subjects between the ages of 8 and 80 years. Measurements were made in 12 different locations.

In one of our studies (2), we calculated the CAC in 120 healthy volunteers between the ages of 15 and 70 (60 men and 60 women). This population was divided into six age groups by 10 year intervals. The measurement zone was the midline of the forehead about 3 cm from the base of the nose. None of the subjects included in this study presented actinic elastosis. Measurements were performed under hygrometric conditions (85%) at the same ambient temperature, 25°C. During measurement different physiologic parameters, including skin temperature, age, and sex, were recorded.

B. Age-Related Variations

The results presented by Tosti et al. showed an age-related decrease in the coefficient of restitution: $r = 0.819$ for the forehead, $r = 0.75$ for the back of the hand, and $r = 0.860$ for the inside of the thigh. This decrease was even

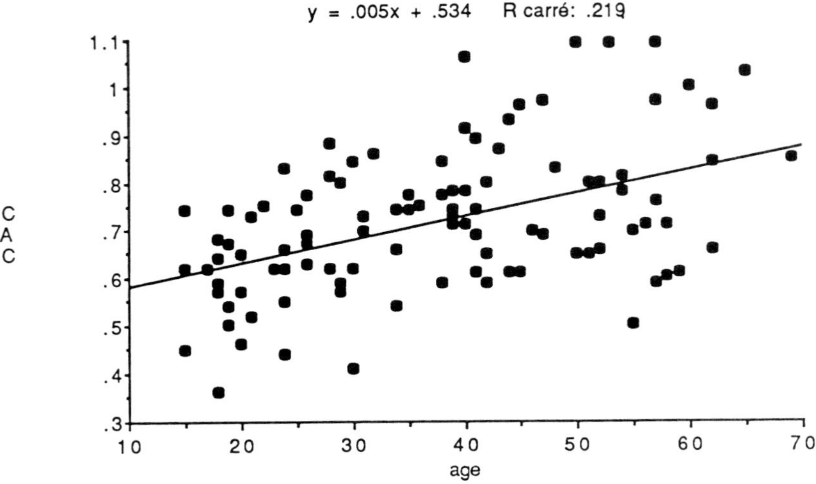

Figure 6 In vivo relationship between CAC (cutaneous absorption coefficient) and age. When age decreases, the elasticity increases.

more marked for sun-exposed zones. The authors also pointed out that the coefficient of restitution varied according to the location of the measurement zone. Thus e values for the forehead or back of the hand were lower than those for the other regions.

The results of the second study showed a significant correlation between the mean age of the sample as a whole and the CAC, $r = 0.48$ ($p < 0.0001$). The relationship between the two parameters was linear (test $F: p < 0.0001$). The CAC increased with age (Fig. 6) but elasticity decreased. Variations in the CAC according to age group are shown in Figure 7. The CAC increased up to a maximum of 0.77 in the 40–50 year group.

If the subjects are divided into two groups according to sex, the relationship between age and CAC is significant ($p < 0.01$) and linear ($p < 0.025$) in both groups. The mean CAC was 0.67 ± 0.02 in women versus 0.76 ± 0.02 ($p < 0.025$) in men. This difference can only be attributed to age differences between the two groups. The mean age was 39 ± 2 years in the male group versus 36 ± 2 in the female group. This difference was not statistically significant.

C. Effects of Physiologic Parameters

A strong correlation was noted between the cutaneous temperature measured at the test site and the CAC. When this relationship was expressed mathe-

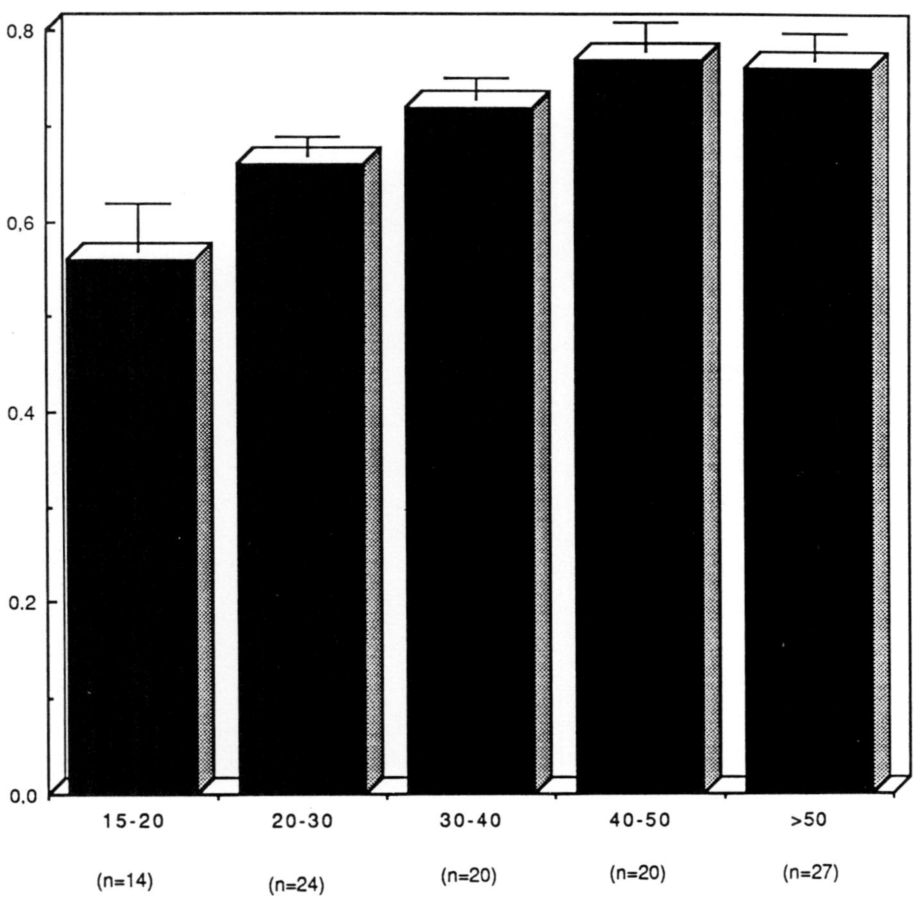

Figure 7 Evaluation of CAC according to different age intervals.

matically, a decrease in temperature was observed concomitant with a loss of elasticity. The relationship between temperature and CAC was significant only in the female group. This observation can be attributed to the greater variations in physiologic activity in women.

IV. DISCUSSION

It is generally accepted that the mechanical properties of the skin depend on four main parameters: age, sex, skin thickness, and location. Some studies

(2–5) showed that these parameters are also interdependent, which complicates the interpretation of results obtained with in vivo techniques designed to measure the mechanical characteristics of skin. The results of ballistometry presented here show that the capacity of the skin to absorb mechanical impact decreases with age.

The small amount of kinetic energy brought to bear suggests that the resulting mechanical impact propagates over a short distance over the surface of the skin and does not extend beyond the dermis. Under these conditions, two parameters can influence the propagation of impact. First, at the level of the skin surface (stratum corneum), the cohesion of horny cells and the presence of water or other agents in intercellular spaces is an important factor. Second, at the level of the epidermis and dermis, ballistometric measurements directly reflect the density of elastic fibers and the geometry of the collagen network.

Since this is an in vivo method, however, it is difficult to determine the individual role of each skin layer in the results obtained. It is also difficult to dissociate the relative role of such parameters as age and thickness. To resolve these problems, further investigation with biochemical and ultrasonic methods are needed. These studies are currently underway.

REFERENCES

1. Tosti A, Campagno G, Fazzini MC, Villardita S. A ballistometer for the study of the plasto-elastic properties of skin. J Invest Dermatol 1977; 69:315.
2. Piérard G, Lapière CM. Physiopathological variations in the mechanical properties of skin. Arch Dermatol Res 1977; 260:231.
3. Piérard GE. Structure et propriétés mécaniques des compartiments adventitiels et réticulaires du derme. Thesis, University of Liège, Belgium 1984; 39.
4. Daly CH, Odland GF. Age-related changes in the mechanical properties of human skin. J Invest Dermatol 1979; 73:84–7.
5. Escoffier C, de Rigal J, Rochefort A, Vasselet R, Levêque JL, Agache P. Age-related mechanical properties of human skin: in vivo study. J Invest Dermatol 1989; 933:353–7.

5

Mechanical Properties of Aged Skin: Indentation and Elevation Experiments

G. E. PIÉRARD

University of Liège
Liège, Belgium

I. INTRODUCTION

Skin may be viewed as a nonlinear, nonhomogeneic, viscoelastic material. Some facets of these properties can be measured by indentation and elevation experiments.

We present a review of the literature, and we use the concepts issued from a report of the committee of standardization of the International Society of Bioengineering and the Skin elaborated in 1980 by Barbenel and Payne.

II. BASIC PRINCIPLES OF INDENTATION

Indentation is regularly used in classic engineering to test the hardness of materials. It was first used to investigate the skin by Schade (1), and since then this technique has been advanced by other workers (2–12).

Schade's original apparatus consisted of a pivoted arm supporting a spherical ball that was indented into the skin. Later developments of the system have used smaller and flat indentors.

The indentation clearly depends on the compression forces and on the resistance of the skin and underlying tissues. Indentation of up to 4 mm may be obtained on the arm (7,11). This is only 1 mm on the forehead (10) or over the tibia (11). Indentation of the skin over muscles may reach 10 mm and depends upon relaxation or contraction of the muscles (11). These rough data identify two markedly different situations:

1. The subcutaneous tissue is much stiffer than the skin and hypodermis. This may be found in such selected sites as the forehead, over the tibia, and most probably over bony prominences. Here the deformation is produced almost entirely by the skin.
2. The subcutaneous tissue has approximately the same stiffness as the skin. This occurs over most body sites where muscles underlie the skin. The indentation depends on both tissues and cannot be allocated precisely to one of the tissues.

There appears to be no way of interrelating the results obtained using different indentor radii or of accounting for differences in skin thickness. However, there is a linear relationship between forces to obtain a defined indentation when muscles are relaxed or contracted (11).

III. BASIC PRINCIPLES OF ELEVATION

In contrast to the indentation methods, the application of a vertical traction force to a membrane and measurement of the resulting elevation of the surface appears to be unique to testing the skin.

There are two distinct approaches to exerting traction: the suction method and the tonometry method using either a disk glued by cyanoacrylate onto the skin or a hollow probe in which the pressure is lowered.

The suction method has been used with different apparatus by a series of authors. Such an approach aimed at two distinct goals, that is, to determine dermoepidermal adherence (13–16) and mechanical properties of the dermis (17–21). The technique of tonometry has been introduced by only a limited number of researchers (22,23) but has yielded a vast body of information about cutaneous pathology (22,24–31).

The elevation due to suction or traction depends on the forces exerted, the body site, and the area of contact between the probe and the skin. Standardization of the methods can only be achieved if the skin under tension is delineated by a guard ring.

There appears to be no mathematical method of interrelating results obtained by different loads and sizes of probes. There is a linear relationship between skin elevation and skin thickness. It is particularly difficult to assess the influence of subcutaneous tethering, but it is certain that tests in which large elevations of the skin occur are strongly influenced by subcutaneous attachments.

IV. BIOLOGIC MEANING OF MECHANICAL MEASUREMENTS DURING AGING

Skin is subjected to forces originating in the body and imposed by the environment. Because forces originating in the body are not measurable, they should be reduced to a minimum to prevent interference with testing. Measuring the overall mechanical characteristics of skin by indentation and elevation methods provides only a rough estimate of the resultant of multiple parameters acting upon the various constitutive elements of the cutaneous tissues. In general terms, they depend mainly on the connective tissue, dermis, and hypodermis, with a possible contribution from the epidermis (32). In the physiologic range of tension, we believe that the structural organization of collagen bundles, their orientation, the anchorage of bundles together, and their relation to elastic fibers and proteoglycans should be considered predominant (33). The anisotropy of skin, related to the natural lines of tension discovered by Dupuytren and Langer, appears related to the architectural organization of the dermis (34). This cannot be evaluated by indentation and elevation test methods.

V. THEORETICAL CONCEPT LINKING CUTANEOUS AGING AND MECHANICAL PROPERTIES

''Cutaneous aging'' is a vague term that encompasses the results of distinct features. It is misleading to consider aging a unique and uniform biologic event. What has been called chronologic or intrinsic aging depends on genetic factors, lapse of time, and the sum of various effects of diseases and desmotropic drugs, as well as physiologic variations and environmental influences with the exception of sun exposure. Photoaging deals with all these features to which chronic exposure to ultraviolet light is added.

All age-related changes in skin obviously have an influence upon mechanical properties. Moreover, mechanical stimuli applied to the skin throughout life affect the structure of the cutaneous tissues, which in turn modifies the mechanical properties (35,36).

Such multiple interrelationships between the variable structure of the skin, the innumerable factors influencing aging, and the complexity of the mechanical properties likely preclude any clear-cut understanding of the problem. Moreover, methodologies used to evaluate the mechanical properties of skin are so diverse in the literature that the data can hardly be compared.

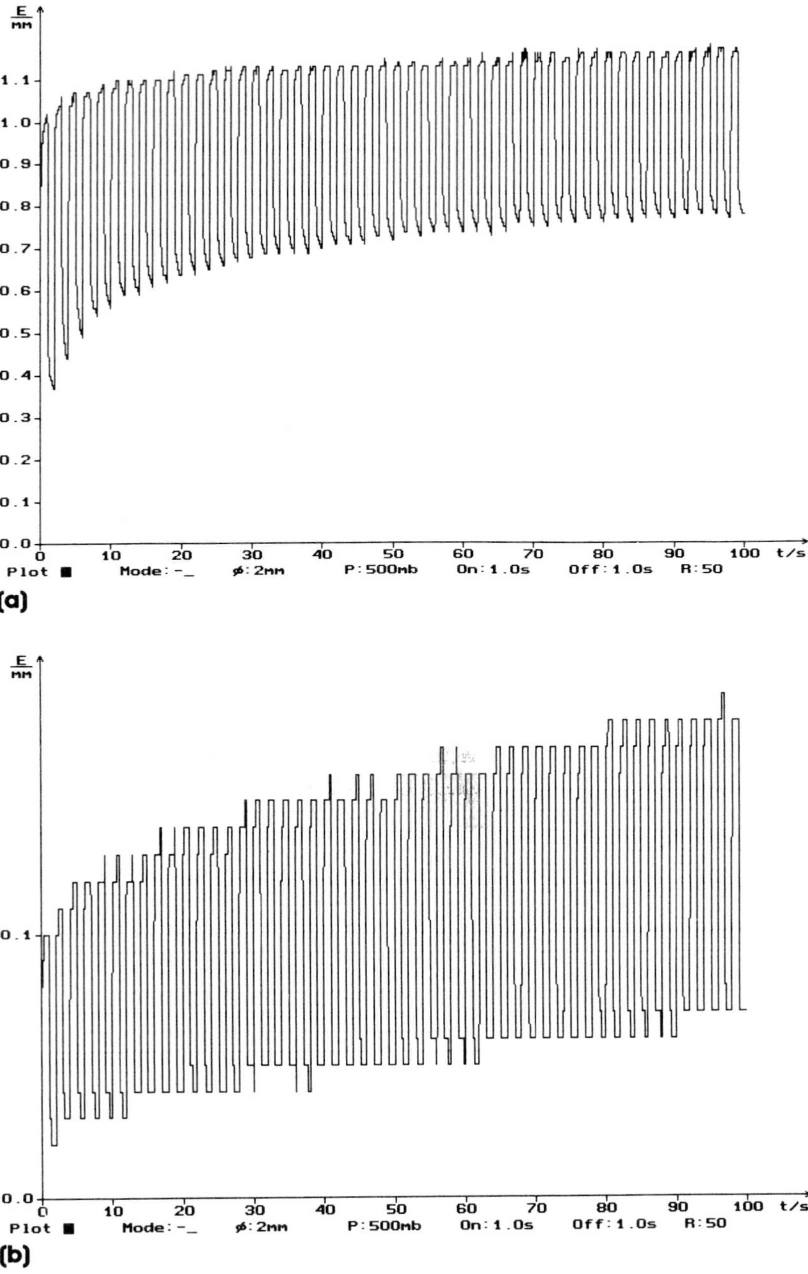

Figure 1 Example in a 74-year old woman of the skin deformation as a function of time during 50 cycles of 1 sec traction—1 sec relaxation. (a) Inner aspect of the arm (chronological aging). (b) Outer aspect of the forearm (photoaging). (c) Inner aspect of the arm after a 6-month treatment with retinoic acid.

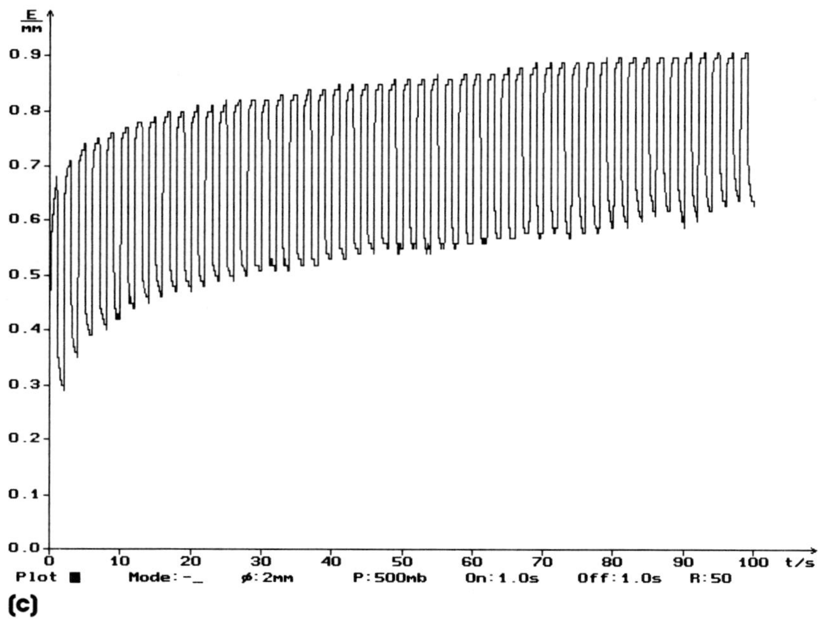

(c)

VI. INDENTATION AND ELEVATION EXPERIMENTS ON AGED SKIN

Ideally, four parameters should be recorded and considered interdependent variables with biomechanical properties. These are age, sex, and skin thickness and texture. Although it is clinically obvious that mechanical properties are different in children and among the elderly, measuring them with different test modes has introduced controversial results (2,3,6,8,12,22,32, 33,37,38). From the available information, it seems that the resistance of the dermis to traction exerted parallel to the skin surface increases with age at least until 60 years. Conversely, the vertical resistance at the dermoepidermal junction and within the dermis and hypodermis progressively decreases.

When looking at the most recent work with sophisticated devices, it appears that the authors agree to consider two main physical parameters: the resistance of skin to deformation and the ability of skin to regain its initial position after deformation.

Indentometry indicates that the resistance to pressure decreases with age. This seems more pronounced in shielded skin than on sun-exposed areas. Subtle differences have been disclosed according to sex, but the data are difficult to interpret (12). The elastic rebound of the skin, also called biologic elasticity, decreases with age in all population groups (11,12,33).

Elevation experiments seem to indicate wide variations in the deformability of skin in aged individuals (22,33,38). Changes in biologic elasticity are more constant, indicating a progressive diminution of this parameter over time (22,33,38).

By computerized elevation method (Cutometer SM 474, Courage Khazaka, Köln, Germany), the time—strain relationship appears altered during aging. The skin deformation plotted as a function of time is markedly increased during chronological aging (Fig. 1 a) compared to photoaging (Fig. 1 b). Topical retinoic acid may in part decrease the skin atrophy as assessed by a decreased skin deformability obtained after a 6-month treatment (Fig. 1 a, c).

REFERENCES

1. Schade H. Untersuchungen zur Organfunktion des Bindegewebes. Z Exp Pathol Ther 1912; 11:369–99.
2. Kirk JE, Kvorning SA. Quantitative measurements of the elastic properties of the skin and subcutaneous tissues in young and old individuals. J Gerontol 1949; 4:273–84.
3. Kirk JE, Chieffi M. Variation with age in elasticity of skin and subcutaneous tissue in human individuals. J Gerontol 1962; 17:373–80.
4. Tregear RT, Dirnhuber P. Viscous flow in compressed human and rat skin. J Invest Dermatol 1965; 45:119–25.
5. Tregear RT. Physical functions of skin. New York: Academic Press, 1966.
6. Parot S, Bourliere F. A new technique for measuring compressibility of skin and subcutaneous tissue. Influence of sex, age and body area. Gerontology 1967; 13:95–110.
7. Vlasblom DC. Skin elasticity. Ph.D. thesis, University of Utrecht, 1967.
8. Kydd WL, Daly CH, Nansen PD. Variation in the response to mechanical stress of human soft tissues as related to age. J Prosthet Dent 1974; 32:493–500.
9. Debelle M. La tonométrie musculaire et ses applications. Ars Med 1977; 32:963–81.
10. Dikstein S, Hartzshtark A. In vivo measurement of some elastic properties of human skin. In: Marks R, Payne P, eds. Bioengineering and the skin. Lancaster: MTP Press, 1979; 45–53.
11. Piérard GE. Evaluation de propriétés méchaniques de las peau par les méthodes d'indentation et de compression. Dermatologica 1984; 168:61–6.
12. Robert C, Blanc M, Dikstein S, Robert L. Study of skin aging as a function of social and professional conditions: modification of the rheological parameters measured with a noninvasive method-indentometry. Gerontology 1988; 34: 384–90.
13. Slowley C, Leider M. Abstract of a preliminary report: the production of bullae by quantitated suction. Arch Dermatol 1961; 83:1029.

14. Kiistala U. Suction blister device for separation of viable epidermis from dermis. J Invest Dermatol 1968; 50:129–37.

15. Lowe LB, Van Der Leun JC. Suction blisters and dermal epidermal adherence. J Invest Dermatol 1968; 50:308–14.

16. Piérard GE, Piérard-Franchimont C, Lapière CM. Alternation des loci minoris resistentiae du derme dans la photosclérose. Dermatologica 1983; 167:121–6.

17. Grahame R. Elasticity of human skin in vivo. Ann Phys Med 1969; 10:130–4.

18. Grahame R. A method for measuring human skin elasticity in vivo with observations on the effects of age, sex and pregnancy. Clin Sci 1970; 39:223–38.

19. Ude P. Ein Vakuum-Elongations-Tonometer zur quantifizierten Bestimmung des Hauttonus. Therapiewoche 1972; 22:4273.

20. Alexander H, Cohen ML, Cook T. In vivo mechanical characterization of human skin. In: Proceedings 10th Int. Conf. Med. Biol. Bioeng., 1973.

21. Cook T, Alexander H, Cohen ML. An experimental method for determining the two-dimensional mechanical properties of living human skin. Med Biol Eng 1977; 15:134–9.

22. Piérard GE, Lapière ChM, Physiopathological variations in the mechanical properties of skin. Arch Dermatol Res 1977; 260:231–9.

23. Hargens CW. The gas bearing electrodynamometer applied to measuring mechanical changes in skin and other tissues. In: Marks R, Payne P, eds. Bioengineering and the skin. Lancaster: MTP Press, 1981; 113–22.

24. Piérard GE, Lapière CM. Skin in dermatosparaxis. Dermal microarchitecture and biomechanical properties. J Invest Dermatol 1976; 66:2–7.

25. Piérard GE, Hermans JF, Lapière ChM. Dynamics of the connective tissue remodeling and of its impaired mechanical properties in scleromyxoedema. J Cutan Pathol 1977; 4:203–4.

26. Piérard GE, Cryns E, Franchimont C. Perspectives d'évaluation par tonométrie de l'effet de cosmétiques sur les fonctions bioméchaniques de la peau. Rev Inst Pasteur Lyon 1978; 11:219–24.

27. Piérard GE, Lapière ChM. Phenytoin dependent fibrosis in polyfibromatosis syndrome. Br J Dermatol 1979; 100:335–41.

28. Piérard GE, Franchimont C, de la Brassinne M, Lapière CM. Photosclerosis induced by long wave ultraviolet light and psoralens. In: Marks R, Payne P, eds. Bioengineering and the skin. Lancaster: MTP Press, 1981; 71–8.

29. Piérard GE, Piérard-Franchimont C, Lapière CM. Les compartiments conjonctifs dans les sclérodermies. Etude de la structure et des propriétés biomécaniques. Dermatologica 1985; 170:105–13.

30. Piérard GE. The Liège experience in the assessment of the variability in the mechanical properties of skin. Bioeng Skin 1987; 2:227–34.

31. Piérard GE. Histological and rheological grading of cutaneous sclerosis in scleroderma. Dermatologica 1989; 179:18–20.

32. Piérard GE. A critical approach of in vivo mechanical testing of the skin. In: Lévêque JL, eds. Cutaneous investigation in health and disease; noninvasive methods and instrumentation. New York: Marcel Dekker, 1988; 215–40.

33. Piérard GE. Structure et propriétés méchaniques des compartiments adventitiel et réticulaire du derme. Thesis of Agregation, University of Liêge, 1984; 1–416.

34. Piérard GE, Laipère CM. Microanatomy of the dermis in relation to relaxed skin tension lines and Langer's lines. Am J Dermatopathol 1987; 9:219–24.

35. Lapière CM. Piérard GE. The mechanical forces, a neglected factor in the age-related changes of the skin. G Ital Chir Dermatol Oncol 1987; 2:201–10.

36. Piérard GE, Lapière CM. The microanatomical basis of facial frown lines. Arch Dermatol 1989; 125:1090–2.

37. Grahame R, Holt P. The influence of aging on the in vivo elasticity of human skin. J Gerontol 1969; 15:121–39.

38. Cua AB, Wilhelm KP, Maibach HI. Elastic properties of human skin: relation to age, sex and anatomical region. Arch Dermatol Res 1990; 282:283–8.

6

Variation in Skin Thickness with Age

JEAN-LUC LÉVÊQUE and JEAN de RIGAL

L'Oréal
Aulnay-sous-Bois, France

I. INTRODUCTION

Skin thickness is an important element of cutaneous physiology. Like most organs, in some way its dimensions reflect its functioning. Skin thickness also reflects the physiologic response to the application or administration of therapeutic agents. This is the case, for example, in chronic treatment with steroids given topically or systemically in which skin atrophy occurs after variable periods. Finally, measurement of skin thickness can be used to evaluate the effects of the sun and ultraviolet radiation. In aging skin, as we shall see later in this chapter, a progressive atrophy reflects a general decrease in cutaneous metabolism. This phenomenon was first described some time ago on the basis of histologic examination of biopsy specimens. More recently, the availability of numerous noninvasive methods has led to the multiplication of measurements at various skin sites and has given rise to a more detailed and precise description of aging skin.

In this short chapter we review the main results describing how skin thickness varies during aging at different skin sites. The results obtained by different methods are compared. Another section concerns the different factors that can influence skin thickness during the aging process (normal status, pathologies, drugs, and others). We begin with a brief review of the noninvasive techniques used to noninvasively measure skin thickness.

II. SKIN THICKNESS MEASUREMENT TECHNIQUES

We do not deal here with in vitro methods in which the thickness of the various skin layers is measured by means of low-magnification microscopic examination of stained histologic sections, which clearly cannot be used for routine studies. It should also be noted that the data obtained using such methods do not provide information on skin in its natural state of equilibrium, since skin sampling leads to some degree of shrinkage. Similarly, we only mention the x-ray method, which can no longer be considered noninvasive and can only be used on certain sites, such as the leg and the arm (1).

The only truly noninvasive and routinely applicable techniques are the skinfold method and A or B mode ultrasound echography. The skinfold method consists of pinching the skin with a caliper and deducing thickness by halving the observed value (2). This method can only be used on sites at which the skin is sufficiently loose to be gripped by the caliper. Another disadvantage is that there is some uncertainty concerning the amount of hypodermal tissue caught within the fold. Finally, the compressibility of the skin varies with age and this can affect the accuracy of measurements (3).

The A mode ultrasound echographic technique was first described in 1979 (4). It consists of measuring the time taken by a high-frequency ultrasound pulse (5–30×10^6 Hz) to cross the skin and return to the emission/reception transducer after being reflected by the dermal/hypodermal interface.

B mode ultrasound echography provides cross-sectional images of the skin. The images are formed by the acquisition of successive echographic lines obtained in A mode. These lines are used to reconstruct an image of the skin in which the various shades of gray represent the amplitude of the echoes detected at each point (5).

III. EFFECT OF AGING ON SKIN THICKNESS

Clinical examination of the skin by simple pinching between the fingers reveals that the skin of the elderly is thin and lacking in tone: the first term that comes to mind in this context is atrophy. But what actually occurs?

The skinfold studies published in 1967 by Ryckewaert et al., together with those of Parot and Bourliere, showed that skin thickness on the back of the hand diminishes gradually throughout the aging process (6,7). We confirmed these findings in 1980 by applying a similar experimental approach to the dorsal surface of the arm. We also found that during the period of maturation (up to the age of about 30 years), skin thickness increases, whereas it decreases thereafter, and that during this period the skin is thicker in men than in women (Fig. 1) (8). This latter result was confirmed in a recent study by Lubach and Kunkler concerning 340 subjects (3). The data showed that skin atrophy becomes marked only after the fifth decade of life and that these changes are clearer on the back of the hand than on the arm.

Despite this general agreement, these data should be interpreted with care given the methodologic limitations mentioned earlier. Indeed, the hypodermis probably contributed to the measured thickness, and the decrease in overall skin thickness may thus have been partly due to the known reduction in hypodermal thickness that occurs at certain sites during aging (9).

With regard to A mode echography, there are two principle studies involving systematic measurements over the entire age range (10,11). Both involved the dorsal skin of the forearm and large numbers of men and women. The results of these two studies (Fig. 2) are in remarkably good agreement, with regard to both mean age group values and variations with age. The

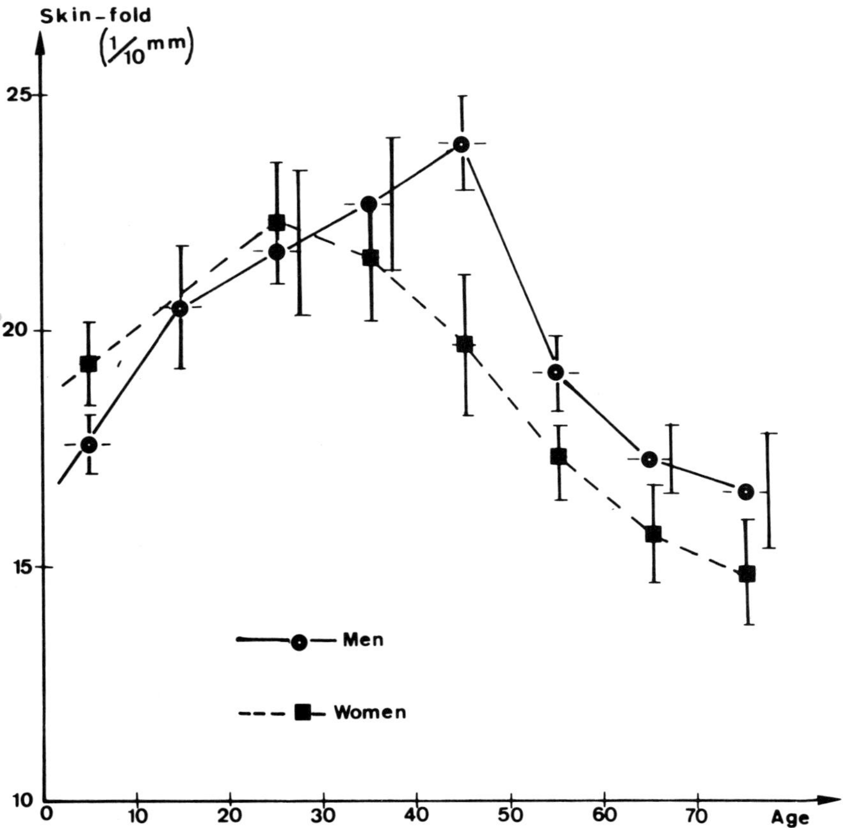

Figure 1 Variation in the skinfold thickness on the forearm (dorsal side) versus age in 141 subjects. (From Ref. 8.)

agreement between studies involving different groups of subjects and investigators underscores the excellent objectivity of this method.

However, interpretation of the results of the two studies differed significantly. The Cardiff team considered that the reduction in skin thickness begins after the maturation period and is progressive. In contrast, according to the L'Oreal team, skin thickness begins to decrease only after the sixth decade of life. These two interpretations illustrate the influence of the statistical methods used with regard to the interpretation of the phenomena recorded. The recent work of Denda and Takahashi (12) extended findings concerning the forearm, the forehead, and the cheeks. They found that (1) skin thickness in men is about 20% greater than in women and (2) there is a linear regression between age and skin thickness of the same order of statistical significance as that reported by Tan et al. (10).

One of the difficulties of the A mode echographic technique is in identifying the echo corresponding to the dermal/hypodermal interface. In addition, measurements made with this technique must be repeated several times to obtain representative values. This latter element should be eliminated in B mode echography because each image obtained corresponds to the sum of at least 100 echographic lines obtained in A mode.

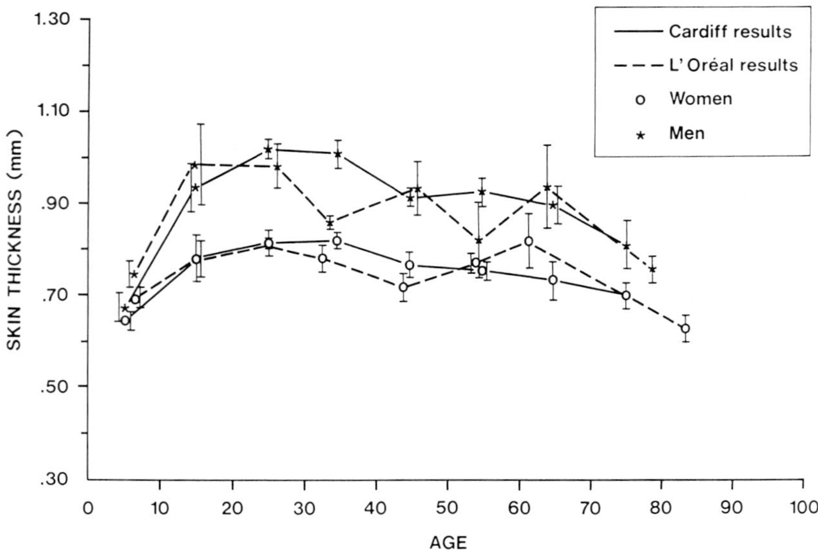

Figure 2   Skin thickness versus age measured by ultrasonography (A mode) of the forearm (ventral side) according to two independent studies (10,11).

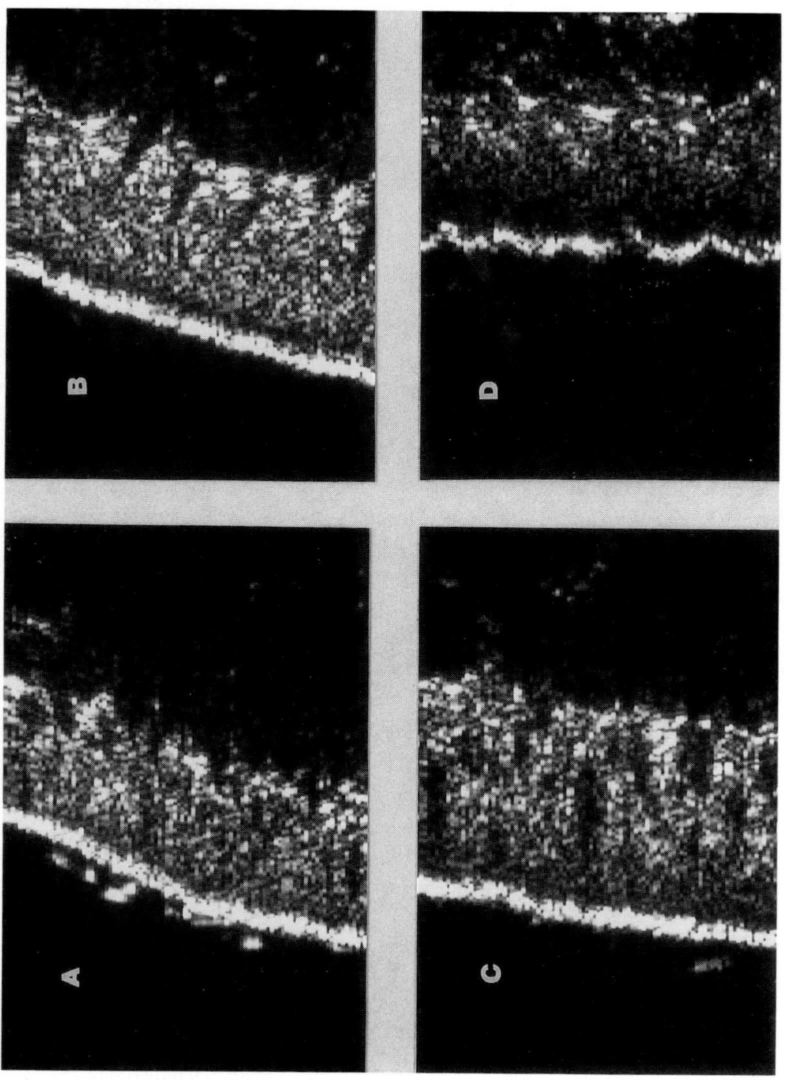

Figure 3 Appearance of the skin in people of different ages. The SENEB, appearing under the bright gel/skin surface interface, is quite invisible in the young but can attain more than half the skin thickness in the aged (see Ref. 14): (A) young; (B) young adult; (C) adult; (D) aged.

Two studies of skin thickness variations with age involving the use of ultrasound imaging (B mode) were published recently (13,14). The results of
the two studies are in agreement on certain points but in disagreement on others. First, they both confirm the differences in thickness between the ventral
and dorsal faces of the forearm. Similarly, they confirm the existence of a
period of maturation during which skin thickness increases between birth and
the end of the second decade of life, with a period of atrophy after the age of
70 years. Between these two periods, both studies agree that skin thickness
remains constant. With regard to the points of disagreement, the main one is
the thickness of the skin of the forearm. The French team advanced a value
of 1.1 mm for the dorsal face and 0.95 mm for the ventral face. The corresponding values published by the U.S. team were 1.5 and 1.3, respectively.
These differences are difficult to explain but show that even with B mode
imaging a degree of standardization is required with regard to identifying the
dermal/hypodermal interface, which can in some cases be confounded with
conjunctive trabeculae adhering along the dermis. On the other hand, we
have no information concerning the type of population investigated in the
U.S. study. In the article by de Rigal and colleagues (14), the important point
concerns the description of a zone, nonechogenic for the ultrasonic waves,
located in the upper dermis. This zone, called the SENEB (subepidermal

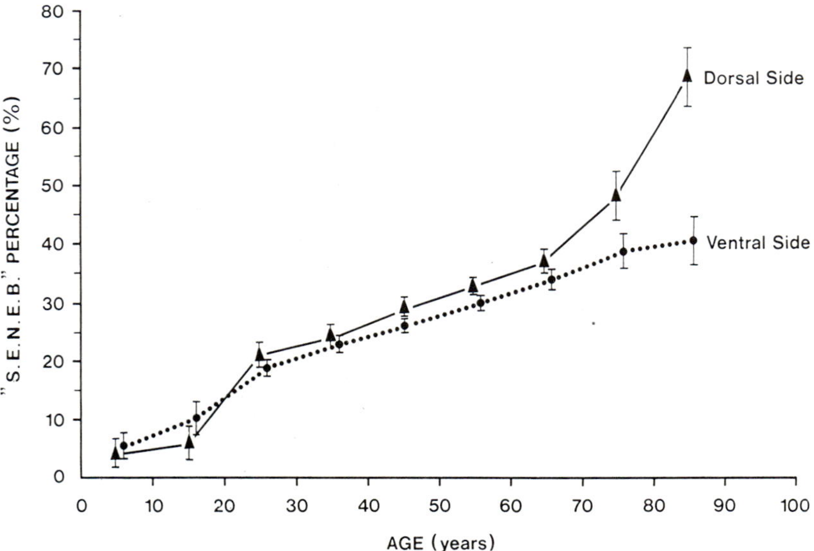

Figure 4 Variation with age in the relative contribution (%) of the SENEB to the
total skin thickness (see Ref. 14).

nonechogenic band), appears as a black band on the photographs. Its thickness would increase as a function of age and would be thicker on the dorsal side of the forearm (exposed) than on the ventral side (protected). The results of this study are summarized in Figures 3 and 4. This band probably corresponds to a zone where the collagen bundles are thin and/or dense and therefore unable to generate echoes. This SENEB appears to be a new and sensitive marker of the aging process at the cutaneous level. The existence of this nonechogenic band was confirmed by Serup (see Chap. 7), who called it the "age band," and by Schatz et al. (13).

IV. FACTORS INFLUENCING SKIN THICKNESS DURING AGING

Among the extrinsic factors that can influence skin thickness, exposure to sunlight is a major factor and can produce an increase of up to 15% in certain cases (15). In exposed areas, such as the neck and the face, data are lacking but it appears that there is no atrophy during aging, at least in persons living in geographic areas where the degree of exposure is high (16). In fact, the relationship between aging, sunlight, and skin thickness has been studied very little. Among the intrinsic (biologic) factors, osteoporosis requires special mention. It has been shown that subjects with this disease of the osseous connective tissue present a skin atrophy of about 15% (Fig. 5) (13). This is of

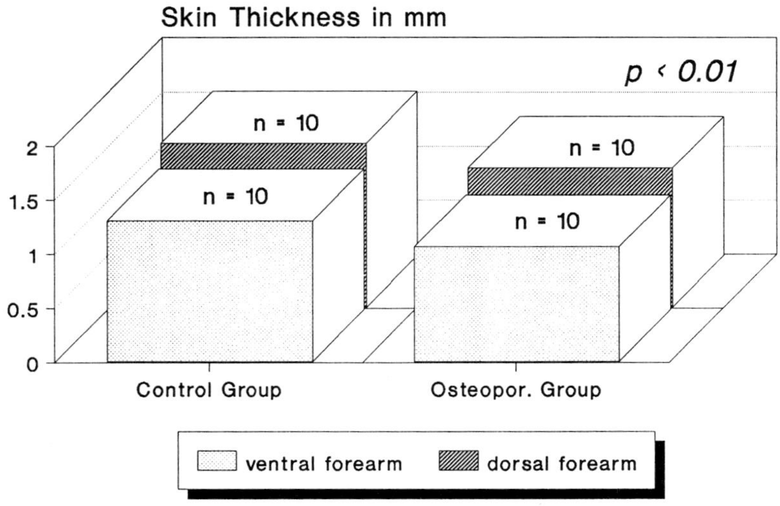

Figure 5 Influence of osteoporosis on skin thickness measured by ultrasonography (B mode) of the forearm. (From Ref. 13.)

great interest because it provides a way of comparing degenerative processes during aging in two distinct tissues.

The influence of hormonal status on the level of collagen present in the skin and skin thickness has been mainly described by Brincat et al. (17,18). They show that postmenopausal women treated with sex hormone implants have a greater skin collagen content and thicker skin compared to a similar group of untreated women. In another study, the skin collagen content and skin thickness were compared in two groups of postmenopausal women with and without rheumatoid disease. The first group had a reduced skin collagen content but an increased skin thickness. The relationships between skin thickness, skin collagen content, bone density, and estrogen deficiency were also demonstrated in a group of women with anorexia nervosa (19). Concerning the effects of growth hormone in aged men, Rudman et al. showed that skin thinning could be reversed by subcutaneous injections of biosynthetic growth hormone (20). We also mention the connective tissue diseases, such as scleroderma, which can be associated with a doubling of skin thickness (21), or the Ehlers-Danlos syndrome, in which the skin thickness is decreased (22).

Similarly, steroids given both topically (23) and orally (24) can induce premature aging of skin, of which atrophy is the main feature (Fig. 6).

Recently, a number of cases have been described in which skin thickness is increased by the topical application of all trans-retinoic acid. This increase in thickness varies between 40 and 80 μm according to different studies and probably results mainly from epidermal acanthosis (25,26).

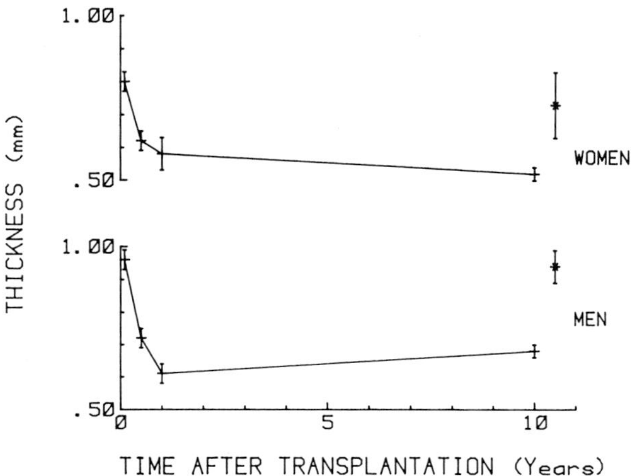

Figure 6   Skin atrophy as a consequence of steroid intake versus time after kidney transplantation. (From Ref. 24.)

Measurement of skin thickness could also be used to provide prognostic information in the gravitational syndrome (27).

V. CONCLUSION AND PERSPECTIVE

The development of noninvasive techniques, particularly ultrasound echography (A and B modes), has made the measurement of skin thickness a routine procedure and has permitted objective monitoring of the skin. In the

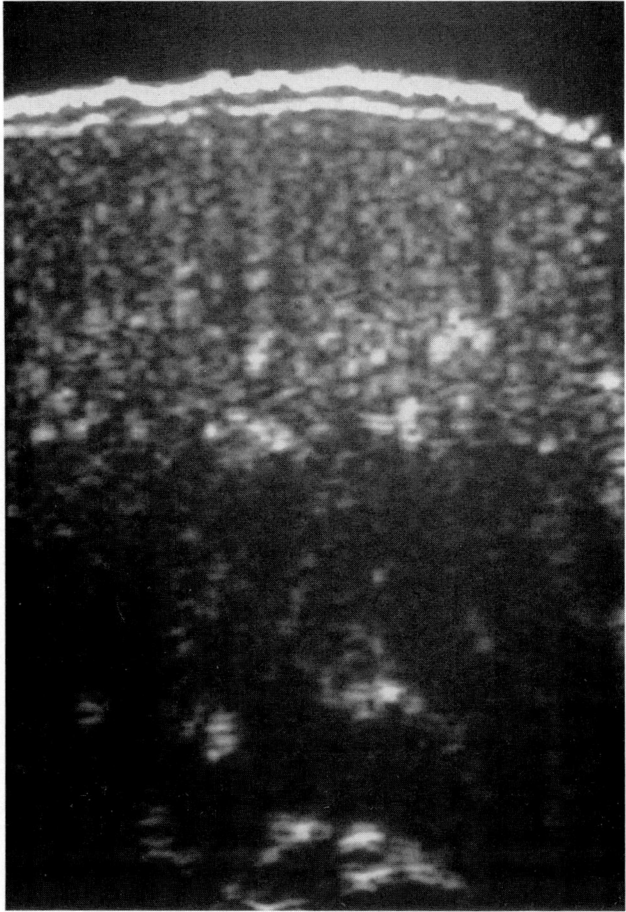

Figure 7 Ultrasonic imaging of the skin of the cheek. The epidermal thickness (distance between the two superficial white lines) is 89 ± 3μm.

context of aging, these methods have already allowed the results obtained by histometric methods to be generalized to a larger number of sites and age categories. With regard to the thickness of the epidermis, present methods lack sufficient axial resolution to obtain accurate readings for all skin sites. Some imaging equipment has provided images of the epidermis in certain sites, such as the back of the hand (it is even possible to measure the thickness of the horny layer) and the face (Fig. 7). The more widespread use of these imaging techniques should soon provide data on variations in epidermal thickness with age. No doubt this future possibility will considerably enlarge the use of ultrasonic techniques in dermatologic research.

REFERENCES

1. Black MM. A modified radiographic method for measuring skin thickness. Br J Dermatol 1969; 81:661.
2. Dykes PJ, Francis AJ, Marks R. Measurement of dermal thickness with the Harpenden skinfold caliper. Arch Dermatol Res 1976; 256:261.
3. Luback D, Kunkler A. Die kombinierte Kompressions-und Dicken-messung (K-D-Messung) einer Hautfalte. Arzt Kosmetol 1984; 14:340.
4. Alexander H, Miler DL. Determining skin thickness with pulsed ultrasound. J Invest Dermatol 1979; 72:17.
5. Querleux B, Leveque JL, de Rigal J. In vivo cross-sectional ultrasonic imaging of human skin. Dermatologica 1988; 177:332.
6. Ryckewaert A, Parot S, Tamisier S, Bourliere F. Variations with age and sex, of skinfold thickness as measured on the back of the hand (French). Rev Fr Etudes Clin Biol 1967; 12:803.
7. Parot J, Bourliere F. A new technique for measuring compressibility of skin and subcutaneous tissue. Influence of sex, age and body area. Gerontologia 1967; 13:95.
8. Leveque JL, de Rigal J, Agache PG, Monneur C. Influence of aging on the in vivo extensibility of human skin at a low stress. Arch Dermatol Res 1980; 269:127.
9. Kurban RS, Bhawan J. Histologic changes in skin associated with aging. J Dermatol Surg Oncol 1990; 908.
10. Tan CY, Statham B, Marks R, Payne PA. Skin thickness measurement by pulsed ultrasound: its reproducibility, validation and variability. Br J Dermatol 1982; 106:657.
11. Escoffier C, de Rigal J, Rochefort A, Vasselet R, Leveque JL, Agache PG. Age-related mechanical properties of human skin: an in vivo study. J Invest Dermatol 1989; 93:353.
12. Denda M, Takahashi M. Measurement of facial skin thickness by ultrasound method. J Soc Cosmet Chem JPN 1990; 23:316.

13. Schatz H, Stoudemayer T, Gabriel K, Kligman AM. Visualization of aging and photodamage in human skin by $20MH_2$ ultrasound. 8th International Symposium on bioengineering and the skin, Stresa, 1990; 32.
14. de Rigal J, Escoffier C, Querleux B, Faivre B, Agache P, Leveque JL. Assessment of aging of the human skin by in vivo ultrasonic imaging. J Invest Dermatol 1989; 93:621.
15. Leveque JL, Porte G, de Rigal J, Corcuff P, Francois AM, Saint-Leger D. Influence of chronic sun exposure on some biophysical parameters of the human skin: air in vivo study. J Cutan Aging Cosmet Dermatol 1988; 1:123.
16. Adhout H, de Rigal J, Privat Y, Leveque JL. Biophysical characterization of solar elastosis (1991 to be published).
17. Brincat M, Moniz CJ, Studd JW, et al. Long-term effects of the menopause and sex hormones on skin thickness. Br J Obstet Gynaecol 1985; 92:256.
18. Pitt P, Dowd O, Brincat M. Reduction of skin collagen with increased skin thickness in post menopausal women with rheumatoid arthritis. Br J Rheumatol 1986; 25:263.
19. Savras M, Treasure J, Studd J, Fogelman I, Moviz C, Brincat M. The effect of anorexia nervosa on skin thickness, skin collagen and bone density. Br J Obstet Gynaecol 1989; 96:1392.
20. Rudman D, Feller AG, Nagraj HS, et al. Effects of human growth hormone in men over 60 years old. N Engl J Med 1990; 323:1.
21. Kalis B, de Rigal J, Leonard F, et al. In vivo study of scleroderma by non-invasive techniques. Br J Dermatol 1990; 122:785.
22. Bramont C, Vasselet R, Rochefort A, Agache P. Mechanical of the skin in Marfan's syndrome and Ehlers-Danlos syndrome. Bioeng Skin 1988; 4:217.
23. Dykes PJ, Hill S, Marks R. Assessment atrophogenicity potential of corticosteroids by ultrasound and by epidermal biopsy under occlusive and non occlusive conditions. In: Christophers E, ed. Topical corticosteroid therapy: a novel approach to safer drugs. New York: Raven Press, 1988; 111.
24. Teillac D, de Prost Y, Debure A, et al. Clinical and biophysical studies of the skin in renal allograft patients. Clin Transplant 1987; 1:195.
25. Lever L, Kumar P, Marks R. Topical retinoic acid for treatment of solar damage. Br J Dermatol 1990; 122:91.
26. de Lacharriere O, Escoffier C, Gracia AM, et al. Reversal effects of topical retinoic acid on the skin on kidney transplant recipients under systemic corticotherapy. J Invest Dermatol 1990; 95:516.
27. Mourad MM, Marks R. Assessment of disease severity and outcome in the gravitational syndrome using pulsed A-scan ultrasound to measure skin thickness. Clin Exp Dermatol 1990; 15:200.

7

High-Frequency Ultrasound Examination of Aged Skin: Intrinsic, Actinic, and Gravitational Aging, Including New Concepts of Stasis Dermatitis and Leg Ulcer

JØRGEN SERUP

Bispebjerg Hospital
University of Copenhagen
Copenhagen, Denmark

I. INTRODUCTION

Ultrasound diagnostics is well established in most specialties. For the examination of skin, special equipment with transducers with high frequency and broad bandwidth are needed. Ultrasound examination of skin is a new discipline. Alexander and Miller in 1979 introduced a high-frequency A mode prototype scanner, which they used for noninvasive measurement of skin thickness (1). This stimulated different centers to develop their own prototypes, and these efforts resulted in commercial development of different advanced ultrasound scanners specially constructed for the examination of skin. Thus, quality devices are now available. Increase in equipment is essential for the methodology to spread.

Basic principles of high-frequency ultrasound and the skin were recently reviewed by Payne (2). With A mode ultrasound, interface echoes are depicted. Based on the known velocity of sound in a given tissue, in vivo distances can be calculated. With B mode scanners cross-sectional images through the different skin layers are obtained (Fig. 1). With C mode scanners the third dimension is added, and such features as in vivo volume can be calculated. M mode scanning is used for the illustration of moving tissue interfaces, such as pulsed waves of arteries.

69

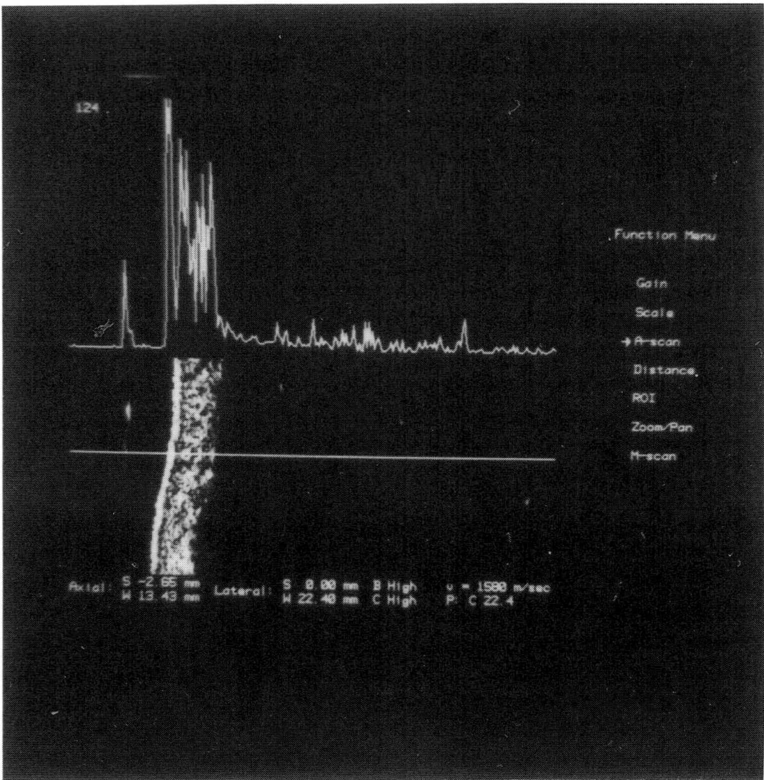

Figure 1 Ultrasound A mode (upper) and B mode (lower) scanning of normal skin of the thigh. The line indicates the selected A mode scan. The epidermis (left) is seen as a bright line with strong reflections. The dermis is also rich in echoes as a result of the regular steric orientation of the fiber network. A hair follicle is seen at the upper margin of the B mode scan.

II. ORIGIN OF ULTRASOUND REFLECTIONS IN VIVO AND INTERPRETATION OF IMAGES

As an acoustic modality, ultrasound follows the general rules for acoustic and optical phenomena. Diagnostic systems are based on pulsed ultrasound, which means that the transducer repeatedly sends out impulses and immediately after "listens" to what is reflected back to the transducer. The ultrasound reflection is determined by the difference in acoustic impedance (products of tissue density and ultrasound velocity in the medium) and the character and angle of the interface, which determine reflection, refraction, and diffraction. Moreover, absorption of the sound energy and scattering in the medium are significant variables that determine the resolution and depth of the viewing field.

Expressed in more practical terms, this means that the characteristics of tissues, including their structure and elastic properties and the smoothness and angle of the tissue interface, are of major importance. Most in vivo structures have an ultrasound velocity between 1450 and 1650 m/s; air and bone have values entirely out of this range. The average velocity in human skin (epidermis and dermis) is about 1580 m/s.

If the skin surface is irregular and covered with scales containing air, most ultrasound energy is absorbed at the surface and the signal must be amplified to depict more profound structures. Obviously, the interface between epidermis and dermis is not smooth, and consequently it is difficult to visualize this interface except on the palms and soles, where the dermis is low in reflectance. Although the interface between dermis and subcutaneous fat is irregular, in most body regions it is acoustically well defined. Compared to other techniques for measurement of skin thickness, ultrasound has the advantage that reflections appear from the smooth part of the interface between the fiber attachments perpendicular to the ultrasound beam, that is, where the skin thickness is biologically better defined.

Reflections from the dermis are determined by the three-dimensional fiber network of this tissue, which is highly reflectant. Disturbances of this network, such as erosion due to tumor invasion or disorganization due to inflammatory edema, result in different echolucent figures. Both in lesions, such as the neurofibromata of Recklinghausen's disease, and in keloids and hypertrophic scars, the reflectance of the dermis is diminished. In this type of lesion histology shows densely packed tissue elements; however, the three-dimensional in vivo structure is either more homogeneous or disorganized compared to the normally well-organized fiber network with its Langer's (cleavage) lines.

Histology is unfortunately not a very good comparative method in the validation of ultrasound. First, during histologic processing the tissue water is extracted and replaced by lipophilic media, and this, together with tissue retraction following biopsy cutting, may create unknown changes in tissue properties and dimensions. Second, with tissue staining those structures with affinity for the stain are observed selectively, and using this desirable artifact, important information may very well be overlooked. With electron microscopy, details of features, such as fiber disorganization, may be better evaluated; however, the higher the magnification the smaller the viewing field, and the sample becomes less representative. With ultrasound almost any body region can be examined noninvasively and repeatedly without interference by such in vivo features as dimension and tissue water. Ultrasound cannot provide the high-resolution information provided by the dermatohistopathology of today; however, it can yield microanatomic information based on a larger and perhaps more representative sample, and other tissue characteristics, such as elastic properties, are included in the structural information.

III. AGE-RELATED SPECIFIC LESIONS FOR ULTRASOUND EXAMINATION

Nonmelanoma skin cancer, particularly basal cell carcinoma, is the most common type of cancer in the human. This type of cancer is strongly age dependent, and exposure to sun is an important risk factor. Cutaneous lymphoma, although not directly a manifestation of aging, is far more common in elderly people. Special tumors, such as Kaposi's sarcoma, have for many years been recognized in elderly people, mainly on the legs and typically as a tumor of relatively slow progression, in contrast to cases associated with the acquired immunodeficiency syndrome.

A number of benign skin lesions, such as seborrheic warts, hemangiomata, and lentigines, are extremely common and normally of cosmetic concern only.

Wrinkling increases with age, particularly on the face and on sun-exposed body sites, and deep furrows and creases may appear. Clinically wrinkled skin is thickened. Peripheral skin, particularly in females, may become very thin and transparent with increased fragility.

In the literature it has been overlooked that stasis phenomena of the legs, stasis dermatitis, and nonarteriosclerotic leg ulcers are obviously strongly age related.

Finally, old skin may become pruritic. This condition may be very inconvenient, and prurigo nodules may appear.

A. Malignant Skin Lesions

In basal cell carcinoma the cancer has its origin in the basal cell layer, and deeper structures may gradually become eroded. By ultrasound imaging the carcinoma is seen as a nonreflectant or low-reflectant tumor mass (see Fig. 2). Quite often the perilesional skin surface is undermined by the tumor, and ultrasound typically shows that a basal cell carcinoma is laterally more extended than was apparent on gross clinical examination. With ultrasound the deeper part of the dermis underneath the tumor can be studied in more detail. Typically, when the tumors are advanced, a good supply with blood vessels is seen. Often a capsule or remnants of the reticular dermis are seen underneath the tumor. The treatment strategy can be decided depending on the ultrasound

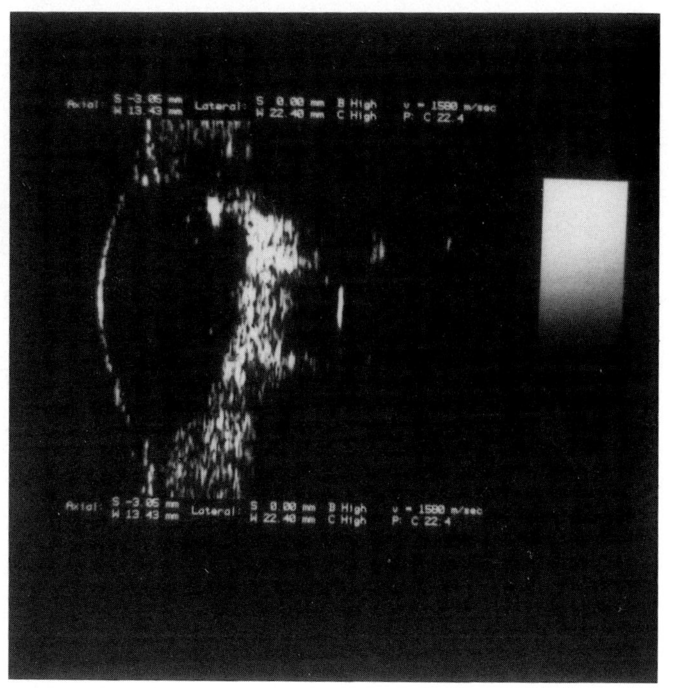

A

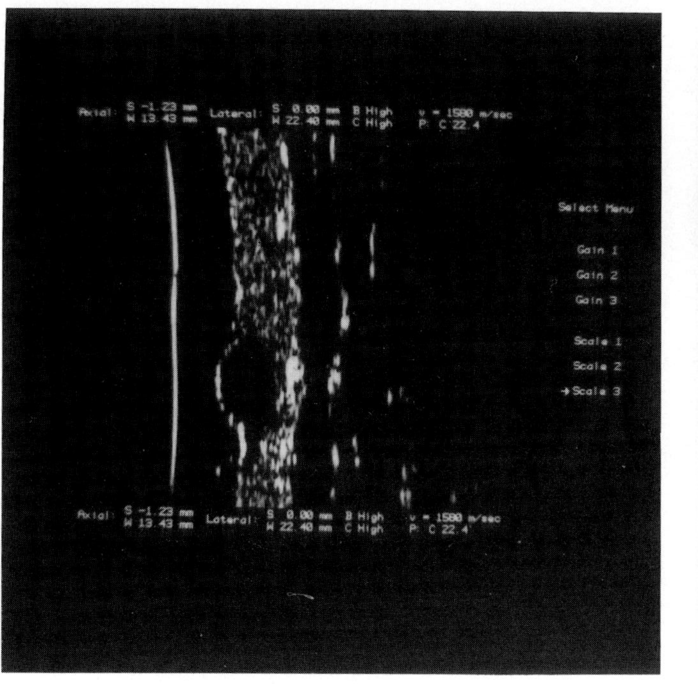

B

Figure 2 A small basal cell carcinoma (A) and a nodular basal cell carcinoma (B). The tumor erodes the fibers of the dermis, and the tumor with its homogeneous structure appears dark and echolucent. Note that basal cell carcinomas tend to progress underneath the epidermis of the perilesional skin. Tumor thickness is easily measured, and the demarcation in depth is similarly easy to assess.

image. If the lesion is superficial, curettage and/or cryotherapy may be chosen. If only a thin capsule is present, plastic surgery and excision may be preferable. If no capsule is seen, Moh's surgery is indicated from the beginning.

Basal cell carcinoma, squamous cell carcinoma, and malignant melanoma have in principle the same internal echo pattern of low reflectance and it is thus not possible to distinguish these tumors with sufficient accuracy by ultrasound. It must be kept in mind that the echo profile of a tumor is strongly dependent on the selection of echo amplification relative to tissue depth. Thus, the internal echo profile of a tumor is not a strictly objective feature unless a common standard is agreed upon.

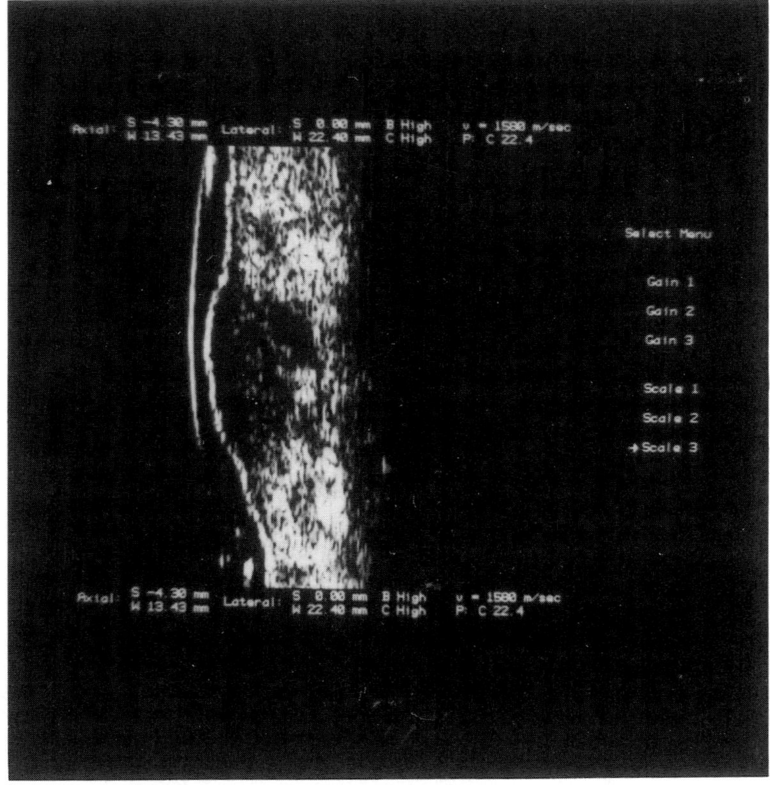

Figure 3 Kaposi's sarcoma. The tumor consists of irregular masses of tumor tissue with no definite tumor capsule and no clear demarcation from the surrounding skin. The tumor tissue is dark and echolucent, with the undisturbed structure of the dermis as a kind of natural contrast medium.

Kaposi's sarcoma may show an entirely different pattern (Fig. 3). In this tumor islands of tumor tissue may be found at different levels within the skin. Obviously, more deeply localized tumor lesions cannot be detected clinically. Thus, ultrasound can be used to determine the treatment. If radiotherapy is chosen, tumor depth is the rational prerequisite in the choice of radiation dose. Cutaneous malignant lymphoma shows a third and very different pattern of progression as evaluated by ultrasound. This lymphoma is called cutaneous because the manifestations representing proliferation and accumulation of pathologic lymphocytes appear and remain within the skin for a long period and therapies directed toward the skin are therefore effective at least in the initial phases. PUVA (methoxsalen + ultraviolet A) treatment has be-

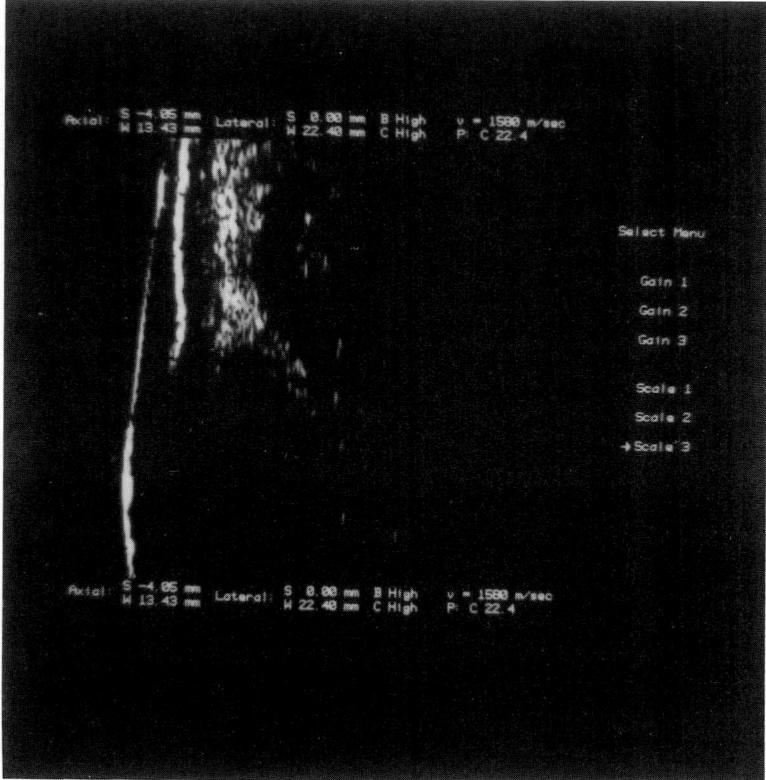

Figure 4 Malignant lymphoma (T cell). A large tumor echolucent on ultrasound, has developed throughout the dermis (lower half), and in the adjacent skin (upper half), the echolucent pathology extends underneath the epidermis in a space corresponding to the papillar dermis.

come standard. In ultrasound it is seen that the tumor infiltrates mainly progress laterally in the papillar dermis, which can be extremely thickened (Fig. 4). Typically a reticular dermis with surprisingly little affection is seen underneath the infiltrate. The thickness of the infiltrate can be measured by ultrasound, and it can be decided whether PUVA treatment is likely to be efficient or whether some other treatment, such as radiotherapy or cytostatics, is preferable.

B. Benign Lesions

Seborrheic warts show a very characteristic ultrasound pattern. The superficial masses of keratotic material strongly absorb ultrasound, and a heavy shadow is created, seen on the image as a dark zone including all profound structures, with straight margins perpendicular to the surface (Fig. 5). If the amplification of the signal is increased, however, a normal dermis pattern appears and it becomes obvious that this pathology is only superficial. This is very typical or pathognomonic for seborrheic lesions. Malignant melanoma, which might be a differential diagnosis, does not show such a phenomenon.

Hemangiomata are variable on ultrasound and may be difficult to discern from surrounding, normal tissues because of a variable internal reflectance from vessels that vary in size. Ultrasound does not now have the resolution to allow a very detailed study of hemangiomata.

C. Other Benign Disorders

Dermatitis may appear in senile skin, particularly in pruritic skin. An echolucent band corresponding to the papillar dermis may be seen. Such an inflammatory band is known from other conditions with dermatitis, including contact dermatitis and atopy. Prurigo nodules are seen as semigloboid tumors in the outer skin (Fig. 6). The lesions are localized surprisingly superficially in the skin, and the reticular dermis appears straight and unaffected. Hyperkeratosis due to scratching may create a shadow. Thus, the cross-sectional image may support the view that inflammation of the outer skin under the influence of scratching develops into more distinct nodules that, being superficial in character, in principle are sensitive to external treatment unless the thickening is gross or the skin inflammation is widespread.

The bullae of pemphigus vulgaris are easily seen by ultrasound, with regular margins, but ultrasound does not have the resolution of histologic or immune techniques for a more detailed description of bullous lesions of the skin, and differential diagnosis is generally not possible by ultrasound (Fig. 7). This is also true of the blisters of herpes zoster.

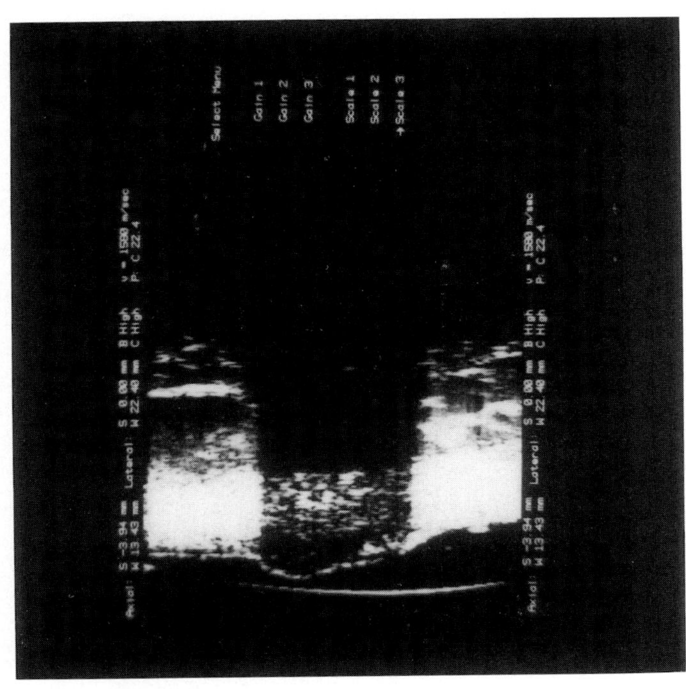

B

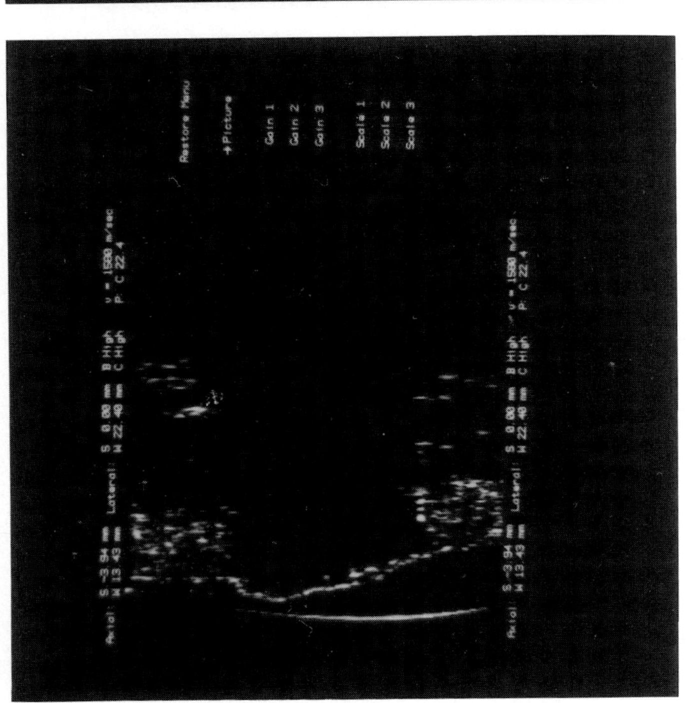

A

Figure 5 Seborrheic wart with a heavy shadow (A). If the gain is increased during the scanning and adjusted to the particular lesion, a normal dermis appears underneath the epidermal wart and the surrounding skin is overgained (B).

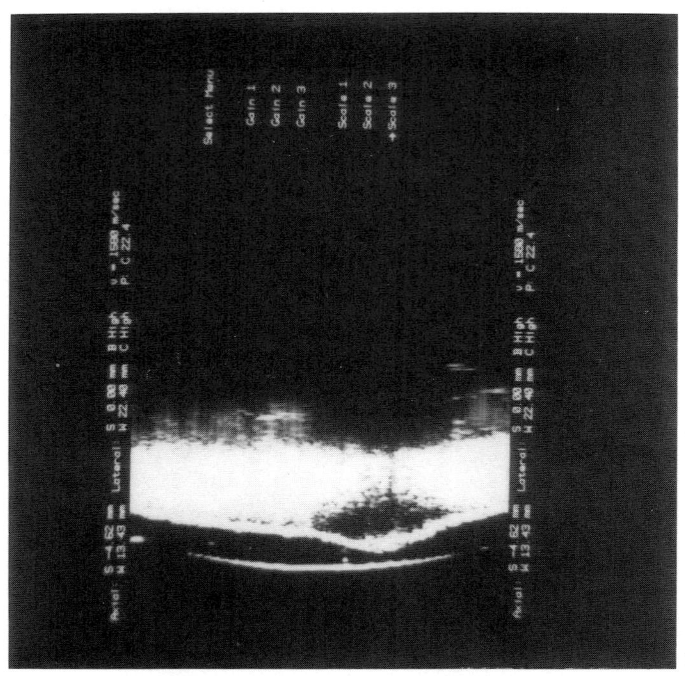

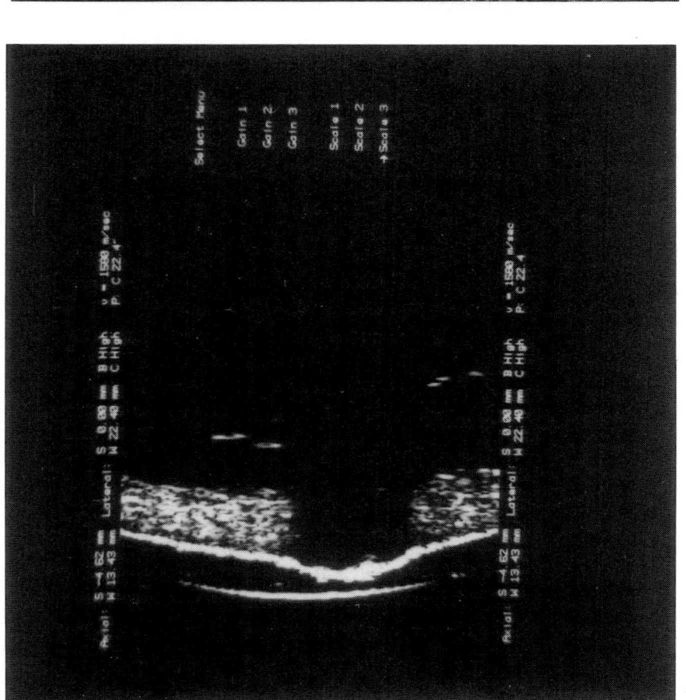

Figure 6 Nodular prurigo (A) with hyperkeratosis and a heavy shadow. With an increase in gain while scanning, the superficial character of the lesion is recognized (B) (see also Fig. 5).

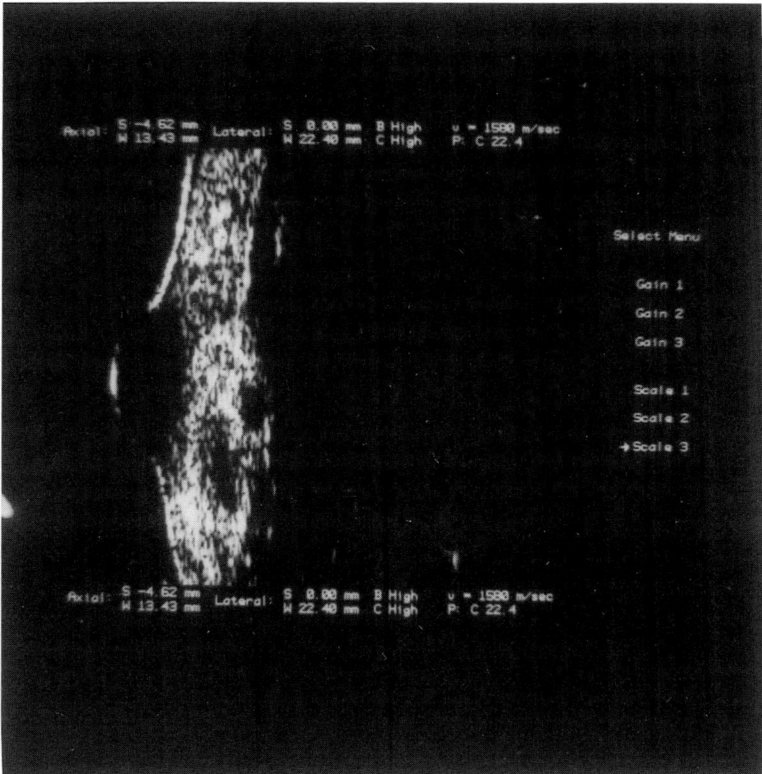

Figure 7 Bullae of pemphigus vulgaris characterized by regular and curved borders. The resolution of ultrasound does not permit differentiation of bullous skin diseases.

IV. INTRINSIC AGING AND ACTINIC DAMAGE

Ultrasound studies show that skin thickness decreases with age. However, it cannot at the moment be concluded whether the decrease in skin thickness occurs linearly or if the thinning is seen mainly in senile skin. Also, it is not known how the thinning takes place in the two sexes or whether the menopause influences the thinning.

It is a general phenomenon that skin thickening and skin thinning relative to internal conditions and endocrine diseases are more pronounced on acral parts of the body, that is, on distal extremities. This is obvious in such conditions as scleroderma, acromegaly, and Cushing's syndrome. Even in psoriasis and localized scleroderma, ultrasound studies have demonstrated that the thickening is more pronounced on the thin skin of extremities (6–9). Thus, the intrinsic thinning of senile skin is mainly expected to occur on distal extremity skin.

Senile skin may become transparent and extremely thin on the dorsum of the hand, and this has been shown to correlate with osteoporosis (10). Ultrasound studies have confirmed, at least in senile skin, that there is a correlation between thin skin and manifestations of osteoporosis (11). Ongoing studies will show whether measurement of skin thickness by ultrasound after menopause can be used to define females at risk who should be treated with estrogens. Postmenopausal osteoporosis is not primarily a disorder of calcium metabolism but a result of deficient bone matrix formation. Decreased formation of connective tissue in bones and in the dermis might develop simultaneously, both as manifestations of aging, and the skin may be a mirror of the bone matrix.

Ultrasound imaging has demonstrated that thinning with increasing age does not affect the papillar and the reticular dermis equally. With increasing age a so-called age band appears in the papillar dermis (12). This band is seen as a dark echolucent zone under the epidermis (Fig. 8). Its structural background is probably progressive thinning and disorganization of the fibril network of the papillar dermis with age. The structural change probably influences the elastic properties of the papillar dermis, which may also show wrinkling. The reticular part of the dermis remains straight. Steric changes of the connective tissue structure of the skin and physical properties are difficult or impossible to demonstrate by conventional histology or electron microscopy. Sun exposure results in thickening of the skin as demonstrated by ultrasound (13). Disorganization and deposition of elastotic material in actinic damage is known, and in actinic damage the age band is more obvious and wider. Intrinsic aging and actinic damage cannot essentially be distinguished by ultrasound since band formation is a common feature. In severe actinic damage, however, the age band may be very broad and the total skin thickness increased; in intrinsic aging the band is narrower and the total skin thickness may be decreased. Such opposite effects on the total skin thickness may explain why ultrasound studies on skin thickness versus age are not quite conclusive, as mentioned earlier.

The age band formation of the papillar dermis has consequences for the clinic. As mentioned, the superficial wrinkling of aged skin affects only the papillar dermis. As part of this superficial dermal atrophy and structural disorganization, the superficial vascular plexus is also involved, with fragility of the vessels. As a result of trauma, ecchymoses easily appear, particularly on distal extremities, and the bleeding makes its way laterally in the atrophic

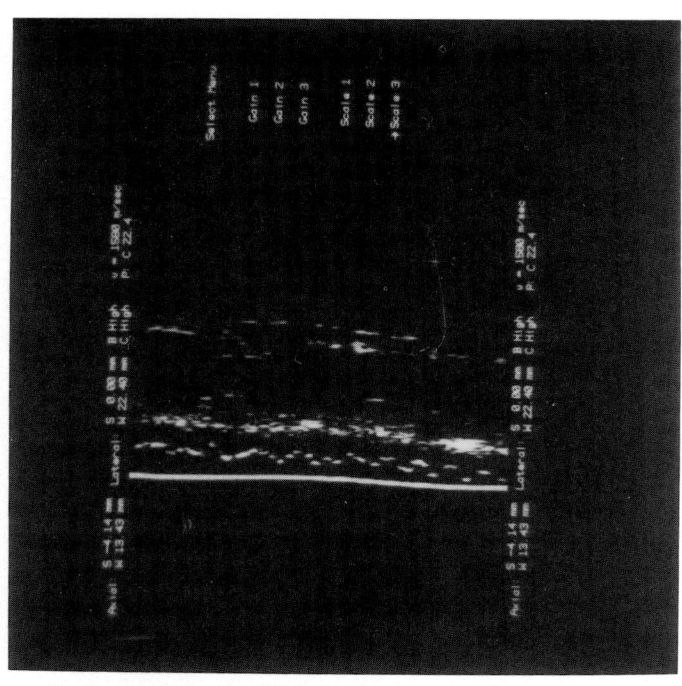

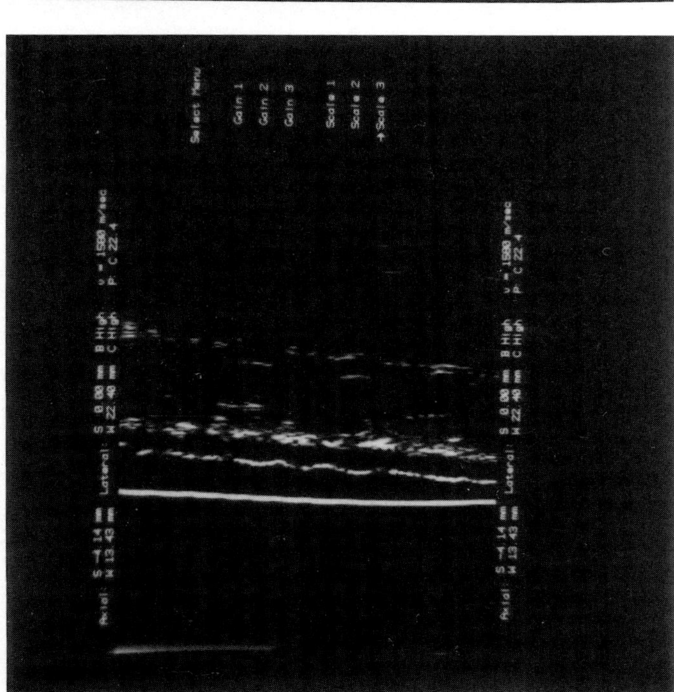

Figure 8 Age band seen as an echolucent band in the outer skin corresponding to the papillar dermis. Fine wrinkling related to age is superficial. The reticular dermis remains straight. The age band is a special space of pronounced atrophy and reduction of mechanical resistance. It is in this space that ecchymoses spread. Gravitational edema of the legs especially distends this space. The entire skin is much thinner (see Fig. 1). The line to the left is the membrane of the probe.

papular dermis, corresponding to the age band seen by ultrasound. Following even a small physical trauma the epidermis and the papillar dermis may break and leave avulsions with sharp and irregular margins; the reticular dermis is normally intact.

Thus, as a result of aging the dermis of the skin becomes a two-compartment system with a fragile papillar dermis, and a better preserved reticular dermis. Ecchymoses and avulsions thus represent a kind of superficial dermatosparaxis.

In neonatal skin ultrasound examination shows that the entire dermis is loose in structure and uniform, but within the first few months dense echo reflections appear throughout the dermis, and this pattern persists until signs of aging appear with alterations of the papular dermis and age band formation (14).

V. GRAVITATIONAL OR VERTICAL AGING

In intrinsic aging, as mentioned, there is an acral or distal vector. During life we are exposed to the influences of gravity, which creates a vertical vector of increased hydrostatic pressure toward the ground. Nonarteriosclerotic ulcers of the so-called venous type appear exclusively on the legs, although forearm and crural skin show analogous lesions. Although some leg ulcers are explained as the sequelae of deep vein thrombosis or aplasia of venous valves, for example, the vast majority of venous leg ulcers cannot clearly be explained, although venous hypertension, deposition of macromolecules in the interstitium, and a mild tissue hypoxia appear common features. It is accepted that edema of the legs and stasis dermatitis represent early clinical stages of venous leg ulcer, and these conditions represent a more widespread abnormality of the lower legs.

The attitude toward venous leg ulcer has been and still is very much focused on the ulcer, rather than on the patient with a leg ulcer, which the considerations just mentioned should indicate.

The ultrasound findings in venous leg ulcer and stasis dermatitis are very distinct and uniform. In skin afflicted with stasis dermatitis, in the perilesional skin surrounding an ulcer, and in the ulcer itself ultrasound imaging shows a pronounced thickening of the skin, particularly distension of the papillar dermis, which is seen as a broad echolucent zone, the stasis band (Fig. 9). This represents gross deformation of the microanatomy, and such a change must have important consequences for the superficial vascular plexus and its supply to the epidermis, as well as the diffusion of oxygen through the tissue and the complete nutritional environment of the epidermal cells. The stasis band is found more widespread on the lower legs.

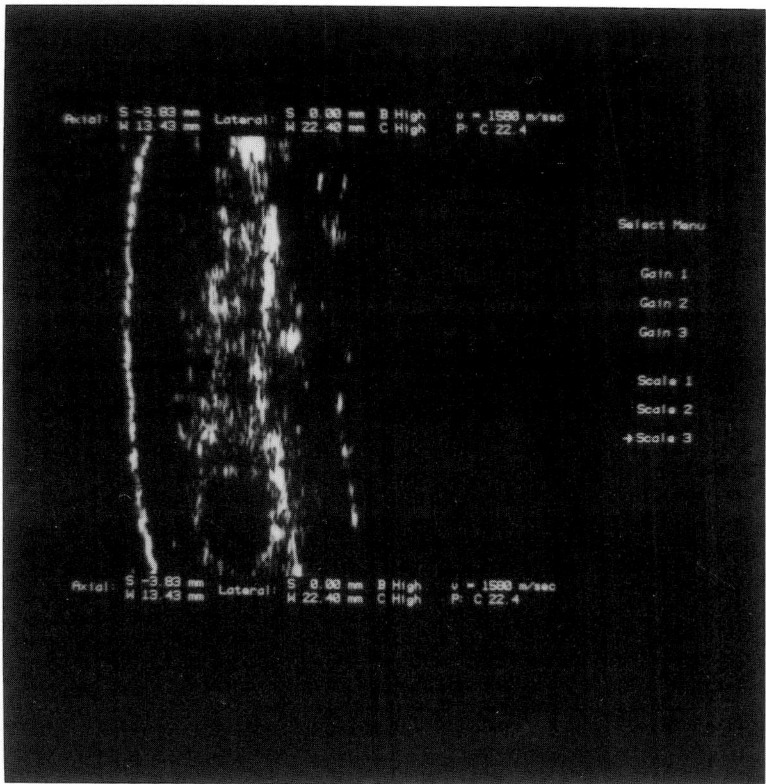

Figure 9 Venous leg ulcer, perilesional skin with stasis and dermatitis. A broad echolucent band is seen corresponding to the papillar dermis. The dermis contains a dilated vein. With such a structure the superficial vascular plexus must be disturbed, possibly with consequences for the survival of the epithelium.

As mentioned, the papillar dermis is mechanically less resistant, and ecchymoses and inflammatory infiltrates tend to make their way laterally into this space. Under the influence of gravity and increased hydrostatic pressure, it is logical that the papular dermis of the legs in particular expands with age.

A recent in vivo study on skin elasticity at 22 different anatomic sites shows that there is normally a vertical vector in skin extensibility, with the tighter skin toward the ground (15). The forces of gravity are normally balanced by such a vertical tissue vector. Thus, patients with stasis dermatitis, stasis band by ultrasound, and later venous leg ulcer may represent a group who do not have this vertical vector of skin and connective tissue resistance to counterbalance the forces and tissue effects of gravity. In the giraffe, the tallest land mammal, the increased mechanical resistance of the legs is concluded important for the prevention of orthostatic vascular complications (16). This hypothesis provides a rationale for compression therapies, and the effects of such treatment can be monitored by the use of ultrasound (17).

Ultrasound examination of legs with arteriosclerotic ulcers has showed thinning of the skin, in contrast to the findings in venous leg ulcer (18).

Although edema formation may be pronounced in lymphedema and thickening of the skin as measured by gross ultrasound, a stasis band in the papular dermis is not prominent by ultrasound imaging. Clinically, lymphedema does not have a strong association with ulceration, as do venous stasis phenomena. This difference in ulcer potential may be explained by the presence or absence of structural change, seen as the stasis band by ultrasound.

Leg ulcers are a great problem in industrialized societies. It will be necessary to change attitudes and policies in the direction of improvement of diagnosis, with much emphasis on evaluation of early stages and risk factors aiming at prophylactic strategies directed toward the public. Dermatologic ultrasound has much to offer in such a scheme.

VI. CONCLUSION

With recent high-frequency ultrasound equipment, details about skin structure and properties, including the effects of aging, can be obtained noninvasively. A number of age-related lesions and diseases, such as tumors, seborrheic warts, prurigo nodules, and dermatitis, show distinct findings.

As a manifestation of intrinsic aging, an echolucent band appears that corresponds to the papillar dermis, representing structural thinning and disorganization. In actinic damage this band becomes broad. Ecchymoses dissect their way laterally in this loose space. Ultrasound demonstrates that the outer part of the skin may be wrinkled but the reticular dermis is still straight and dense. In gravitational aging, thickening of the skin may be great as a result of the accumulation of edema, particularly in the papillar dermis, where a stasis band is seen by ultrasound. Distension and disorganization of the papillar dermis are probably the main risk factors in venous leg ulcer, clinically preceded by crural edema and stasis dermatitis, in which ultrasound demonstrates identical but less advanced changes.

REFERENCES

1. Alexander H, Miller DL. Determining skin thickness with pulsed ultra sound. J Invest Dermatol 1979; 72:17–9.

2. Payne PA. Applications of ultrasound in dermatology. Bioeng Skin 1985; 1:193–320.

3. Miyauchi S, Tada M, Miki Y. Echographic evaluation of nodular lesions of the skin. J Dermatol (Tokyo) 1983; 10:221–7.

4. Breitbart EW, Müller CE, Hicks R, Vieluf D. Neue Entwicklungen der Ultraschalldiagnostik in der Dermatologie. Aktuel Dermatol 1989; 15:57–61.

5. Hoffman K, el Gammal S, Matthes U, Altmeyer P. Digitale 20MHz-Sonographie der Haut in der präoperativen Diagnostik. Z Hautkr 1989; 64:851–8.

6. Serup J. Localized scleroderma (morphoea): thickness of sclerotic plaques as measured by 15 MHz pulsed ultrasound. Acta Derm atonver (Stockh) 1984; 64:214–9.

7. Serup J. Quantification of acrosclerosis: measurement of skin thickness and skin-phalanx distance in females with 15 KHz pulsed ultrasound. Acta Derm Venereol (Stockh) 1984; 64:35–40.

8. Serup J. Localized scleroderma (morphoea). Clinical, physiological, biochemical and ultrastructural studies with particular reference to quantitation of scleroderma. Acta Derm Venereol (Suppl) (Stockh) 1986; 66:122.

9. Marks R. Device and rule. The Dowling Oration 1984. Clin Exp Dermatol 1985; 10:303–27.

10. McConkey B, Fraser GM, Bligh AS, Whiteley H. Transparent skin and osteoporosis. Lancet 1985; 1:693–5.

11. Schatz H, Stoudemayer T, Gabriel K, Klingman A. Ultrasound: a method to follow progressive skin conditions and treatment effects in dermatology. Zentrbl Haut Geschl 1990; 157:331.

12. de Rigal J, Escoffier C, Querleux B, Faivre B, Agache P, Leveque JL. Assessment of aging of the human skin in vivo. Ultrasound imaging. J Invest Dermatol 1989; 93:621–5.

13. Leveque JL, Porte G, de Rigal J, Corcuff P, Francois AM, Saint Leger D. Influence of chronic sun exposure on some biophysical parameters of the human skin: an in vivo study. J Cutan Aging Cosmet Dermatol 1989; 1:123–7.

14. Petersen S, Serup J. Ultrasound examination of neonatal skin. Biol Neonate, in press.

15. Malm M, Samman M, Serup J. In vivo skin elasticity of twenty-two anatomical sites. Skin Pharmacol, in press.

16. Hargens AR. Gravitational cardiovascular adaptation in the giraffe. Physiologist 1987; 30:15–7.

17. Mourad MM, Marks R. Assessment of disease severity and outcome in the gravitational syndrome using pulsed A-scan ultrasound to measure skin thickness. Clin Exp Dermatol 1990; 15:200–5.

18. Mandy P. An investigation into the effect of peripheral vascular disease on skin thickness. Bioeng Skin 1988; 4:323–32.

8

Direct Observation of Capillary Modifications in the Aged

TERENCE JOHN RYAN

Churchill Hospital
Oxford, England

I. INTRODUCTION

The purpose of this chapter is to illustrate the network of capillaries that can be perceived by looking at the surface of the skin. In particular, the changes that occur with aging are described. In so doing it should be emphasized that the capillary bed one is examining in the upper dermis is not only the source of nutrition of the epidermis but also contributes to skin color and thus to the function of display. Besides nutrition, it contributes to moisturization and provides the cells that recognize foreign material invading the epidermis. It is part of the body's system for thermoregulation, and it contributes to the vascular capacity of the entire organism, contributing significantly to peripheral resistance and the control of blood pressure.

Macroscopically, it is easy to see how blood supply contributes to the function of display, such as the flush or blush of embarrassment and anger or the pallor of fear. The rosy cheek is often described as the bloom that characterizes good health. Aging is associated with changes in the macroscopic appearance of the skin, including, on the face, broken veins and red noses or, on the legs, the commonly observed star bursts and other vascular anomalies.

In considering the function of protection of the skin and the way in which the blood supply contributes to the health of the epidermis, such as its function as a barrier, it is important that the blood supply be readily available and thus closely applied to the epithelium to enhance its viability. However, blood supply is not the only vasculature needed by the epidermis. There is also a lymphatic system (1), which must not be too far away if important cells, such as the Langerhans' cell, are to carry information to the lymph nodes. There are disease states in which even these vessels are visible at the surface. Information concerning aging in this system is lacking; probably pre-lymphatic pathways are the most disrupted (Fig. 1).

With respect to thermoregulation, systems that shunt blood away from the visible superficial capillary bed are important, particularly at the peripheries. At the same time, heat loss often depends on an increase in the rapidity of flow through such shunts as more blood is brought to the peripheries. Lux-urious perfusion is not necessarily equated with increased nutritional blood supply and thus with an increase in flow through the visible capillary bed. Thermoregulation is often claimed to be the reason that the skin has such a rich vasculature, but it is probably more important that the skin must engen-der such richness to meet the needs of repair. Thus there are studies that show that the skin in diabetes (2) may be well perfused at rest but is quite unable to meet the demands for increased supply following a period of ischemia (re-

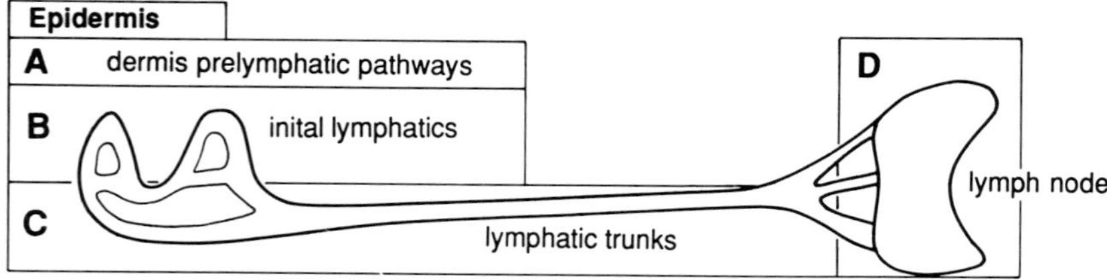

Four regions of lymphatic function

A   Prelymphatic pathways depend on dermal organisation.
     This is severely attenuated in old age.

B   Initial lymphatics. (No information about aging,
                          possible increase in basal lamina
                          impeding entry and responsiveness
                          to mechanical forces)
C   Lymphatic trunks (fibrosis occurs with aging)

D   Lymph nodes   (fibrosis and attenuation is a
                        feature of aging.)

Figure 1   The lymphatic system is also a vascular system affected by aging. It should not be ignored and can be observed directly.

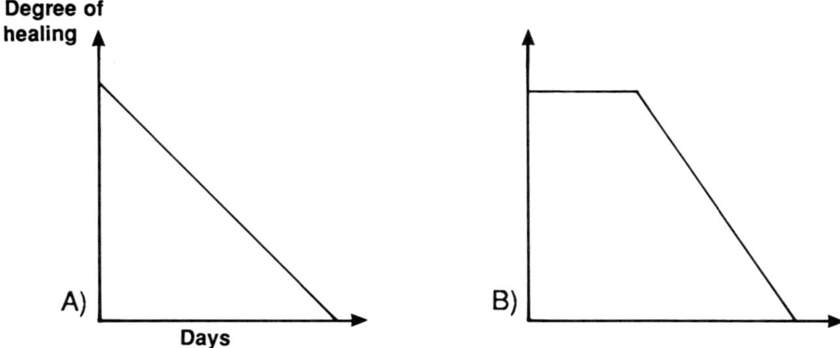

Figure 2   Rates of wound healing are influenced by blood supply. (A) Young tissues: immediate recruitment of blood supply and immediate healing. (B) In atrophic skin there is often an initial delay in the onset of healing while new vessels are recruited.

active hyperemia), and consequently wound healing is severely impaired. On wounding it is necessary to immediately recruit an increase in blood supply (Fig. 2). This can only occur where vascular beds are significantly richer than required for the function of an uninjured organ at rest. It is a feature also of skin affected by liposclerosis in gravitational or venous disease of the leg, which it is well perfused at rest with fast circulation times but reactive hyperemia is impaired and repair following even minor wounds is defective.

The skin is the largest organ of the body and, as such, has a large capillary bed that contributes to the overall vascular capacity and peripheral resistance. It is argued that essential hypertension, as opposed to renovascular disease, is associated with and may in part be caused by loss of the capillary bed. If this is so, then atrophy of the skin must be regarded as one component or cause of hypertension.

II. CORRELATION OF CAPILLARY MORPHOLOGY WITH THE DEMANDS OF THE EPIDERMIS

Insofar as aging incorporates both growth and degeneration, the blood vessels of the skin should be seen as behaving phasically, initially proliferating, later maintaining a prolonged steady state, but eventually showing slow regression. Ultimately in old age, a substantial loss of capillaries is observed in many organs and the skin is perhaps the most obvious of these (3). Such phasic behavior is exaggerated or accelerated in wound healing or in such conditions as the strawberry nevus (4) or pyogenic granuloma. New vessel formation can be switched to a maximum, and this usually lasts days or weeks, known as the plateau phase. Regression occurs over a period of months or years. Even in extreme old age, an atrophic capillary bed can be stimulated by injury to produce new capillaries, but the response depends on both the local angiogenic stimulus and the requirement that the arterial system dilate to provide adequate perfusion.

III. STRUCTURE OF THE CAPILLARY IN THE DERMIS

The normal blood supply to the skin is that most commonly observed in healthy skin. It consists of capillaries, mostly sited within the papillae of the upper dermis and therefore perpendicular to the surface. They have the shape of a hairpin loop and tend to present only their peaks to view. They are supplied by a deeper arterial system, and the overall pattern resembles a cande-

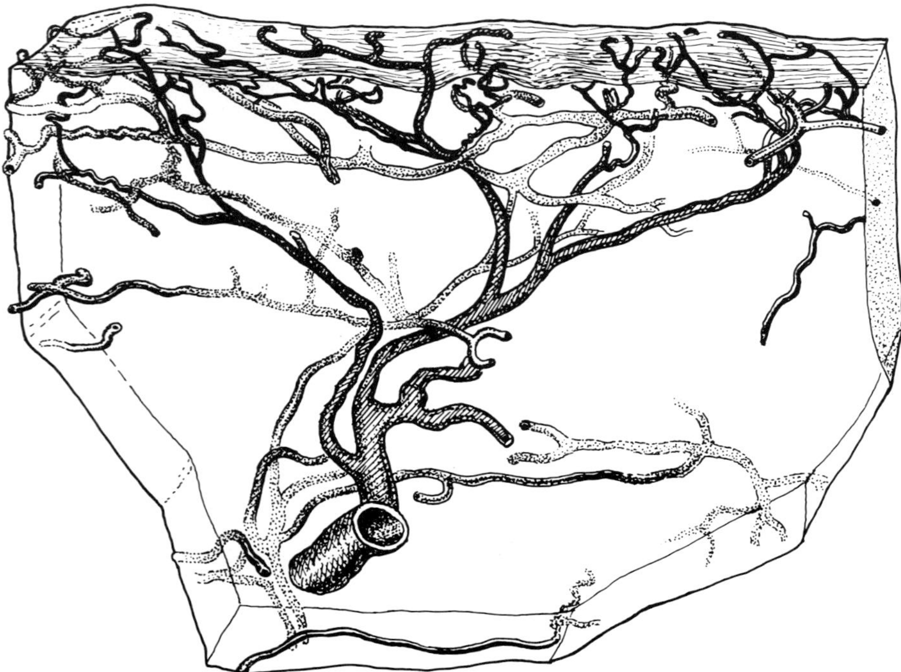

Figure 3 Drawing by Spaltholz (nineteenth century) of the normal capillary and arteriolar system of the skin with the shape of a candelabra.

labra (Fig. 3) that drains into a rich subpapillary venous plexus. It is this latter that provides most of the color seen at the surface of the skin. Because the papillary vessels are the nutritional capillaries, they provide the tissue fluid that lies in the upper dermis and acts as an obscuring veil overlying the subpapillary venous plexus (Fig. 4). The number of papillary vessels at the surface is approximately 60–70 per mm^2. Several observers have noted that the capillary density is consistently rich in the palms and the soles but never exceeding the figure of 70 per mm^2. In a comparison of 20 body sites, taking skin biopsies in elderly cadavers, Pasyk et al. (5) noted that the head and neck had significantly more vessels than other sites and that the lower leg was particularly sparse. Aged skin, with its overall atrophy, also shows great variations in anatomy, modified by repetitive injury and repair, including such

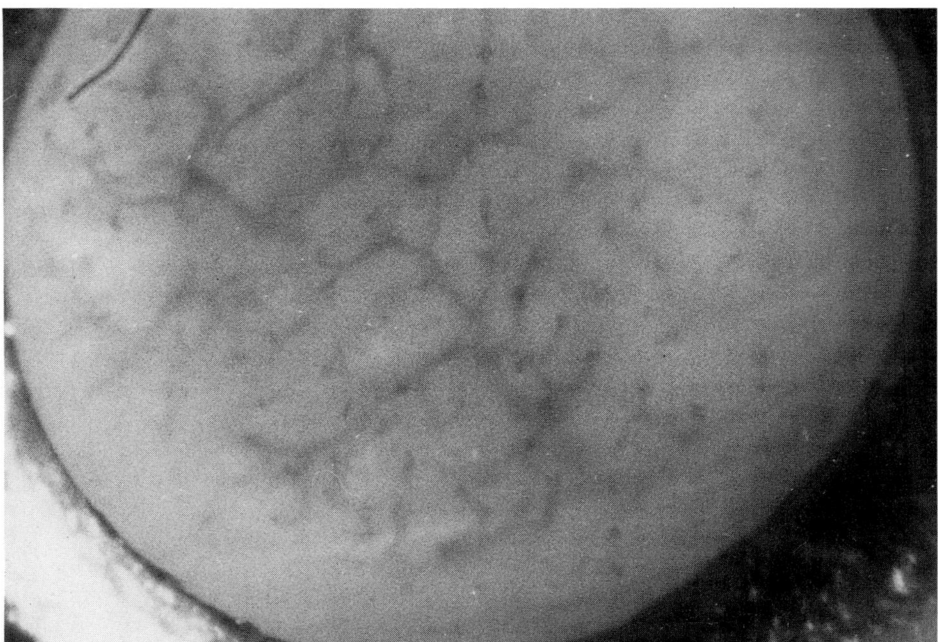

Figure 4 The blood supply of the upper dermis in normal skin. In the center of the field the vessels are visible because tissue fluid has been dispersed (see Fig. 12); in the peripheries of the field the tissue fluid obscures all the vessels. The diameter of the steel loop is 2 mm. The papillary loops and the subpapillary venous plexus are visible.

factors as peripheral vascular disease and gravitational venous responses affecting the capillary bed (1). In older skin the papillary loops are often diagonally oriented, and with increasing sparseness of the papillary loops, the subpapillary venous plexus may become more visible (Fig. 5). Regional variation is considerable, and thus the nailfold capillaries are always horizontally disposed and the richness of the vasculature of the cheek is a consequence of a rather more dense, horizontal, subpapillary venous plexus (Fig. 6), to some extent replacing the perpendicular hairpin loops of the papillary system. Certain sites of continued microinjury due to surface abrasion or intermittent shearing forces due to stretch, such as may occur over the elbows or knuckles, tend to preserve the papillary system. Often vessels at these sites are more elongated and tortuous and less inclined to atrophy in old age. When there is an increased demand by the epidermis, as occurs in wound healing or in diseases like psoriasis, the papillary vessels tend to elongate and

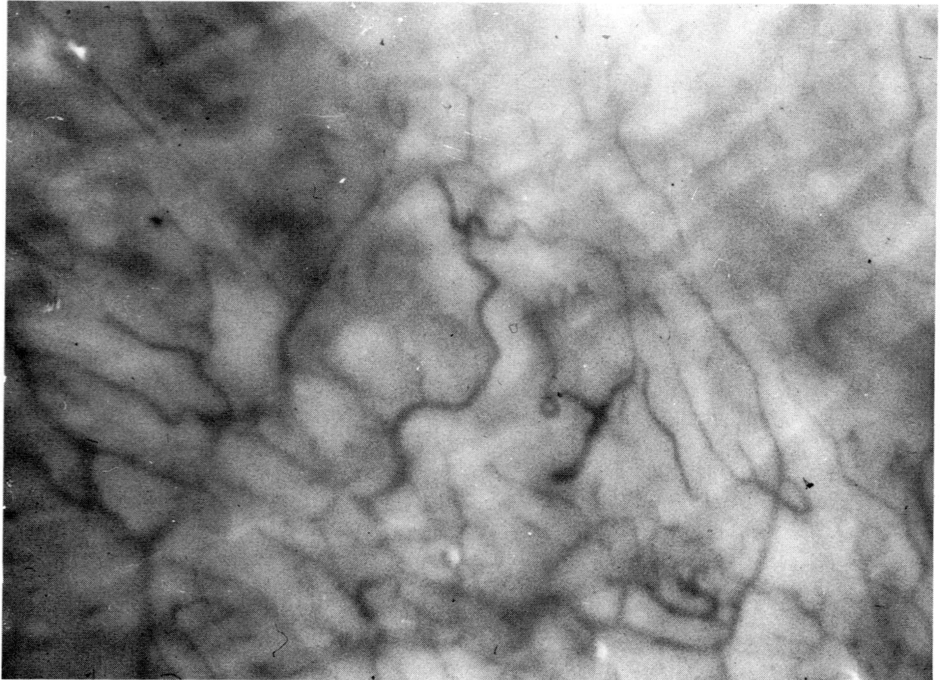

Figure 5 Atrophic skin of old age: no papillary vessels are visible, and only a sparse and attenuated subpapillary plexus is revealed. This is easily visible, however, because there is increased transparency as a result of the atrophy of the upper dermis.

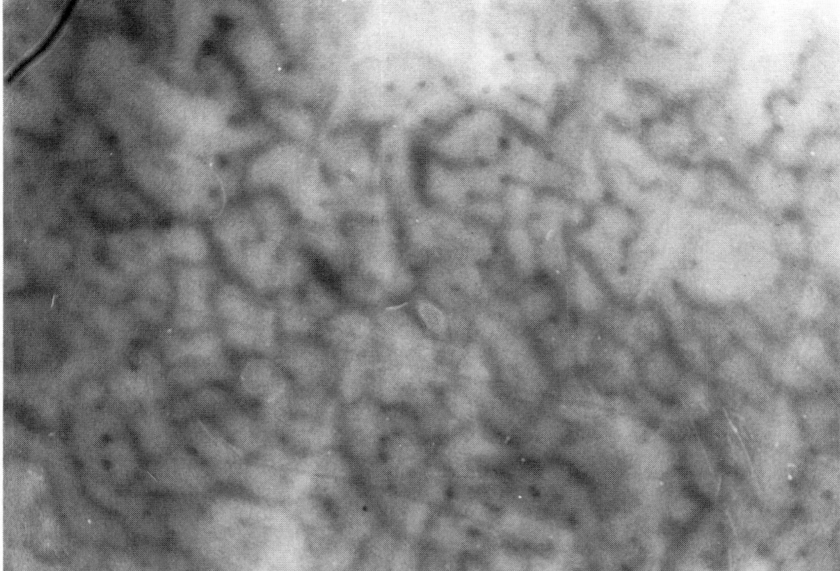

Figure 6 Sparse papillary vessels and rich dilated horizontal subpapillary plexus characterize red cheeks.

become more tortuous (6,15,22) and have been likened to the tortuosity of cotton in cotton wool balls. A feature of such vessels is that they are closely applied to the epidermis, projecting into the papilla and almost completely surrounded by epidermis. In contrast, in old age, atrophy of the papillary system results in a distancing of the capillary endothelium from the epidermis, which has implications for its nutrition (Fig. 7).

One way of considering or describing the richness of the capillary bed supplying the epidermis is to plot the capillaries as a Gaussian (normal) distribution curve (Fig. 8) (6). In health, there are few atrophic or hypertrophic-forms and a large component of hairpin loops. In hyperplasia, such as wound healing or psoriasis, there is increased tortuosity and a lesser component of atrophy. In the aged, there is the overall marked reduction in capillaries but also greater heterogeneity, so that there are both more hypertrophic and more atrophic forms. Most of the anomalies seen in old age lead to the dilated and atrophic patterns. Angiomata and various forms of telangiectasia are mostly not generous nutritional systems but are dilated, slow flowing, and relatively impermeable. The epidermis overlying such vessels is often thinner but able to make a well-knit and firm stratum corneum.

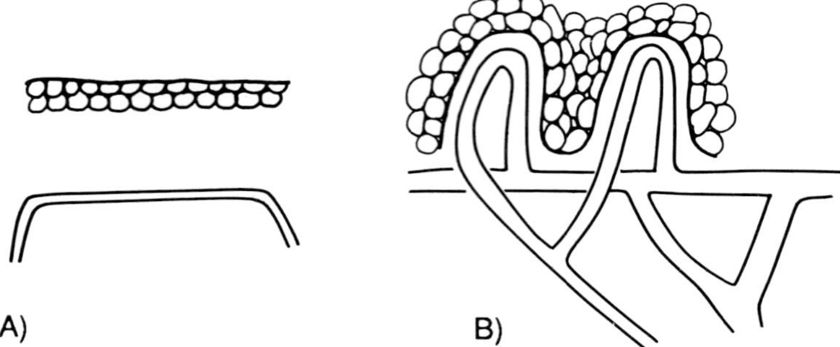

Figure 7   One difference between rich and atrophic nutritional beds is their distance from the tissues they supply. (A) Atrophic blood supply and separation from epidermis. (B) Hyperplastic blood supply: intimate contact with epidermis.

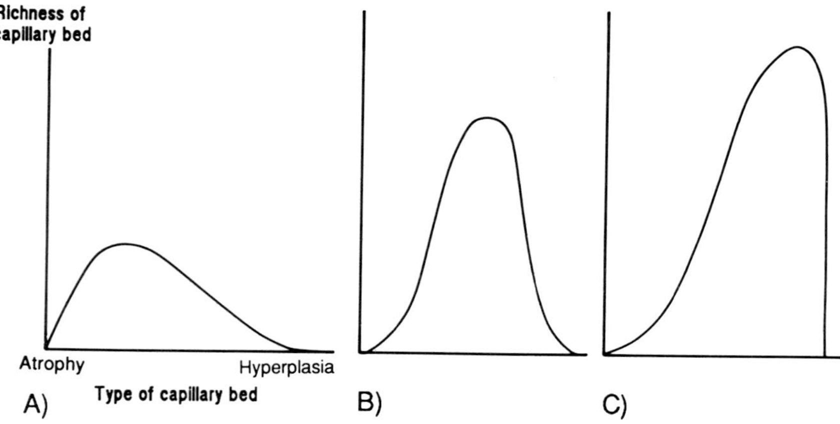

Figure 8   Distribution curves of papillary vascularization in normal, atrophic, and hyperplastic states. (A) Aging: reduction in capillary bed, more atrophy, but wide scatter of vessel types. (B) Normal adult: little atrophy, no hyperplasia, but uniformity. (C) Hyperplasia of repair or psoriasis: more vessels, more hyperplasia, but no atrophy.

IV. RETICULATE ERYTHEMAS

The markings visible at the surface of the skin are determined in part by the distribution of the arterioles (Fig. 9). Children, in particular, when cold, often show a mixture of pink, blue, and white areas in a reticulate pattern, known as cutis marmorata. With aging this patterning becomes less obvious except in disease states, in which it may become exaggerated. It is then known as livedo reticularis. It has always been recognized that this pattern is determined by perfusion and the distribution of the arterials to the skin as well as to the degree with which they are vasoconstricted. Extreme vasodilatation usually produces a homogeneous flush. Braverman et al. (7), in a very detailed study, recently confirmed that the distribution of arterioles influences flow patterns, as picked up by the laser Doppler, but it is important also to realize that these flow patterns, depend on blood rheology and the many factors that impair or facilitate flow through the capillary bed, such as rouleaux formation or white cell trapping (8). One needs an explanation of why all these factors have the most obvious effect on skin color in the young and that the skin in the aged mostly shows very few of these patterns. One explanation is the recent concept (9) that blood flow through the capillary bed is affected by the number of bifurcations in the system, especially

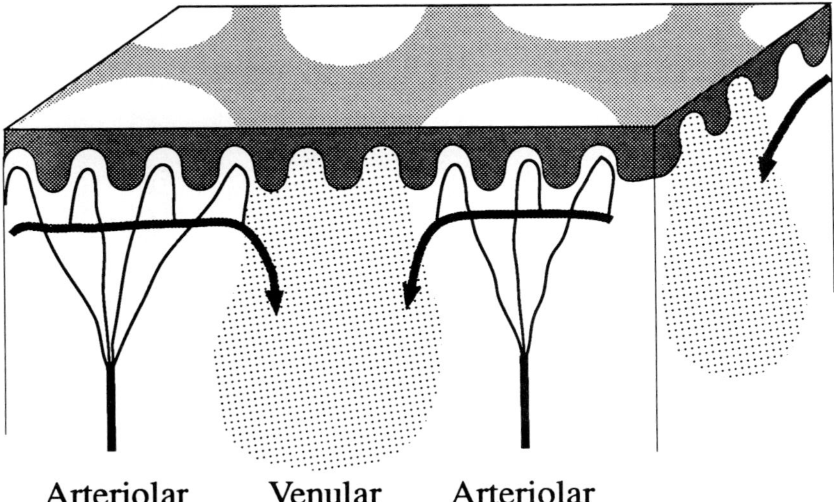

Figure 9 Reticulate markings visible at the surface of the skin are determined by the distribution of arterioles.

bifurcations distal to the sites of maximum autonomic nervous control (Fig. 10). The phenomenon of vasomotion is one that determines that all sections of the vascular bed show intermittent opening up versus shutting down, and this gives rise to the waveforms picked up by the laser Doppler flowmeter. When laser Doppler flowmetry is combined with observation of capillaries using videomicroscopy (10), it can be seen that there is often no correlation between the stops and starts in the capillary bed and the vasoconstrictor versus vasodilator changes occurring in the arterials supplying the bed. It is probable that local factors, such as the changes in blood flow, that are a consequence of rapid changes in permeability and rises in hematocrit, all of which occur as a result of changes in rouleaux formation or white cell stickiness, all contribute to an enormous range of possible stops and starts anywhere in the capillary bed. The waveforms that result from this appear chaotic. Such chaos occurs because there are too many possibilities. At every bifurcation there is always a choice for blood to go in one or two directions, and the more bifurcations, the greater the number of choices. I emphasize this because there is a great difference between aged and young systems. The reduction in the overall capacity of the capillary bed results in fewer bifurcations and thus fewer choices. The dominant influence comes from the autonomic control of the arterial system.

In the young adult, the reticulate markings of the skin, so obvious when cold, are of varying size, as might be expected by the varying distribution of the arterials supplying the skin. If one examines the reticulate markings in the newborn one finds that they are mostly the same size, because at birth the number of arterials per unit area of the skin is approximately the same in all

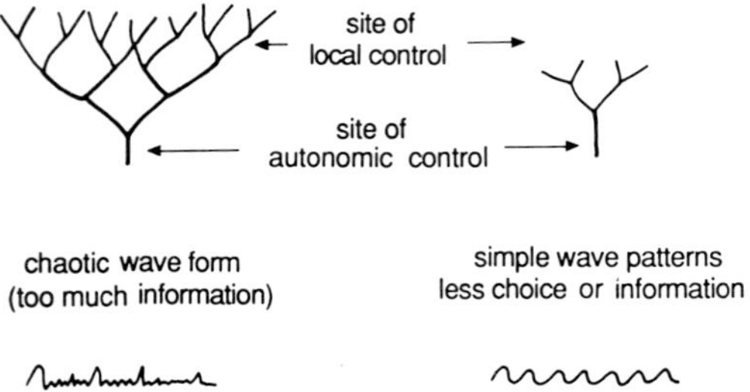

Figure 10 Few bifurcations in atrophic vascular beds provide fewer choices for blood flow, and wave patterns dependent on local factors are simplified. The richer the capillary and the more bifurcations, the more choices are available and the more local control determines flow patterns. In atrophy, local control is relatively less and autonomic control proportionally more dominant. Flow pattern waveforms show less information.

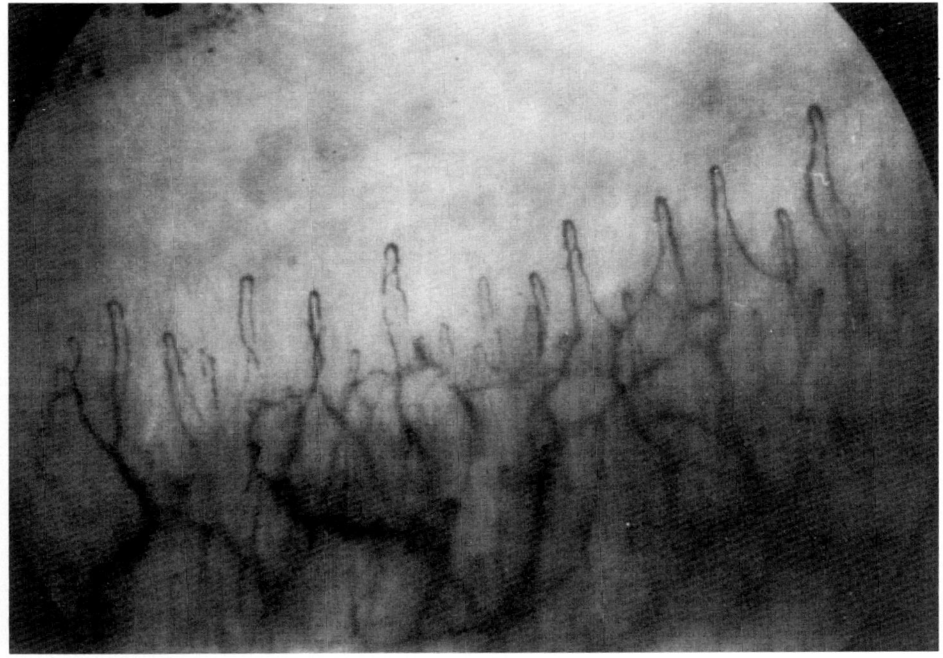

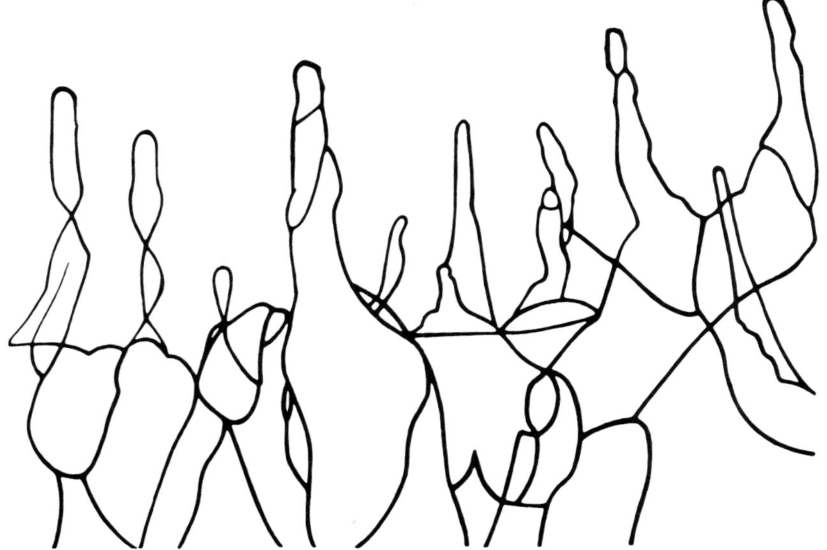

Figure 11 (A) Transparent and horizontally disposed capillary network in the human nailfold. (B) The drawing emphasizes the numerous cross-communications. There are anastomotic channels even in the papillary vessels. (From H. R. Maricq, with permission.)

areas, but after the first years of life, no new arterioles are made and as the limbs in particular elongate, the area of skin supplied by an artery increases. To meet the demands of the epidermis the capillary bed grows more bifurcations. One consequence is that livedo is most obvious on the thighs.

V. TECHNIQUES FOR EXAMINING A CAPILLARY BED OF THE SKIN

Early observers used microscopes with short working distances and/or depth focus. It was the nailfold capillary that was the most easily observed (11), but the vessels there are horizontally disposed and may not be wholly representative of capillaries found elsewhere. The introduction of long working distances allowed better visualization of capillaries (12) in any part of the body surface (13). The magnification required is usually no more than about × 50, and for a general view of the distribution of the capillary bed, × 12–20 may be sufficient. Good illumination is helpful, sometimes with green filters to produce greater contrast between pink and red, and the skin is made transparent by various oils, such as paraffin oil. The typical appearance of the nailfold is illustrated in Figure 11 from the work of Maricq (12). The regular horizontal distribution of the hairpin loops at the distal edge of the nailfold can be easily seen. One feature of elderly skin is that of apical dilatation, which can be found in approximately 25% of the elderly. It is difficult to know when these become pathologic. Micropools or microaneurysms have been thought to be more common in patients with arteriosclerosis (14), but they are also features of cold-sensitive disorders and they may be a temporary feature of abnormal repair (15). The elderly leg and foot show the greatest heterogeneity of vascular form (20). Overall there tends to be a reduction in the number of capillaries to between 20 and 30 per mm^2. The network of rather sparse capillaries shows numerous, more horizontally disposed vessels, and some of these must trek long distances to provide a supply (16). Ryan has always emphasized that it is the red blood column that is observed. Empty capillaries are invisible. By obstructing outflow with a steel ring, superficial capillaries fill more completely. The steel ring can also be used to push away upper dermal tissue fluid, and this, too, increases the visibility of the capillaries (Fig. 12) (6).

A. Dynamic Capillaroscopy Without Dyes

A microscope television system was introduced by Bollinger et al. (17). Essentially this is a high-magnification system for short working distance and suitable only when the capillary bed can be immobilized. Consequently most information has come from the nailfold. Fagrell et al. (18) further developed the system, particularly for the lower limb. The importance of this was that capillary blood cell velocity could be measured in a single capillary and correlated with such phenomena as arterial pulsation or the effects of the autonomic nervous system or respiration. By recording blood flow on a video, various modalities can be analyzed and successive examinations preserved for the sequential analysis of the effects of therapy. Some of the greatest interest has been generated by combining these techniques with the laser Doppler flowmeter and analyzing the rhythmic variations in skin microcirculation. Techniques like postocclusive reactive hyperemia and cooling have helped to distinguish between local and systemic influences (10).

Transparency of the skin. This is a feature of atrophy in which there is thinning of both epidermis and upper dermis. It is a feature of steroid overusage, and so-called preatrophy due to steroids has been equated with an early demonstration of a greatly visible subpapillary plexus (21). It occurs spontaneously in essential telangiectasis. The feature of a dilated and easily visible horizontal subpapillar venous plexus can be reversed by the daily application of retinoids. In a comparison of the effect of retinoids on skin thickness with the effects of epidermal abrasion (mild with an abrasive powder), it was observed that greater changes occur with the abrasion (19). Several studies of skin thickness in post-menopausal women have recorded the influence of hormones and the "normal" thinning that characterizes female as opposed to male skin.

B. Dynamic Capillaroscopy with Dyes

By injecting intravital fluorescent dyes, it is possible to enhance images and to analyze the plasma layer as well as the erythrocyte column. Dyes inoculated intradermally can also be used to enhance the visibility of the superficial lymphatic plexus (Fig. 13).

VI. AGE-ASSOCIATED DISEASE

In considering the capillary bed in the aged, one cannot afford to ignore common associated phenomena, such as arterial occlusive disease, hypertension, diabetes mellitus, or venous incompetence. Nor can one ignore the accumulated scars of the environment, such as the difference between chronically sun-exposed skin and nonexposed skin or the effects of a temperate climate with its chronic cooling and consequent perniosis. An examination of the skin in old age reveals a diversity of vascular anomalies, with areas of extremely sparse vasculature mixed with bizarre vascular shapes, some visible to the naked eye and others present as red spots or plaques, the irregular patterns being identifiable with a low magnification (Fig. 14).

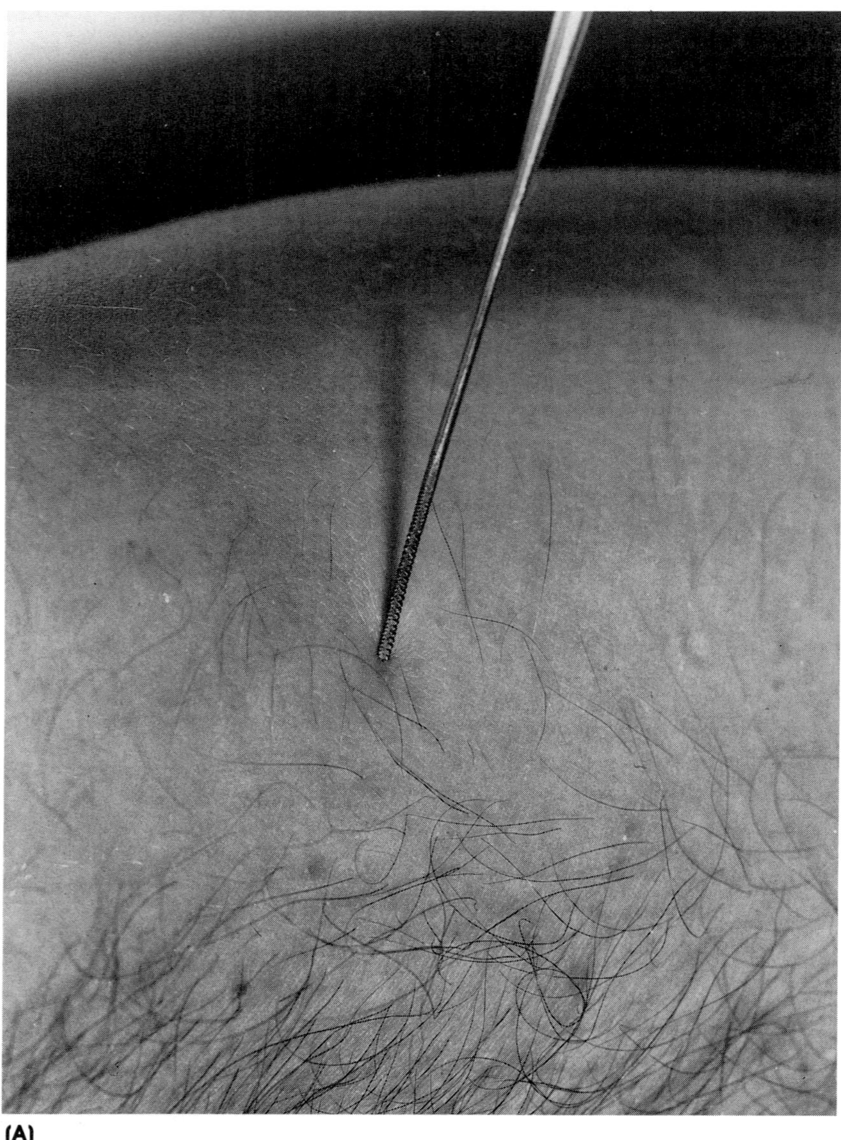

(A)

Figure 12   The use of a steel probe (Jobson Horne) to disperse tissue fluid and to enhance the visibility of vessels in the upper dermis.

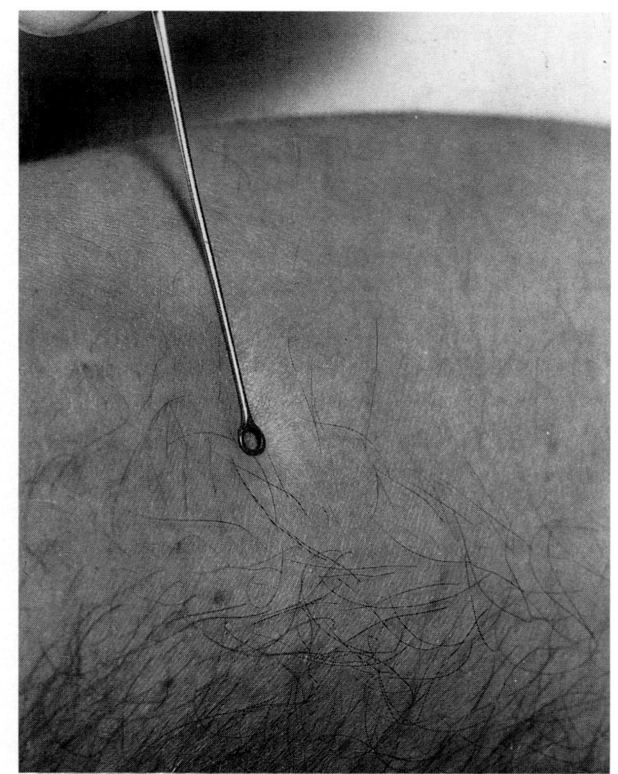

(B)

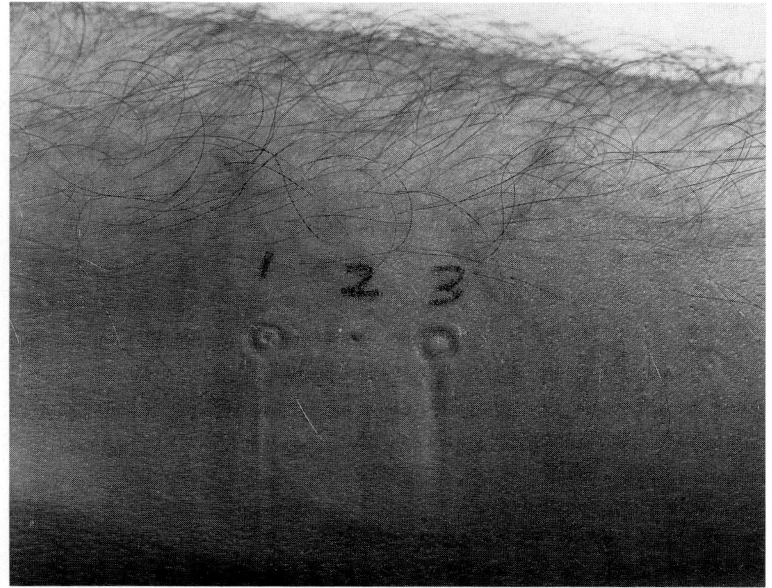

(C)

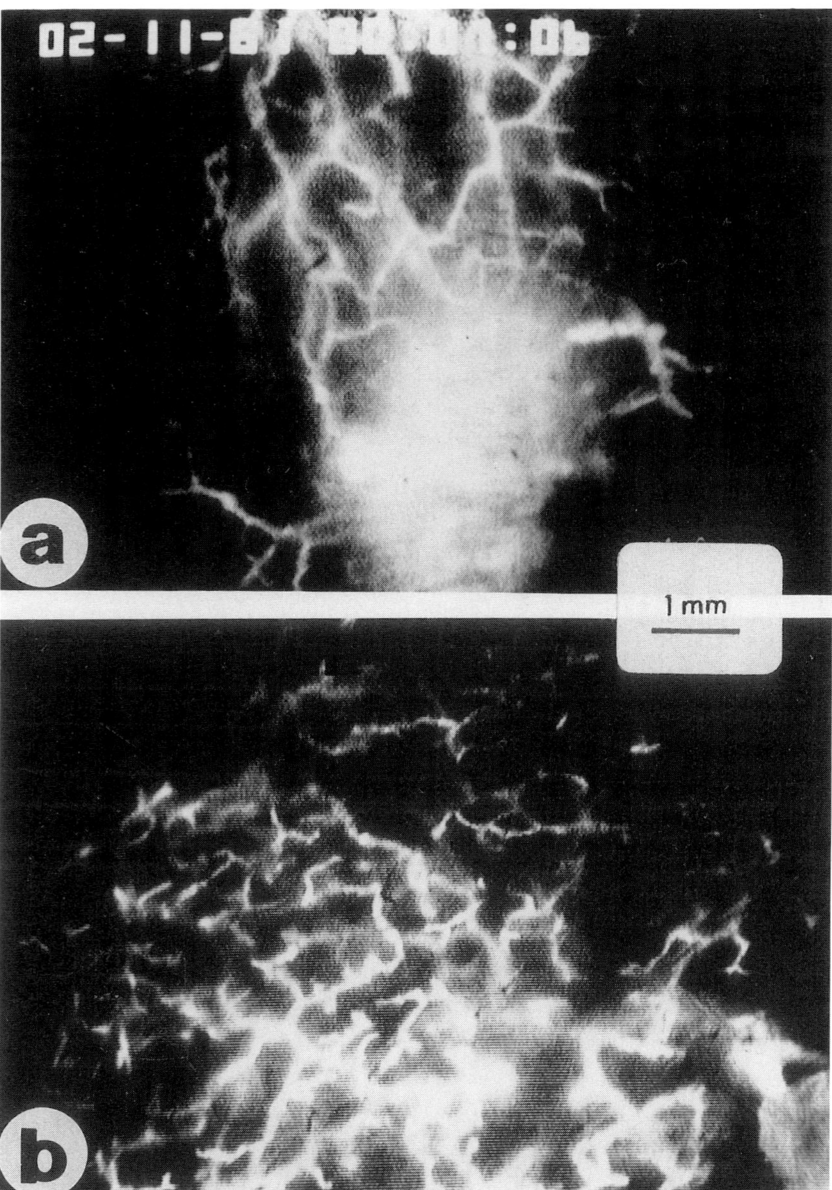

Figure 13 Protein-bound fluorescent dyes inoculated into the upper dermis are cleared by the lymphatics and can be used to enhance the visibility of the skins' lymphatic system. (From Bollinger, with permission.)

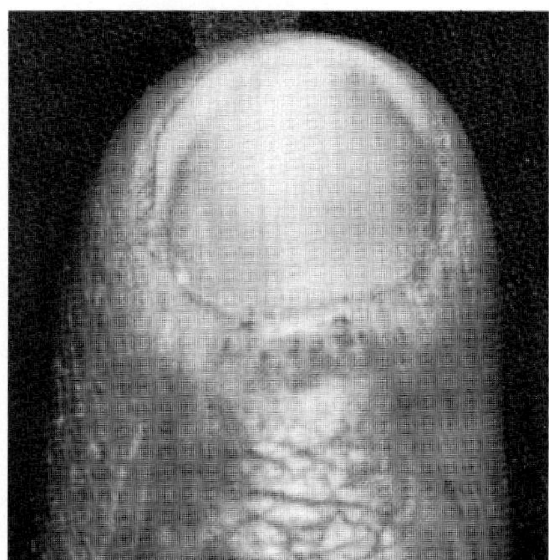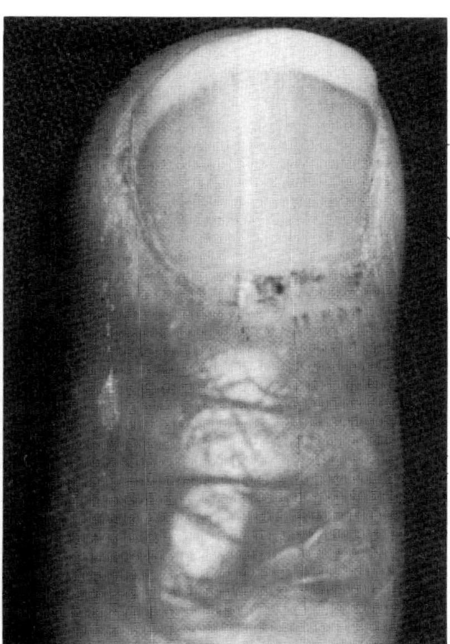

Figure 14 Grossly irregular patterns of upper dermal vascularization are characteristic of many pathologies in which there is an angiogenic stimulus in a background of atrophy or scarring. It has long been recognized by the naked eye in the nailfold of such diseases as scleroderma and dermatomyositis.

REFERENCES

1. Ryan TJ. The structure and function of lymphatics. J Invest Dermatol 1989; 93:185–245.
2. Rayman G, Williams SA, Spencer PD, Smaje LH, Wise PH, Tooke JE. Impaired microvascular hyperaemic response to minor skin trauma in type 1 diabetes. Br Med J 1986; 292:1295–8.
3. Ryan TJ. The microcirculation of the skin in old age. Gerontol Clin 1966; 8:327.
4. Pasyk KA. Vascular birthmarks. In: Ryan TJ, Cherry GW, eds. classification of haemangiomas. London: Oxford University Press, 1987; 1–54.
5. Pasyk KA, Thomas SV, Hassett CA, Cherry GW, Faller R. Regional differences in capillary density of the normal human dermis. J Plast Reconst Surg 1989; 83:939–47.
6. Ryan TJ. A study of the epidermal capillary unit in psoriasis. Dermatologica 1969; 138:459–72.
7. Braverman IM, Keh A, Goldming D. Correlation of laser doppler wave patterns underlying microvascular anatomy. J Invest Dermatol 1990; 95:283–6.

8. Ryan TJ, Copeman PWM. Microvascular pattern and blood stasis in skin disease. Br Dermatol 1969; Dermatol 8:563.

9. Intaglietta M. Vasomotion and flow modification in the microcirculation. Prog Appl Microcirc 1989; 15:1–102.

10. Bollinger A, Fagrell B. Clinical capillaroscopy. Toronto: Hogrefe and Huber, 1990, 166.

11. Davis E, Landau J. Clinical capillary microscopy. Springfield, Il: Charles C. Thomas, 1972.

12. Maricq HR. Nailfold capillary photography. Prog Appl Microcirc 1986; 11: 11–27.

13. Gilje O. Capillaroscopy in the differential diagnosis of skin disease. Acta Derm Venereol (Stockh) 1953; 33:303–17.

14. Knisely MH, Barnes RH, Satterwhite WM Jr. In vivo observations of the bulbar conjunctival blood vessels and blood of functioning people 60 years of age and over. Gerontol 1957; 12:429–36.

15. Ryan TJ, Kurban AK. New vessel growth in adult skin. Br J Dermatol 1970; Suppl. 5; 82:92–98.

16. Ryan TJ. The epidermis and its blood supply in venous disorders of the leg. Trans St Johns Hosp Dermatol Soc (Lond) 1969; 55:51.

17. Bollinger A, Butti P, Barras JP, Trachsler H, Siegenthaler W. Red blood cell velocity in nailfold capillaries of man measured by a television microscopy technique. Microvasc Res 1974; 7:61–72.

18. Fagrell B, Fronek A, Intaglietta MA. Microscope television system for studying flow velocity in human skin capillaries. Am J Physiol 1977; 233:H318–21.

19. Marks R, Hill S, Barton SP. The effects of an abrasive agent on normal skin and on photo-aged skin in comparison with topical tretinoin. Br J Dermatol 1990; 123:457–66.

20. Fagrell B. Vital capillaroscopy—a clinical method for studying changes of skin microcirculation in patients suffering from vascular disorders of the leg. Angiology 1972; 23:284–98.

21. Katz HI, Prawer SE, Mooney JJ, Samson CR. Pre-atrophy: Covert sign of thinned skin. J Am Acad Dermatol 1989; 20:731–5.

22. Ryan TJ. The microcirculation in psoriasis: blood vessels, lymphatics and tissue fluid. In: Baden HP, ed. The chemotherapy of psoriasis. International encyclopaedia of pharmacology and therapeutics, sec. 10. Oxford: Pergamon Press, 1990; 145–84.

9

Laser Doppler-Measured Cutaneous Blood Flow: Effects with Age

ANDREAS J. BIRCHER

University of Basel
Basel, Switzerland

KATHLEEN V. ROSKOS

SRI International
Menlo Park, California

HOWARD I. MAIBACH and RICHARD H. GUY

University of California—San Francisco, School of Medicine
San Francisco, California

I. INTRODUCTION

Many physiologic and biochemical changes occur in human skin with increasing age. These include modifications in the epidermal barrier function and immunologic defense, a decrease in glandular functions, and significant alterations in the cutaneous microvasculature (1–3). In the literature several direct (venous occlusion plethysmography and xenon[133] clearance) and indirect (skin temperature and transcutaneous pO_2) methods have been used to measure cutaneous blood flow (CBF) and to characterize these changes. More recently, new noninvasive technologies based on optical principles that allow direct measurement of the cutaneous microcirculation have been increasingly employed.

Of these, photopulse plethysmography (PPG) and laser Doppler flowmetry (LDF) have been most widely used (4). These two techniques operate on different optical principles, yet are both totally noninvasive, the data being collected via probes held to the skin surface by adhesive tape. PPG, introduced in the late 1930s (5,6), essentially measures the local blood volume as determined by the extent of absorbed infrared radiation by hemoglobin (7). The application of the laser Doppler principle to assess CBF was introduced in 1975 (8). In LDF, a laser light source and the Doppler effect are used to generate an output proportional to the erythrocyte flux through the microvessels under investigation (9–12). Since its introduction this technique has been widely employed to study the vascular physiology of various tissues (13), the effects of topically and systemically applied pharmacologic agents (14), and the response of skin diseases to therapeutic interventions (15). Both PPG and LDF permit fast and semiquantitative measurement of CBF; however, because of the ease of handling and sophisticated technology, LDF has been widely used to assess microcirculation in most human tissues (13).

A detailed knowledge of the age-related physiologic and pathologic changes in CBF and the microvasculature reactivity of various age groups are of considerable importance (e.g., with respect to the absorption of drugs from topical formulations and transdermal drug delivery systems), but systematic investigations of CBF in young and aged skin are few.

The microvasculature in the dermis undergoes considerable alteration with age: there is a reduction in vertical length and diameter of the capillary loop and a decreased density of the capillary network, especially of the vertically ascending subset. Nevertheless, the dermal capillary pressure remains unchanged despite increases in arteriolar pressure (16,17). Whether this reduction in the capillary network results in diminution of the vascular response (3) remains unresolved and controversial. Some of the measurable differences in CBF (as determined by LDF) may be explained in part by the small tissue volume in which the measurement is made and the heterogeneity of the cutaneous microvasculature (18,19). These inconsistencies in LDF blood flow measurements may be simply circumvented by the acquisition of multiple standardized readings through the use of a special probe holder (20) or the application of a special multifiber probe (21,22). In addition, care must also be exercised on initial positioning of the laser probe to take the heterogeneous distribution of the capillaries into consideration (19). This is accomplished by direct observation of the laser Doppler wave pattern upon initial placement. Other factors possibly influencing CBF may be elevated blood pressure or underlying subclinical disorders, such as diabetes mellitus, atherosclerosis (23), and anemia (24).

II. BASELINE BLOOD FLOW

In a study of 120 male and female individuals aged 10 to >70 years, fingertip blood flow of the nondominant hand was not significantly dependent on age or gender (Table 1) (24). Also, an examination of 45 healthy volunteers from four age groups (<20 years, 21–30 years, 31–40 years, and >40 years) revealed no significant differences in CBF of the fingertip (25). In contrast, in another large investigation of 201 subjects from four age groups (10–29 years, 30–49 years, 50–69 years, and 70–89 years) (26), age-related changes

Table 1 Comparison of Baseline Cutaneous Blood Flow Between Age Groups

Groups (*n*)	Subjects (*n*)	Age range (years)	Anatomic location	Age-related blood flow difference	Reference
7	11	10–19	Fingertip	NS[a], decreased in >60 years old	Hatanaka et al. (24)
	26	20–29			
	19	30–39			
	10	40–49			
	17	50–59			
	20	60–69			
	19	>70			
4	4	<20	Fingertip	NS	Zeghal et al. (25)
	26	21–30			
	12	31–40			
	3	>40			
4	65	10–29	15 Sites	NS, decreased in older age groups at sites with higher perfusion	Ishihara et al. (26)
	49	30–49			
	50	50–69			
	37	70–89			
2	13	24–29	Leg, foot, toe	NS	Kvernebo et al. (27)
	11	61–74			
2	10	27–49	Not mentioned	NS	Fagrell (28)
	10	52–84			
2	4	26–29	Forearm	NS	Bircher (unpublished)
	5	66–74			
2	16	22–29	Toe	Significant increase in old versus young	Kvernebo et al. (31)
	10	60–75			
2	9	21–29	Leg	NS	Kvernebo et al. (31)
	5	62–70			
3	56	10–39	Fingertip	Significant decrease in old versus young	Oimomi et al. (34)
	43	40–69			
	40	70–89		NS, middle versus young	

[a]Not significant.

in CBF in anatomic areas with a high CBF were found. In particular, a clear although not significant trend toward lower CBF values in older individuals was found in the acral sites of the body with many arteriovenous shunts (lip, fingertip, nose, and forehead). In subjects aged 70 years and above, CBF was also decreased in the earlobe, the cheek, and the palm (Fig. 1). In sites with

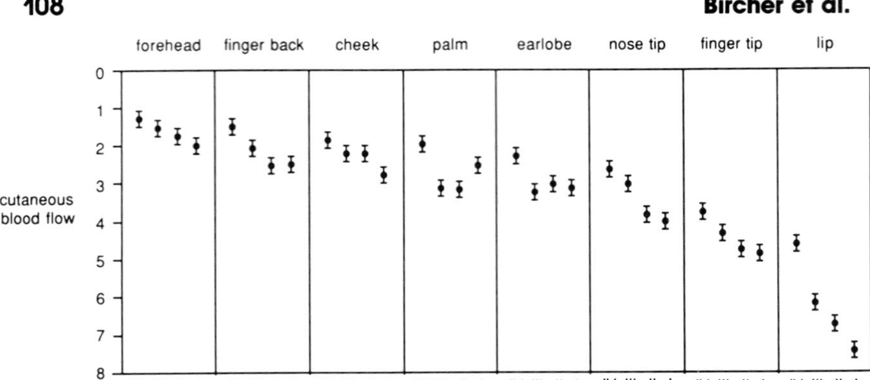

Figure 1 Resting blood flow at different anatomic sites in four age groups (I = 10–29, II = 30–49, III = 40–69, IV = 70–89 years). (Redrawn from Ref. 25.)

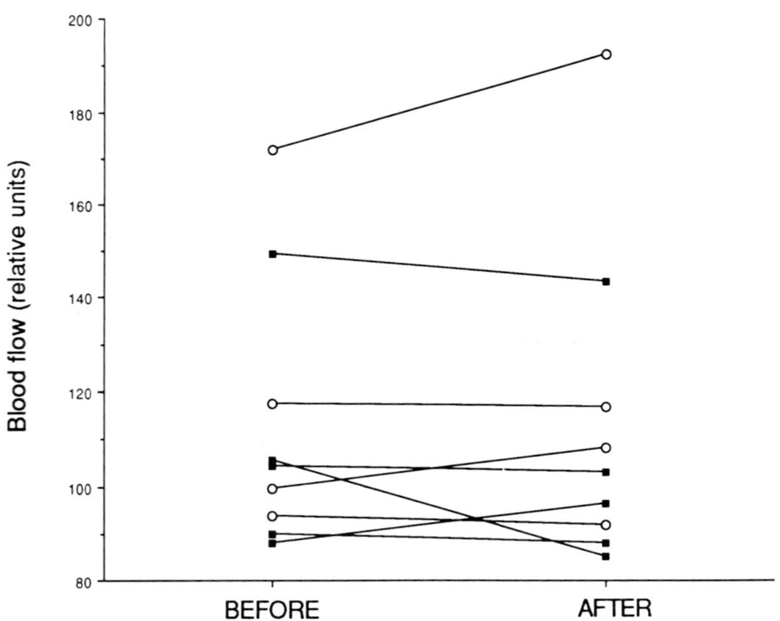

Figure 2 Resting LDF values recorded in young (circles) and old (squares) subjects. Each data point represents the mean of eight measurements. There was no age-related difference in either the baseline or the stability of blood flow in a 60–90 minute period.

low CBF (trunk and extremities), however, there were no obvious variations in CBF with age.

Resting CBF has also been measured at various points on the lower limb of healthy young ($n = 13$, 24–29 years) and healthy old subjects ($n = 11$, 61–74 years) in a recumbent position. Again, comparable CBF values were obtained and no discrimination between the age groups was possible (27). Similar results were observed when measurements were made in a supine and sitting position with a multifiber probe in a young ($n = 10$, 27–49 years) and an old ($n = 10$, 52–84 years) age group. Also, no discrimination was possible for either position between the two groups (28).

We also found (unpublished data) no age-related variation in the stability of baseline CBF over short time periods. The baseline or resting CBF in forearm skin did not differ significantly between young ($n = 4$, 26–29 years) and old ($n = 5$, 66–74 years) individuals. Moreover, there was also no age-related difference in the stability of CBF at the beginning and at the end of a resting period of 60–90 minutes (Fig. 2).

III. STIMULATED BLOOD FLOW

Several stimuli that have the ability to affect the cutaneous blood vessels (i.e., temperature, occlusion, and vasoactive chemicals) have been used to investigate age-dependent differences in the reactivity of the skin microvasculature (Table 2). Data indicate that stimulated CBF values are more reproducible and show less variation than baseline CBF measurements. They are, therefore, more likely to detect small differences in the response of the microvasculature. For example, investigation of the CBF response to thermal stimulation allowed healthy individuals to be correctly differentiated from patients with vascular disease (28,29).

A. Temperature

The effect of temperature on CBF and on the volume of circulating erythrocytes in forearm skin was measured in 60 male subjects from three age groups: young (20–39 years), middle-aged (40–59 years), and old (60–79 years) (23). Three different temperatures were achieved by placement of the subject's forearm in a water bath at 30, 35, and 40°C. LDF values were not different within or between the age groups at the two lower temperatures. At 40°C, however, a significantly ($p < 0.03$) higher CBF was observed for the young compared to the two older groups (Fig. 3). The erythrocyte volume did not significantly change within or between the age groups at 30 and 35°C but significantly increased with higher temperatures in all three groups. This

Table 2 Comparison of Stimulated Cutaneous Blood Flow Between Age Groups

Groups (n)	Subjects (n)	Age range (years)	Anatomic location	Blood Flow stimuli	Age-related blood flow difference	Reference
3	20	20–39	Forearm	30, 35, 40°C	Significant increase in young versus middle and old at 40°C	Richardson (23)
	20	40–59				
	20	60–79			NS at 30 and 35°C	
2	23	Mean 23	9 Sites	35°C	Significant increase in young at 2 sites (35°C)	Bartek et al. (30)
	25	Mean 74		44°C	Significant increase in young at 4 sites (44°C)	
4	13	10–29	Fingertip	10°C	NS in >50 years old	Ishihara et al. (26)
	16	30–49				
	8	50–69				
	19	70–89				
2	16	22–29	Toe	Occlusion	NS	Kvernebo et al. (31)
	10	60–75				
2	9	21–29	Leg	Occlusion	NS	Kvernebo et al. (31)
	5	62–70				
2	6	20–30	Forearm	Nicotinate	Significant increase in young (R_{max})	Guy et al. (32)
	6	63–80				
2	6	20–36	Forearm	Nicotinate	NS	Roskos et al. (33)
	7	64–86				
3	43	10–39	Fingertip	Standing up	Significant decrease old versus young	Oimomi et al. (34)
	41	40–69			NS middle versus young	
	28	70–89				
2	30	10–49	Back	Sodium lauryl sulfate	NS	Ishihara et al. (26)
	17	50–89				
2	11	10–49	Back	Ultraviolet B	NS	Ishihara et al. (26)
	8	50–89				

result indicates decreased response of the cutaneous microvasculature to thermal stimuli with increasing age. To assess the influence of diseases (diabetes mellitus, atherosclerotic vascular disease, and hypertension) that may affect the dynamic response of the microvessels, subjects were monitored for blood pressure, as well as plasma glucose, triglycerides, and cholesterol. Systolic

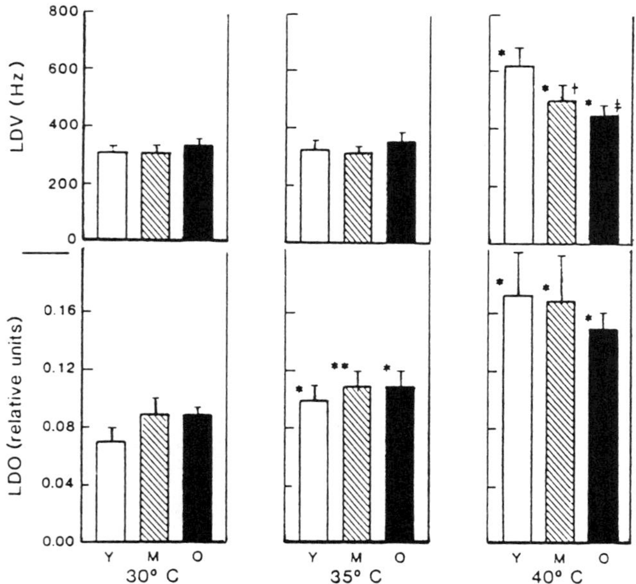

Figure 3 LDF values (LDV) and erythrocyte volume (LDO) measured at three temperatures in young (open), middle-aged (hatched), and old (solid) men. Values are given as mean ± SEM.
*,**Significant within-group temperature effect.
†Significant young versus middle-aged.
‡Significant young versus old.
(Reprinted by permission from Ref. 23.)

blood pressure was significantly higher in the old group, and glucose and cholesterol levels were significantly increased in the middle-aged and old groups. However, multiple regression analyses showed that age alone was the significant factor that determined the response of the microcirculation to thermal stimulation.

This higher response of CBF to heat in young individuals has also been found at other anatomic locations (30). At a laser probe holder temperature of 35°C (temperature restricted to the area of probe attachment), CBF measured on the face and the pulp of the big toe was significantly higher ($p < 0.05$) in healthy young ($n = 23$, average 23 years) than in healthy old subjects ($n = 25$, average 74 years). At 44°C, further significant differences in CBF were measured at the cubital fossa, the knee, and the toe. No temperature-related CBF differences between age groups were observed at the wrist, the dorsal finger, the finger pulp, or the ankle.

As stated, baseline CBF in the finger pulp decreased with increasing age (26). In a similar group of subjects the effect of cold water at 10°C on finger pulp blood flow was investigated. A decrease in CBF was present in all individuals. It was greater in subjects older than 50 years, and restoration was poorest in the oldest group (>70 years). However, compared to the important fall in CBF to cold stimuli in patients with chilblains, a cold-induced skin disorder, or systemic lupus erythematosus, the age-related changes in healthy individuals were small.

B. Postocclusive Hyperemia

Postocclusive hyperemia in healthy young and old control individuals was examined in a study investigating patients with peripheral vascular disease (31). Resting CBF values measured in supine position at the toe were significantly ($p < 0.05$) higher in elderly than in young controls (Table 1). CBF in leg skin in the same subjects, on the other hand, was not different. No age-related differences were found in (1) the extent of the hyperemic response after occlusion or (2) the time of onset or the time of peak response of CBF at either measuring site (31).

C. Pharmacologic Stimuli

In two studies examining the age-related response of the microvasculature to a topically applied pharmacologic agent, only minor differences in the reactivity of the microcirculation between young and old age groups have been found.

In a first study (32), a potent vasodilator (100 mM aqueous methyl nicotinate, MN) was applied via a saturated paper disk for 15 s to the forearm in young ($n = 6$, 20–30 years) and old ($n = 6$, 63–80 years) subjects. Following topical application, MN rapidly penetrates the epidermis and acts upon the dermal capillaries. Because finite doses of MN are applied, the measured vasoresponse passes through a maximum and then decays. Several parameters were examined, but only the magnitude of the CBF response (R_{max}) was significantly ($p \leq 0.05$) different between the age groups. However, the methodology and the data analysis did not differentiate between possible changes in either microcirculation sensitivity or epidermal barrier function.

A more detailed investigation (33) involved four concentrations (2.5, 5, 10, and 25 mM) of MN in a young ($n = 6$, 20–34 years) and an old ($n = 7$, 64–86 years) age group, and the individual kinetic processes of local skin absorption, cutaneous reactivity, and elimination of MN were analyzed using a pharmacokinetic-pharmacodynamic model. The parameters chosen to characterize the dose-response behavior were the time of response onset, the time

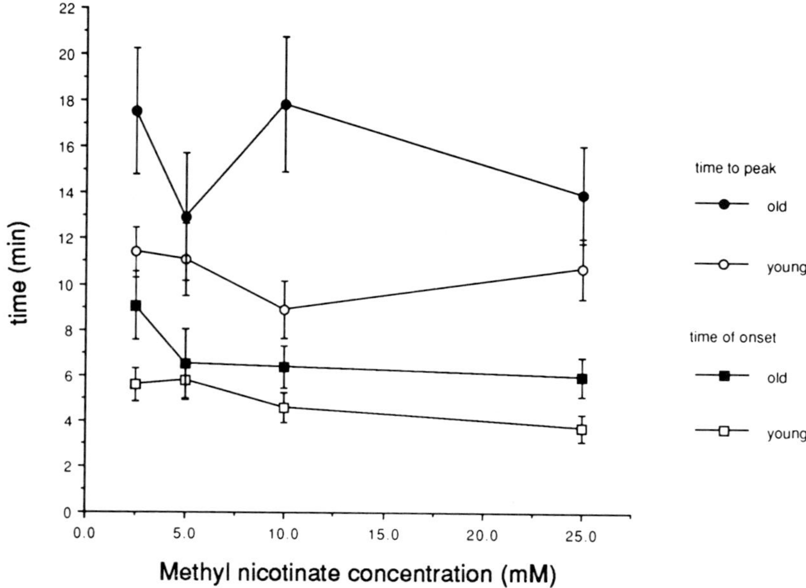

Figure 4 Time of onset of action (squares) and time of maximum response (circles) as a function of applied methyl nicotinate concentrations. Values are given as mean ± standard error of the mean (Redrawn from Ref. 33.)

to reach R_{max} of the vasodilatory response and the time for the response to decay to 75% of R_{max}, the peak value (R_{max}), and the area under the response-time curve. Using the pharmacokinetic-pharmacodynamic model to evaluate the individual sensitivity and the efficiency of the microcirculation, no significant differences in the capillary response to MN were found between the age groups. For the old individuals, however, there was a trend to a slower reaction represented by longer time periods (Fig. 4).

D. Other Stimuli

CBF in the fingertip skin following standing up and a Valsalva maneuver was determined in three age groups (young, 10–39; middle, 40–69; old, 70–89 years) to evaluate autonomic nerve function (34). Baseline CBF in a sitting position was significantly ($p < 0.05$) lower in the old compared to the young age group (Table 1); furthermore, the vascular responses to the two stimuli were significantly (standing up: $p < 0.05$; Valsalva: $p < 0.005$) attenuated in the old group. It was concluded that this simple test method may be useful to evaluate autonomic nerve function in elderly individuals and in patients with neurologic diseases.

Some studies indicate that the extent of skin irritation induced by sodium lauryl sulfate applied to the skin surface may depend on gender (35) and ethnicity (36). Between a young ($n = 30$, 10–49 years) and an old ($n = 17$, 50–89 years) group, however, there was no difference in CBF to occlusive patch tests with three concentrations of sodium lauryl sulfate (26).

In similar young and old age groups, the LDF-determined erythematous response to increasing doses of ultraviolet B was measured. Lower CBF values in the older group were apparent, particularly after higher doses of irradiation (>0.234 J/cm^2).The number of individuals in this experiment, however, was not sufficient to allow statistical analysis (26).

IV. CONCLUSIONS

Although the histologic structure of the cutaneous microcirculation changes considerably with age, the function of the capillaries, as measured by LDF, remains largely intact. In most studies reviewed here, significant age-related variations in resting baseline CBF at different anatomic sites are not found. Typically, however, CBF tends to be lower in older cohorts. Several stimuli of CBF, such as postocclusive hyperemia, topical methyl nicotinate, and chemical and physical irritation, do not permit distinction between young and old individuals in a reliable manner. The most obvious and reproducible age-related differences were seen in the dynamic response of CBF to a thermal challenge. Some predisposing factors for atherosclerosis, such as hypercholesteremia or subclinical vascular disease, may influence CBF in eldery subjects; these individuals should be excluded from studies comparing CBF responses in normal populations of young and old cohorts.

REFERENCES

1. Gilchrest BA. Skin and aging processes. Boca Raton, FL: CRC Press, 1984.
2. Kligman AM, Takase Y. Cutaneous aging. Tokyo: University of Tokyo Press, 1988.
3. Cerimele D, Celleneo L, Serri F. Physiological changes in aging skin. Br J Dermatol 1990; 122(Suppl 35):13–20.
4. Guy RH, Tur E, Maibach HI. Optical techniques for monitoring cutaneous microcirculation. Int J Dermatol 1985; 24:88–94.
5. Hertzman AB. Photoelectric plethysmography of the fingers and toes in man. Proc Soc Exp Biol Med 1937; 37:529–34.

6. Hertzman AB. The blood supply of various skin areas as estimated by the photoelectric plethysmograph. Am J Physiol 1938; 124:323–40.

7. Challoner AVJ. Photoelectric plethysmography for estimating cutaneous blood flow. In: Rolfe P, ed. Non invasive physiological measurements, Vol 1. New York: Academic Press, 1979; 125–51.

8. Stern MD. In vivo evaluation of microcirculation by coherent light scattering. Nature 1975; 254:56–8.

9. Stern M, Lappe DL, Bowen PD, et al. Continuous measurement of tissue blood flow by laser Doppler spectroscopy. Am J Physiol 1977; 232:H441–8.

10. Bonner RF, Clem TR, Bowen PD, Bowman RL. Laser-Doppler continuous real-time monitor of pulsatile and mean blood flow in tissue in microcirculation. In: Chen SH, Chu B, Nossal R, eds. Scattering techniques applied to supramolecular and non-equilibrium systems, NATO, ASI Series B73. New York: Plenum Press, 1981; 685–702.

11. Holloway GA, Watkins DW. Laser Doppler measurement of cutaneous blood flow. J Invest Dermatol 1977; 69:306–9.

12. Watkins D, Holloway GA. An instrument to measure cutaneous blood flow using the Doppler Shift of laser light. IEEE Trans Biomed Eng 1978; 25:28–33.

13. Shepherd AP, Öberg PÅ. Laser-Doppler blood flowmetry. Boston: Kluwer Academic, 1990.

14. Bircher AJ, Guy RH, Maibach HI. Skin pharmacology and dermatology. In: Shepherd AP, Öberg PÅ, eds. Laser-Doppler blood flowmetry. Boston: Kluwer Academic, 1990; 141–74.

15. Bircher AJ, Maibach HI. The assessment of the cutaneous microcirculation by laser Doppler and photoplethysmographic techniques. In: Maibach HI, Lowe NJ, eds. Models in dermatology, Vol. IV. Basel: Karger, 1989; 209–31.

16. De Lacharrière O, Kalis B. Measurement of cutaneous microcirculation in dermatology and dermatopharmacology. In: Leveque J-L, ed. Cutaneous investigation in health and disease. New York: Marcel Dekker, 1989; 385–420.

17. Stüttgen G, Ott A. Senescence in the skin. Br J Dermatol 1990; 122(Suppl 35):43–8.

18. Johnson JM. The cutaneous circulation. In: Shepherd AP, Öberg PÅ, eds. Laser-Doppler blood flowmetry. Boston: Kluwer Academic, 1990; 121–39.

19. Braverman IM, Keh A, Goldminz D. Correlation of laser Doppler wave patterns with underlying microvascular anatomy. J Invest Dermatol 1990; 95:283–6.

20. De Boer EM, Bezemer PD, Bruynzeel DP. A standard method for repeated recording of skin blood flow using laser Doppler flowmetry. Dermatosen 1989; 37:58–62.

21. Salerud EG, Nilsson GE. Integrating probe for tissue laser Doppler flowmeter. Med Biol Eng Comput 1986; 24:415–9.

22. Östergren J, Schöps P, Fagrell B. Evaluation of a laser Doppler multiprobe for detecting skin microcirculatory disturbances in patients with obliterative arteriosclerosis. Int Angiol 1988; 7:37–41.

23. Richardson D. Effects of age on cutaneous circulatory response to direct heat on the forearm. J Gerontol 1989; 44:89–94.

24. Hatanaka H, Matsumoto S, Ishikawa K, et al. Fundamental studies on the measurement of skin blood flow by a Periflux laser Doppler flowmeter and its clinical application. Rinsho Byori 1984; 32:1025–8.

25. Zeghal K, Geslin P, Maurel A, Lagrue G, Lhoste F. La vélocimétrie laser-Doppler: nouvelle technique d'évaluation de la microcirculation. Presse Med 1986; 15:1997–2000.

26. Ishihara M, Itoh M, Oshawa K, Kinoshita M, Satoh Y. Cutaneous blood flow. In: Kligman AM, Takase Y, eds. Tokyo: University of Tokyo Press, 1988; 167–81.

27. Kvernebo K, Slagsvold CE, Stranden E, Kroese A, Larsen S. Laser Doppler flowmetry in evaluation of lower limb resting skin circulation. A study in healthy controls and atherosclerotic patients. Scand J Clin Invest 1988; 48: 621–6.

28. Fagrell B. Peripheral vascular disease. In: Shepherd AP, Öberg PÅ, eds. Laser-Doppler blood flowmetry. Boston: Kluwer Academic, 1990; 201–13.

29. Del Guercio R, Leonardo G, Arpaia MR. Evaluation of postischemic hyperemia on the skin using laser Doppler velocimetry: study on patients with claudicatio intermittens. Microvasc Res 1986; 32:289–99.

30. Bartek JP, Drobny E, Dovgan D, Evans E, Rendell M. Skin blood flow determined by laser Doppler flowmetry: comparison of young and old subjects. Clin Res 1989; 37:973A.

31. Kvernebo K, Slagsvold CE, Stranden E. Laser Doppler flowmetry in evaluation of skin post-ischaemic reactive hyperaemia. J Cardiovasc Surg 1989; 30:70–5.

32. Guy RH, Tur E, Bjerke S, Maibach HI. Are there age and racial differences to methyl nicotinate-induced vasodilation in human skin? J Am Acad Dermatol 1985; 12:1001–6.

33. Roskos KV, Bircher AJ, Maibach HI, Guy RH. Pharmacodynamic measurements of methyl nicotinate percutaneous absorption: the effect of aging on microcirculation. Br J Dermatol 1990; 122:165–71.

34. Oimomi M, Hatanaka H, Maeda Y, et al. Autonomic nervous function determined by changes of periflux blood flow in the aged. Arch Gerontol Geriatr 1986; 5:159–63.

35. Lammintausta K, Maibach HI, Wilson D. Irritant reactivity in males and females. Contact Dermatitis 1987; 17:276–80.

36. Berardesca E, Maibach HI. Racial differences in sodium lauryl sulphate induced cutaneous irritation: black and white. Contact Dermatitis 1988; 18:65–70.

10

Indirect Assessment of Changes in Skin Microcirculation with Age

JEAN-LUC LÉVÊQUE and JEAN de RIGAL

L'Oréal
Aulnay-sous-Bois, France

PIERRE G. AGACHE

University Hospital,
Besançon, France

I. INTRODUCTION

Several authors have described the morphologic changes that occur in the various cutaneous circulatory networks during the aging process (1,2). The overall character of these modifications involves increased twisting and dilatation of the vessels. The capillary network becomes less dense and presents a number of collapsed and disorganized loops. This paucity has several consequences at the physiologic level, in particular with regard to temperature homeostasis. Several indirect methods can be used to illustrate the paucity of the skin microcirculation in the elderly subject. They are based on the clearance of products applied to the skin, such as ^{22}Na-labeled molecules (3) and dyes, such as fluoresceine (4); other products are used to induce edema (5). All these methods show that the time of clearance is increased approximately twofold in elderly skin (see Chap. 15). The more direct methods also show differences, but mainly in terms of the cutaneous response to physiologic (e.g., heat) or pharmacologic challenge (e.g., esters of nicotinic acid), which shows more clearly the changes that occur in the microcirculation (see Chap. 9).

In this chapter we shall deal with a new experimental approach to these phenomena, based on the fact that blood pressure is far lower in the capillaries than in the larger vessels. It is therefore possible to distinguish the various circulatory networks by varying the pressure applied by experimental probes placed on the skin surface.

II. CHARACTERISTICS OF THE METHODS USED

We have used both laser Doppler (LDV) and photoplethysmographic (PPG) techniques to measure the skin microcirculation. Another parameter related indirectly to the concentration of hemoglobin in the upper dermis is the skin color, particularly its red component.

With regard to the methods available for measuring the skin microcirculation (LDV and PPG), it should be remembered that they are not specific to a given circulatory network. Indeed, the red light used in LDV (675 nm) and the infrared used in PPG (900 nm) penetrate deeply within the skin, and the light reemitted at the skin surface therefore contains information on the deep (subdermal plexus), middepth (dermal plexus), and superficial circulation. It should also be noted that the two methods measure different phenomena. As its name indicates, LDV records changes in the frequency of the light waves reflected by the red cells; the signal shown by the apparatus is therefore proportional to mean blood flow, that is, nV, where n is the mean number of red cells circulating and V is the mean velocity. Because the physical parameter measured is the frequency of the light reemitted, it is important to remember that the signal obtained with LDV is theoretically independent of the light energy reflected.

In contrast, PPG records changes in the amplitude of the light reflected. This modulation is due to periodic changes in the volume of blood flow resulting from systolic pressure variations. The variations recorded are related to blood flow, arterial pressure changes, arterial dilation, and so on. The signal delivered by PPG is therefore a parameter of amplitude dependent on the light energy emitted by the apparatus and reemitted by the skin. The PPG signal amplitude depends on both the periodic variations of the blood flow and the total amount of blood present in the skin, which decrease the reemitted light. Capillary loops that are nonpulsatile only provide an indirect contribution to the PPG signal by decreasing the amount of light reemitted by the skin.

III. EXPERIMENTAL APPROACH

The principle of the experimental approach is based on the work done by Landis on blood pressure in the various circulatory networks (Table 1) (6). Blood pressure decreases as the diameter of the vessels decreases and as they

Table 1 Blood Pressure in the Different Vessels

Vessels	Blood pressure (mm Hg)
Large arteries	100
Small arteries	40–100
Capillaries	20–40
Small veins	10–20
Large veins	0–10

Source: According to Landis (6).

approach the skin surface. In the capillaries, blood pressure is very low and this explains why the skin blanches when pressed. The aim of this work was to record variations in the PPG signal and skin color as a function of the pressure exerted by the measurement probe at the skin surface. As the pressure is increased gradually, different circulatory networks are blocked—first the capillary loops and then other networks of larger diameter in which blood pressure is higher. The experiments concerned three age groups of volunteers: 3–12 years ($n = 16$), 20–57 years ($n = 18$), and 60–92 years ($n = 25$). The pressure applied was varied by using brass rings placed on the recording heads of the apparatus. LDV measurements were performed only in the 20–57 year age group.

IV. EXPERIMENTAL RESULTS AND DISCUSSION

Figure 1 shows the decrease in the LDV signal with increasing pressure applied to the skin. As mentioned, the LDV signal does not depend on the intensity of the light signal; the gradual decrease thus reflects a decrease in blood flow within the various circulatory networks under the influence of the brass weights.

Figure 2 shows the variations in the luminance of the skin, measured using our Trilumen apparatus (7), as a function of the pressure applied to the forehead in the three groups of volunteers. It is noteworthy that the parameter increases in the three groups, reflecting skin blanching. The intergroup variations in luminance are not very large, whereas the interindividual variations in the 3–12 years age group are relatively wide (see Table 2). Skin blanching occurs with pressures of approximately 25 mm Hg and more.

Figure 3 shows the curves representing the variations in the PPG signal as a function of the pressure applied in the three groups of subjects. The maximum signal occurs with a pressure of approximately 20 mm Hg and then

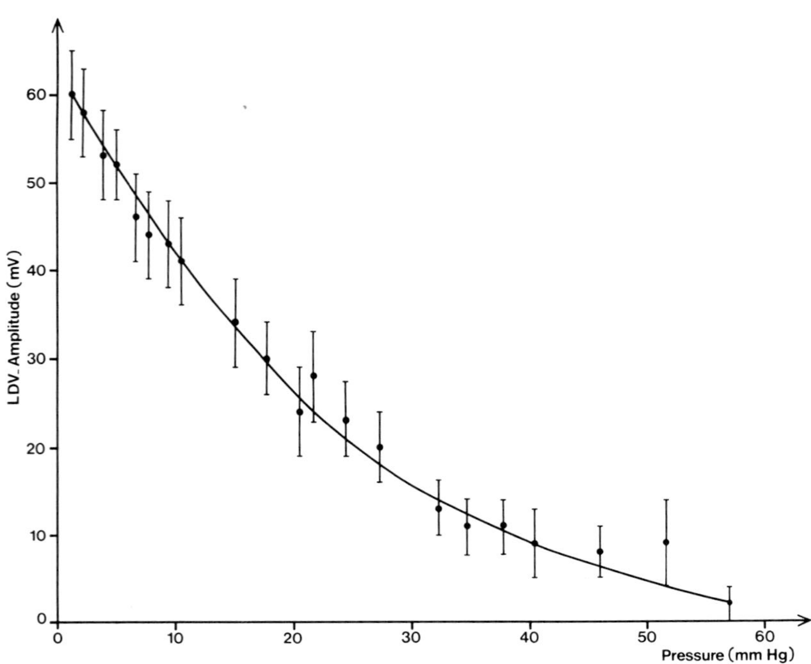

Figure 1 Decrease in the LDV signal versus the increasing pressure applied to the skin (mean ± standard error of the mean, SEM; $n = 18$).

falls to zero at pressures that are higher as age increases. The values of the signals corresponding to P_0 and P_{max}, as well as the variations in amplitude between P_0 and P_{max}, are shown for the three groups of volunteers in Table 3. The increase in the amplitude of the PPG signal between P_0 and P_{max} is probably because in the range of low pressures used blood is expelled from the superficial circulatory system (capillary loops and veins), in which it circulates at very low pressure. The decrease in light absorbance results in an increase in the PPG signal.

Above a P_{max} of about 20 mm Hg, the signal decreases for the same reasons as in the LDV technique. It is noteworthy that the pressure of 20 mm Hg corresponds closely to that reported by Landis for capillary loops (Table 1).

We checked that the use of recording heads of different sizes for the PPG measurements did not influence the shape of the curves and that the maximum signal obtained with this technique was not due to a modification of the distance between the various circulatory networks and the recording head. This phenomenon can be compared to those occurring when the blood pres-

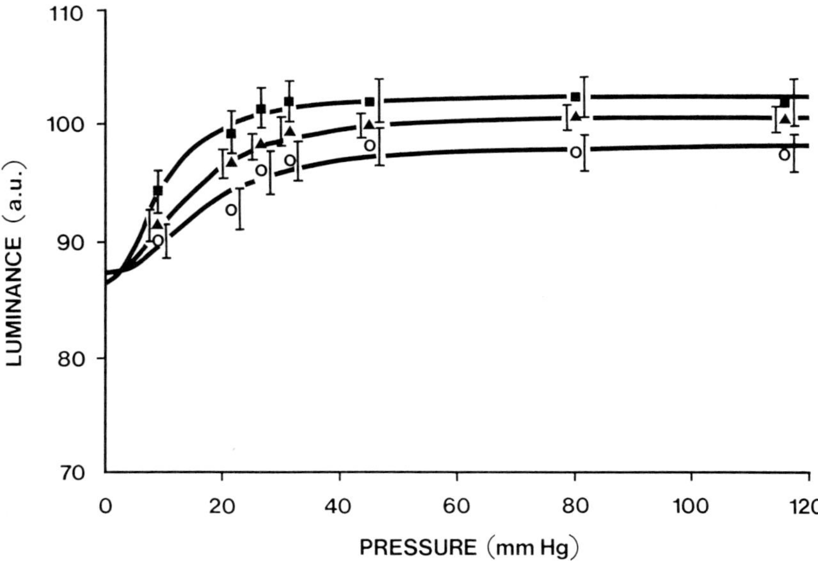

Figure 2 Variation in the luminance of the forehead skin as a function of the pressure applied to the skin: adults, $n = 18$ (squares); young, $n = 16$ (triangles); aged, $n = 25$ (circles).

sure is measured through a pneumatic tensiometer. When the average pressure ($P_{max} + P_{min}$ divided by 2) is reached, the oscillometric index (oscillation amplitude) is maximum. This phenomenon corresponds either to a lower damping of the tissues surrounding the arteries or to cancellation of the transmural pressure (pressure across the vessel wall). This phenomenon does not obligatorily correspond to a maximum of blood flux as is shown under our experimental conditions by the PPG.

Table 2 Skin Luminance (Arbitrary Units)

	P_o	$P > P_{max}$	%		Δ	
Young	86.4 ± 2	101.5 ± 3	17.5	NS	15.1	NS
Adult	86.4 ± 4	103.2 ± 4	19.4	a	16.8	a
Aged	87.2 ± 6	98.2 ± 7	12.6		11	

[a] $P < 0.01$.

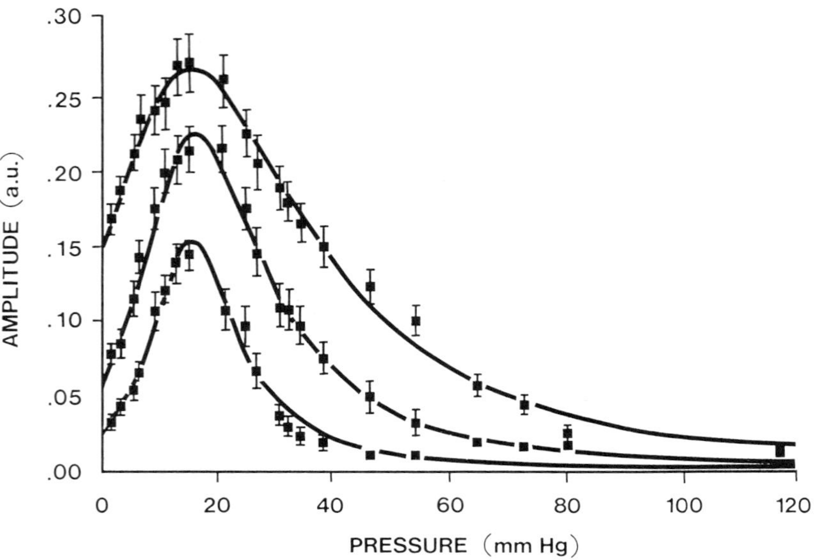

Figure 3 Variation in the photoplethysmographic amplitude versus increasing pressure applied to the skin. The lower curve corresponds to the young, the higher to the aged, and the middle to the adults.

The parameters characteristic of the three populations (Table 3) show that they differ according to the amplitude of the PPG signal. At P_0 and P_{max}, however, the differences are impossible to interpret in terms of skin microcirculation since the nature of the PPG signal is too complex (with a role for arterial pressure, skin thickness, pigmentation, heart rate, and so on). In contrast, the variations in this parameter between P_0 and P_{max} are representative of the richness of the low-pressure microcirculatory network in the upper

Table 3 Photoplethysmography: Amplitude (Arbitrary Units)

	P_o	P_{max}	%	Δ
Young	25 ± 4	150 ± 10	500	125
Adult	65 ± 8	228 ± 30	251	163
Aged	150 ± 10	266 ± 40	77	116

[a] $P < 0.01$.

dermis for the three populations studied. It is worth noting that no PPG amplitude at P_0 or P_{max} is related to the average blood pressures of the individuals in the three groups, which were 9.5 ± 0.2, 13.1 ± 0.2, and 14.9 ± 0.4 cm Hg (8), respectively.

Whether they are expressed as relative or absolute values, these differences diminish in elderly subjects, and the difference between adult and young subjects is only significant when the values are expressed as relative differences. It is interesting to note that young subjects aged under 12 years are by definition immature.

The results presented in Table 2 also show that the luminance parameter varied little between the three groups but that here, too, the relative and absolute variations were always lower in elderly subjects than in adults and young subjects. Skin color depends mainly on the density of the various pigments in the epidermis and on the quantity of blood present. Clearly, the application of pressure to the skin does not change pigment density; the relative and absolute variations in skin luminance between the three groups therefore represent the richness of the microcirculation and confirm the results obtained with the PPG technique.

V. CONCLUSION

The gradual loss of elements of the skin microcirculation (mainly capillary loops) has been widely described. The various techniques available for the measurement of blood flow within the skin are poorly adapted to studying this phenomenon experimentally. This is, of course, because they do not measure blood flow directly but also because they are not specific to any element of the skin microcirculation. Efforts are currently being made to improve the methods by the use of shorter wavelength light (9) and ultrasound (10).

Nonetheless, the highly indirect techniques based on the measurement of relative and absolute variations of skin color or the PPG signal permit the gradual loss of microcirculation in the superficial dermis with age to be quantified. As is often the case in studies of skin aging, it is not the measurement of a given parameter that reflects physiologic changes but rather variations in the response of the skin to constraints or stimuli.

ACKNOWLEDGMENT

The authors are very indebted to S. Navier for her excellent experimental work.

REFERENCES

1. Montagna W, Carlisle K. Structural changes in aging skin. J Invest Dermatol 1979; 79:47–53.
2. Ryan TJ. Cutaneous circulation. In: Lowell A Goldsmith, ed. Biochemistry and physiology of the skin, Vol. 2. New York: Oxford Univeristy Press, 1983; 817–37.
3. Christopher E, Kligman AM. Percutaneous absorption in aged skin. In: Montagna W, ed. Advances in biology of the skin, Vol. VI. New York: Pergamon Press, 1964; 163–75.
4. Lund F, Lund S, Dynamic fluorescein angiography by rapid sequence still photo recording a new technique for assessement of circulation time and adequacy of skin blood flow in the limbs. In: J. and D H. Lewis, ed. Bibliotheca Anatomica 11. Karger, Basel, New York; 1973; 13–18.
5. Kligman AM. Perspectives and problems in cutaneous gerontology. J Invest Dermatol 1979; 79:39–46.
6. Landis E. Microinjection studies of capillary blood pressure in human skin. Heart 1930; 15:209–28.
7. Leveque JL. Physical methods to measure the efficiency of cosmetics in humans. Cosmet Technol 1984; 99:43–6.
8. Leveque JL, Corcuff P, de Rigal J, Agache P. In vivo studies of the evolution of physical properties of the human skin with age. Int J Dermatol 1984; 23:322–9.
9. Duteil L, Bernengo JC, Shalla W. A double wavelength laser Doppler system to investigate skin microcirculation. IEEE Trans Biomed Eng 1985; 32:439–44.
10. Payne PA. Applications of ultrasound in dermatology. Bioeng Skin 1985; 1:293–320.

11

Influence of Age on Transcutaneous Oxygen Pressure

PIERRE G. AGACHE, ALAIN LUCAS, and AUDE AGACHE

University Hospital
Besançon, France

I. INTRODUCTION

Under normal conditions there is a faint but continuous outflow of oxygen from the skin surface, which reflects the diffusion of oxygen from the bloodstream across vessel walls and superficial skin tissue. Through local hyperemia this flow can be measured with a polarographic probe (1,2). Pediatricians were the first to use this technique to record and monitor systemic arterial pressure in premature neonates (3–5). In adults it has been currently used for some years by angiologists and vascular surgeons to evaluate the prognosis of peripheral thrombotic arterial disease either by simply measuring the basal transcutaneous oxygen pressure ($tcPO_2$) or by assessing its degree of increase following oxygen breathing or increasing blood pressure through dependency (6–9). The technique also demonstrated a decreased skin oxygen perfusion following cigarette smoking as a result of a reduction in the oxyhemoglobin content of red blood cells (10). More recently it has been used to assess the state of skin tissues peripheral to leg ulcers in venous insufficiency (11,12).

In adult clinical studies, $tcPO_2$ was mostly measured in lower limbs, principally on the dorsum of the foot close to the first toe web. Only in neonate monitoring was the probe placed on the anterior chest below the clavicle. In all studies the skin surface was heated to 43–45°C before measurement because the tcPO$_2$ at 37°C, the highest temperature of normal skin (in fact, on the lower limb in adults it is often below 20°C) (13), is barely measurable, being between zero and 5 mm Hg (14) and, furthermore, is variable. Heating the skin beyond 42°C induces a maximum skin vasodilation to a constant level and allows tcPO$_2$ to settle by 60–80 mm Hg. Incidentally, the energy required to raise the skin temperature to 44°C is inversely related to skin blood flow and consequently can be used as an index of skin perfusion (15).

Our main interest in measuring tcPO$_2$ over a wide range of ages was to obtain control groups mostly for aged people with vascular disease.

II. MATERIALS AND METHODS

We used a Radiometer TCM2 tcPO$_2$ monitor with digital display. Before each measurement the device was calibrated in relation to atmospheric pressure and allowed to equilibrate for 20 minutes.

Our subjects, all devoid of apparent vascular disease, ranged from 20 to 92 years of age. Measurements were made on the dorsum of the foot and the leg above both medial and lateral malleoli while the subject was recumbent. A total of 75 subjects entered the study. They were divided in seven age groups (20–29, 30–39, 40–49, 50–59, 60–69, 70–79, and 80–92).

The reproducibility of the measurement was checked in three subjects whose tcPO$_2$ was assessed on 5 consecutive days on the dorsum of the foot. Mean values ± standard errors of the mean (SEM) were 73.3 ± 4.0, 82.2 ± 4.8, and 82.8 ± 5.2 mm Hg (9.75 ± 0.53, 10.93 ± 0.64, and 11.01 ± 0.69 kPa) in subjects 1, 2, and 3, respectively (mean coefficient of variation, 5.9%).

III. RESULTS

A. Dorsum of the Foot

There was a steady and significant decrease in tcPO$_2$ over the adult life span ($p < 0.05$), with significant scattering in each age group. The decrease fit a linear regression ($p < 0.0001$, $r = 0.56$) according to the equation tcPO$_2$(mm Hg) = (88.6 − 0.33) × age [kPa: (11.8 − 0.04) × age]. The standard deviations were 3.7 (4%) and 0.06 (19%) for the intercept and the slope, respectively.

B. Medial and Lateral Supramalleolar Areas

The same trend was observed in both medial and lateral malleolar areas. The equations were tcPO$_2$ (mm Hg) = (90.8 − 0.38) × age [kPa: (12.1 − 0.05) × age] and (89.2 − 0.36) × age [kPa: (11.9 − 0.05) × age], respectively.

C. Pooled Data

No significant difference was found between the three areas with respect to either absolute values in each age group or the rate of the decrease with age. Accordingly, the data were pooled and the overall changes in $tcPO_2$ were plotted versus age (Fig. 1). The difference between the 20–39 and 40–59 year pooled groups on the one hand and between the 40–59 and 60–79 year groups on the other were significant ($p < 0.05 + < 0.001$, respectively). A significant difference was also seen between the 70–79 and 80–89 year groups.

In general the $tcPO_2$ was lower in males but the difference was significant only in the 50–79 year range (Fig. 2). No significant difference was found between the sexes in the rate of $tcPO_2$ decrease with age (slope: -0.31 ± 0.06 in males and -0.37 ± 0.01 in females), but the intercept of the regression line was higher in females (92.6 ± 4.0 versus 83.6 ± 3.6 mm Hg, $p < 0.01$). Accordingly, the two regression lines can be considered parallel.

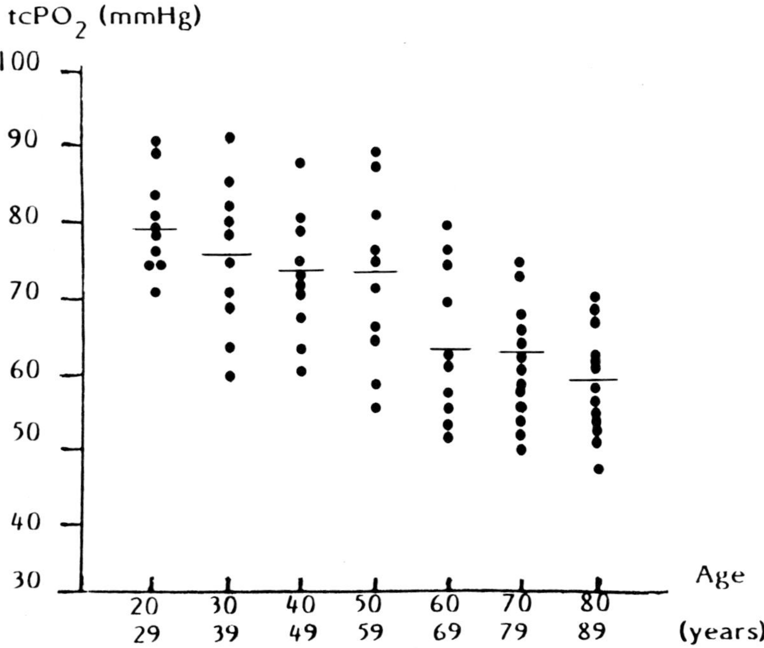

Figure 1 $tcPO_2$ versus age.

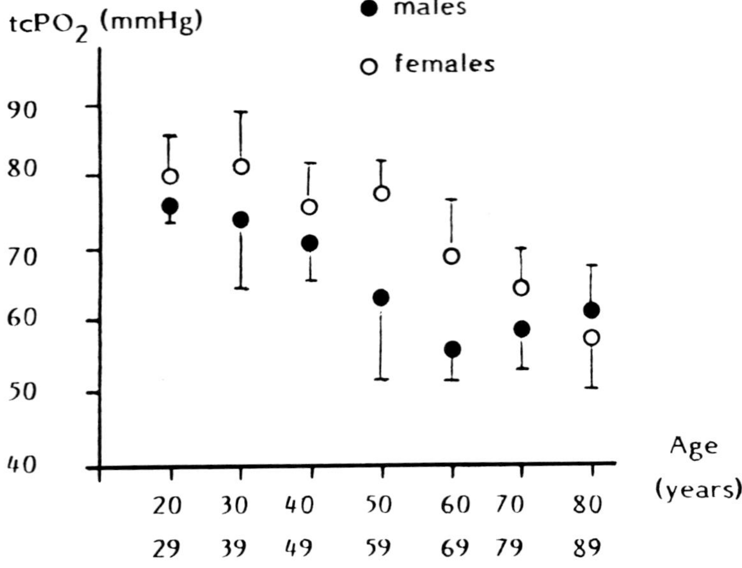

Figure 2 tcPO$_2$ versus age and sex.

IV. DISCUSSION

A decrease in tcPO$_2$ with increasing age was first described by Gøthgen and Jacobsen in 20 patients aged 19–80 years (16). By linear regression analysis they found tcPO$_2$ (kPa) = (10.4 − 0.035) × age (r = 0.406), which is close to our results. Also, Vayssairat et al. (8) in 32 subjects aged 21–90 years found a negative correlation with advancing age (r = 0.37; $p < 0.05$). Other authors (6,9,17) confirmed the lower values of tcPO$_2$ in people over 50 years compared to young adults.

Gøthgen and Jacobsen placed the electrode in the subclavicular position, whereas in our study it was on the lower extremity. The ratio of limb to trunk tcPO$_2$ was called the regional perfusion index by Hauser and Shoemaker (6) and found to be in the range 0.90–0.95. When this ratio is applied to our data, they fit the data of Gøthgen and Jacobsen.

Although in our regression analysis of tcPO$_2$ versus age the departure from linearity was not significant in either sex or for the three areas, the data suggest (Figs. 1 and 2) that the variation in tcPO$_2$ with age may not be uniform and accelerates from 60 years onward. To our knowledge no information is available in the literature on this point.

Also in our study females had higher values than males except in the 80–92 age group. The difference was significant at the 0.01 level or more only between 50 and 80 years. However, in another group of 27 normal subjects aged 20–35 years (14 males and 13 females), we also found higher $tcPO_2$ values in females at the 0.05 level (18). As shown by the regression lines, no difference was found in the rate of $tcPO_2$ decrease between the sexes. Accordingly, the lower (nonsignificant) $tcPO_2$ value in females over 80 years compared to males is only a random variation.

Our finding that $tcPO_2$ decreases with aging from 20 years onward is not surprising. The transfer of oxygen from the blood to the skin surface occurs in the subpapillary plexus and papillary loops (19–21), and it is known that such vasculature is progressively resorbed with aging (Chap. 8). Also it is known that skin rosiness regresses with age probably as a result of the same phenomenon (Chap. 8).

Physiologic studies have demonstrated that four main factors influence $tcPO_2$, namely skin blood flow (15,22), arterial blood oxygen pressure (16, 23,24), arterial pressure (25,26), and the permeability of the superficial skin to oxygen (19,27). At 44°C the oxyhemoglobin dissociation curve is shifted to the right and the ability of red blood cells to bind oxygen is reduced. Accordingly, the oxygen concentration in plasma is strongly increased. Hence the assessed $tcPO_2$ is not the oxygen flux occurring under normal conditions but under maximal hyperemia and optimal oxygen supply (2). In such a situation the limiting factors are the vasculature available in the skin and the pressure of the blood entering the skin. The latter is linearly related to the arterial pressure upstream, which in fact tends to rise with aging.

In older people there is fall in both arterial PO_2 (16) and skin temperature (13), with subsequent restraint in oxyhemoglobin dissociation and an increased distance from the subpapillary plexus to the skin surface through regression of papillary loops (Chap. 8). These phenomena can explain the decrease observed in skin blood flow (Chaps. 9 and 10) (28,29), despite a rise in arteriolar pressure (Chaps. 9 and 10). A reduction in the oxygen transfer capacity of stratum corneum as observed for other substances (30), associated with xerosis or an increase in renewal time (31), may also support in part a decreased $tcPO_2$. Such phenomena are unlikely to take place before the age of 60 years, however, and other factors should be involved in younger people. A thickening of stratum corneum is improbable, but only this, together with a thicker epidermis that augments the epidermal oxygen consumption, can explain the lower $tcPO_2$ in males compared to females while the skin blood flow remains identical (28). Finally, the main factor seems to be the progressive reduction of the skin superficial vascular bed, both in length and volume, as shown by capillaroscopy (Chap. 8). Such a reduction could be disclosed by

$tcPO_2$ because it is carried out in an extreme situation and is not detected by plethysmography or laser Doppler flowmetry, which although very sensitive deal with more usual conditions in which skin blood perfusion is far from its maximum while largely exceeding the metabolic needs of the skin (32).

From the linear regression equation, $tcPO_2$ would fall by 4 mm Hg (5%) in a decade and consequently the subepidermal vascular bed would shrink in the same proportion according to the preceding hypothesis. Could this have any influence on skin function, as $tcPO_2$ also reflects the oxygen supply to skin tissue? Not in young or even middle-aged people, but a 20% reduction like that in the seventies, associated with a decrease in skin blood flow at normal skin temperatures (28), that is, related to other causes, could impair the resistance to skin ischemia due to pressure in recumbency, giving way to decubitus ulcers occurring more readily than in younger people. Thermoregulatory processes could also be impaired in both cold—old people are often colder than young people in winter—and in summer, when heat stroke is known to occur more often in old age.

REFERENCES

1. Clark L. Measurement of oxygen tension: a historical perspective. Crit Care Med 1981; 9:690–2.
2. Lubbers D. Theoretical basis of the transcutaneous blood gas measurement. Crit Care Med 1981; 9:721–33.
3. Huch R, Huch A, Lubbers DW. Quantitative polarographische Sauerstoffsruckmessung auf der Kopfhaut der Neugeboren. Arch Gynekol 1969; 207:443–51.
4. Huch R, Lubbers DW, Huch A. Quantitative continuous measurement of partial oxygen pressure on the skin of adults and newborn babies. Pflugers Arch 1972; 337:185–98.
5. Rooth G. Transcutaneous oxygen tension measurement in newborn infants. Pediatrics 1975; 55:232–5.
6. Hauser C, Shoemaker W. Use of a transcutaneous $tcPO_2$ regional perfusion index to quantify tissue perfusion in peripheral vascular disease. Ann Surg 1983; 197:337–43.
7. Mustapha N, Redhead R, Jain S, Wielogorski J. Transcutaneous partial oxygen pressure assessment of the ischemic lower limb. Surg Gynecol Obstet 1983; 156:582–4.
8. Vayssairat M, Mathieu JF, Priollet P, Vellay P, Pines JC, Housset E. Mesure transcutanée de la pression artérielle d'oxygène. Une nouvelle méthode d'exploration fonctionnelle en pathologie vasculaire. Presse Med 1984; 13: 1683–6.
9. Bilesimo M, Didier JP, Casillas JM, Javelas S, Lucet A. Exploration du reflexe veino-artériolaire chez le sujet jeune et âgé par l'enregistrement de la $tcPO_2$. J Mal Vasc 1989; 14:19–25.

10. Lucas A, Agache P, Risold JC, Cuenot C. Variations de la tcPO_2 en fonction de la consommation de tabac chez le sujet sain. J Mal Vasc 1989; 14:363–4.

11. Borzykowski M, Krähenbühl B, Harms M. Mesure non invasive de l'oxygénation cutanée des ulcères de jambe. Med Hyg 1981; 39:170–81.

12. Stacey MC, Burnand KG, Layer GT, Pattison M. Transcutaneous oxygen tensions in assessing the treatment of healed venous ulcers. Br J Surg 1990; 77:1050–4.

13. Howell TH. Skin temperature readings in aged subjects. In: Kligman AM, Takase Y, eds. Cutaneous aging. Tokyo: University of Tokyo Press, 1988; 159–65.

14. Evans NTS, Naylor PRD. The systemic oxygen supply to the surface of human skin. Respir Rhysiol 1967; 3:21–37.

15. Enkema L Jr, Holloway GA, Piraino DW, Harry D, Zick GL, Kenny MA. Laser-Doppler velocimetry vs heater power as indicators of skin perfusion during transcutaneous O_2 monitoring. Clin Chem 1981; 27:391–6.

16. Gøthgen I, Jacobsen E. Transcutaneous oxygen tension measurement. I. Age variation and reproducibility. Acta Anaesthesiol Scand Suppl 1978; 67:66–70.

17. Dowd GSE, Linge K, Bentley G. The effect of age and sex of normal volunteers upon the transcutaneous oxygen tension in the lower limb. Clin Phys Physiol Meas 1983; 4:65–8.

18. Atallah M, Lucas A, Agache P. Unpublished data, 1988.

19. Kimmich HP, Kreuzer F. Model of oxygen transport through the skin as basis for absolute transcutaneous measurement of PaO_2. Acta Anaesthesiol Scand Suppl 1978; 68:16–19.

20. Grønlund U. Evaluation of factors affecting relationship between transcutaneous PO_2 and probe temperature. J Appl Physiol 1985; 59:1117–27.

21. Huch A, Franzeck UK, Huch R, Bollinger A. A transparent transcutaneous oxygen electrode for simultaneous studies of skin capillary morphology, flow dynamics and oxygenation. Int J Microcirc Clin Exp 1983; 2:103–8.

22. Eickhoff J, Jacobsen E. Correlation of transcutaneous oxygen tension to blood flow in treated skin. Scand J Clin Lab Invest 1980; 40:761–5.

23. Dautzenberg B, Carter H, Sors C. Mesure de la PO_2 par voie transcutanée. Rev Fr Mal Respir 1981; 9:327–35.

24. Severinghaus J. Current trends in continuous blood gas monitoring. Biotelem Patient Monit 1979; 6:9–15.

25. Eickhoff J, Ishihara S, Jacobsen E. Effect of arterial and venous pressures on transcutaneous oxygen tension. Scand J Clin Lab Invest 1980; 40:755–60.

26. Wyss CR, Matsen FA, King RV, Simmons CW, Burgess EM. Dependence of transcutaneous oxygen tension on local arteriovenous pressure gradient in normal subjects. Clin Sci 1981; 60:499–506.

27. Hansen TN, Sonoda Y, McIlroy MB. Transfer of oxygen, nitrogen, and carbon dioxide through normal adult human skin. J Appl Physiol 1980; 49:438–43.

28. Ishihara M, Itom M. Oshawa K, Kinoshita M, Sato Y. Cutaneous blood flow. In: Kligman AM, Takase Y, eds. Cutaneous aging. Tokyo: University of Tokyo Press, 1988; 167–81.

29. Tsuchida Y. Age-related changes in skin blood flow at four anatomic sites of the body in males, studied by xenon 133. Plast Reconstr Surg 1990; 85:556–61.
30. Roskos KV, Maibach HI, Guy RH. The effect of aging on percutaneous absorption in man. J Pharmacokinet Biopharm 1989; 17:617–30.
31. Plewig G, Marples RR. Regional differences of cell sizes in human stratum corneum. Part II. Effects of age and sex. J Invest Dermatol 1970; 54:19–23.
32. Martineaud JP, Seroussi S, eds. Physiologie de la circulation cutanée. Paris: Masson, 1977.

12

Measurement of Skin Relief by Two- and Three-Dimensional Profilometry

YANG XIE

Laboratoire de Biophysique Cutanée
Faculté de Médecine
Besançon, France

JEAN MIGNOT

Laboratoire de Métrologie des Interfaces Techniques
Institut Universitaire de Technologie
Besançon, France

I. INTRODUCTION

The skin is the covering of the human body. It not only acts as a barrier, but its role is also studied in terms of its chemical, biologic, and structural components; its pathologies, and its surface, namely its relief and the different annexes that can be found there.

The main characteristic of the skin surface is the existence of actual relief. This relief has been known to exist for a very long time in the plantopalmar zones, but it is only recently that it seemed interesting to analyze the other zones.

The characteristic relief of these zones is of interest to anthropologists, but it is much less so to general practitioners since this relief distinguishes itself from other parts of the body and remains insensitive to a fair number of outside aggressions. As opposed to the others, the relief of the other parts of the body, although they vary from one zone to another, presents many particular characteristics and varies under the influence of numerous parameters.

These factors can be exterior:—exposure to diverse influences, humidity, mechanical restrictions, temperature, or chemical agents,—or interior:—aging, diseases, and the effect of drugs.

II. SKIN SURFACE RELIEF

A. Palmoplantar Regions

Fingerprints characterize an individual and have been studied mainly by means of "drawings" (1–4). The lines, loops, and branches are characteristics of an individual and are constantly the subject of new methods of image analysis.

Although it is not the subject of the present study, the structure of dermaglyphs lends itself to the same analytic methods as those designed for the study of the surface relief of the other parts of the body. Figure 1 is a typical image of a dermaglyph, and Figures 2 and 3 show two ways of quantifying the distribution of peaks or valleys:

1. Studying the superficial distribution of the furrows by making use of the image given by television camera and an appropriate numeric treatment intended to reproduce the privileged directions. Thus, the decomposition of furrows into elementary segments makes it possible to obtain a two-dimensional study of the repartition of the characteristic furrows of this zone.

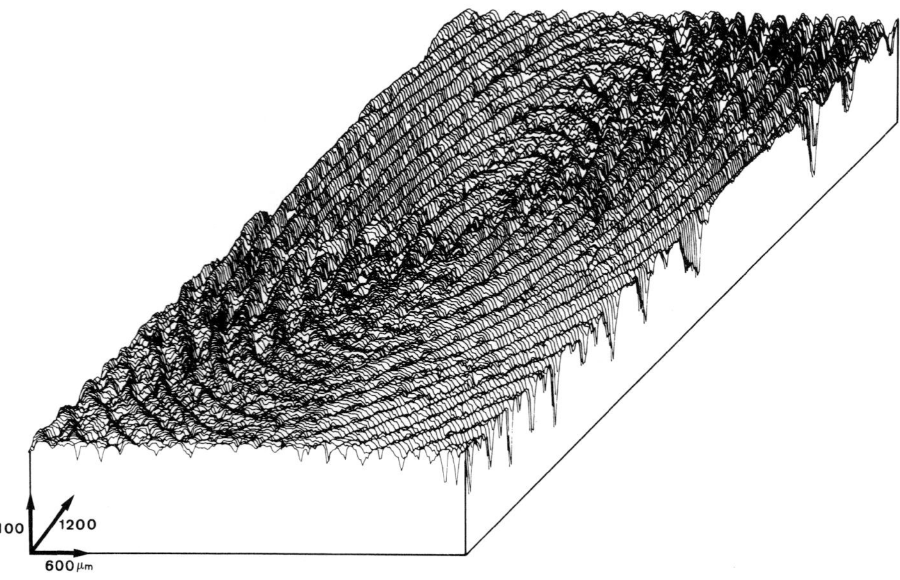

Figure 1 Image of a dermaglyph.

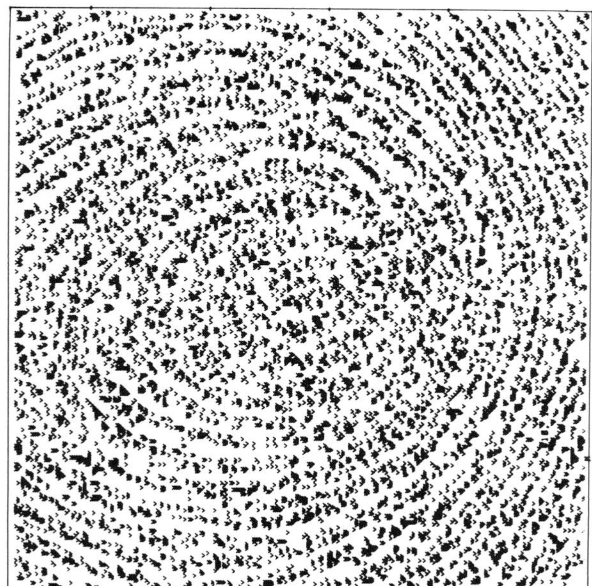

Figure 2 Fingerprint: particular points.

2. Using a detector to facilitate the three-dimensional representation, then analysis of the surface being studied. Such a study (Fig. 3) of the palmoplantar zones seems thus far not to have been the subject of work of this nature.

B. Relief of Other Skin Areas

The relief of all the areas of the human body, excluding the palmoplantar zones, is composed of plateaus crossed by valleys. These valleys can be separated into principal furrows that cover great distances and are very deep (about 100 µm) and secondary furrows, more superficial and running through one or two plateaus. However, this classification is very arbitrary: after a certain distance a primary fold can become secondary, and vice versa (Fig. 4).

In each area of the body, this relief appears virtually specific. On the forehead, for example, the relief is distributed according to two perpendicular axes; on the elbows and knees the valleys often have nonsystemized curvilinear shapes, representing a privileged axis. These different examples of the surface of the skin relief show the variability of the relief according to the zone that is being studied and the anisotropic character of this surface. This

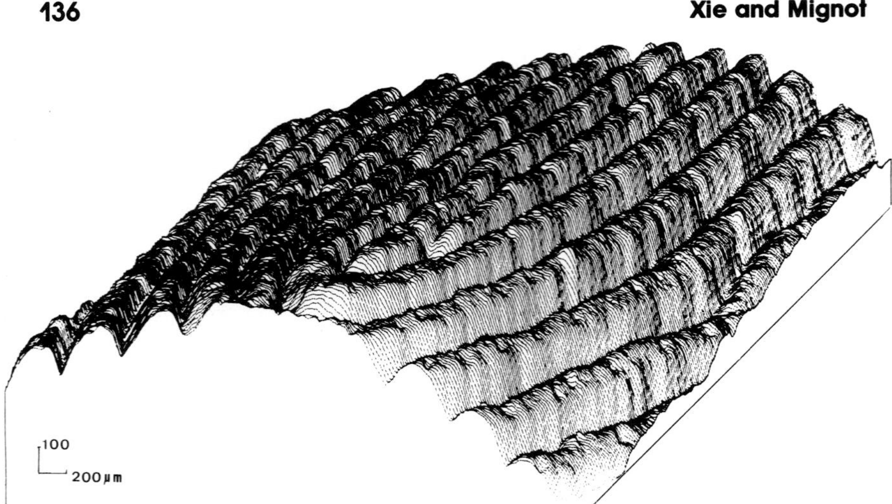

Figure 3 Three-dimensional analysis of dermaglyphs.

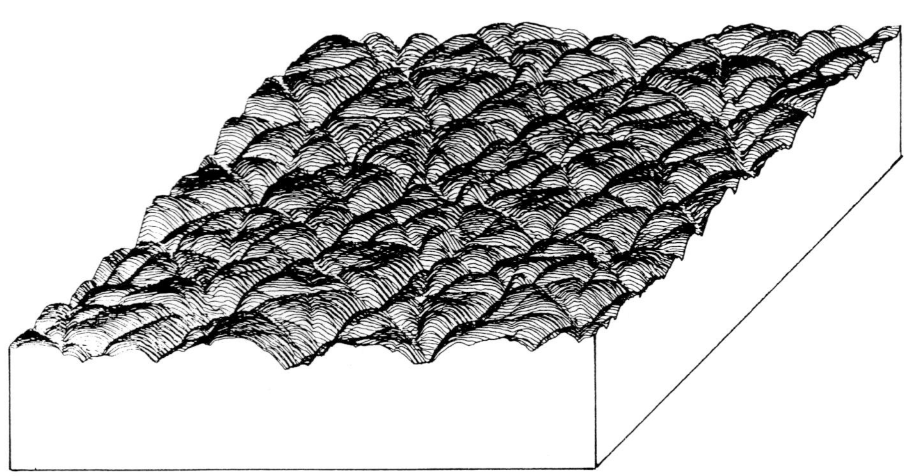

Figure 4 Skin surface: principle and secondary furrows.

anisotropy justifies the transition from a two-dimensional to a three-dimensional study.

III. MEASURING SKIN RELIEF

A. Tactile Sensors

To quantify skin relief, researchers first used profilometric techniques designed to measure mechanical surfaces. This method is based on the use of a mechanical profilometer (5) whose measuring instrument, the fine tip of a diamond pyramid, follows the local variations in relief (Fig. 5). In this way a profile representing the surface cut by a plane perpendicular to the surface is extracted from the relief. This is done by shifting the stylus at a constant speed on the surface during study. However, this technique cannot be applied directly to the skin, because the pressure that results from the contact with the diamond stylus is much too great. In fact, if the diamond-tipped stylus ends in a spherical cap with a radius of about 5 μm, the minimum stylus force that brings about the plastic deformation of the analyzed material is given by

$$N = 23.2 \left(\frac{r}{E}\right)^2 \sigma_0{}^3$$

where r is the radius of the tip of the stylus, E Young's modulus, and σ_0 the flow stress of the skin.

In the skin surface the minimum force that brings about the plastic deformation is theoretically less than 4×10^{-4} N. Although in the appliances that are used the stylus force is weak ($<10^{-3}$ N), the local deformation of the analyzed surface is to be avoided, all the more so if the surface is that of the skin. It is also necessary to use an artifice to avoid this deformation.

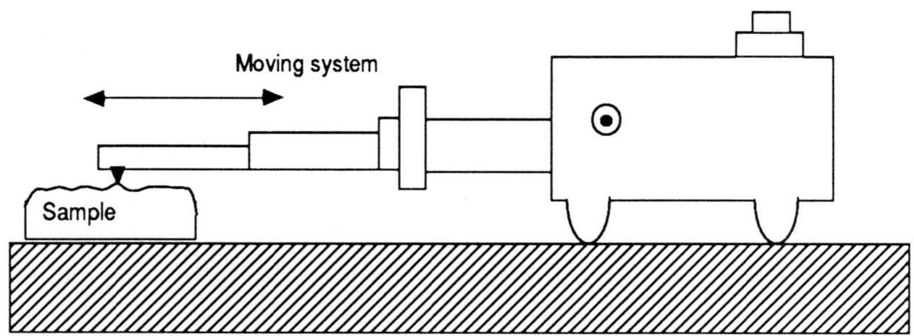

Figure 5 Mechanical profilometer.

B. Replica Technique

The use of the fingerprint technique to measure skin relief dates back 30 years (6–8). This totally painless method, which can also be used for wounds, is quick and yields a very accurate reproduction. The method consists of obtaining a siliconized rubber replica of the skin surface (7, 8). The replica takes about 1 minute to harden. This imprint reproduces the negative image of the surface to the smallest detail. As a result of its insufficient hardness, this material cannot withstand contact with the stylus. It is also necessary to make a second imprint on the supple replica using material that can attain sufficient hardness (epoxy resin). It is therefore this second imprint that is then analyzed by the measuring instrument instead of the skin itself.

The advantage of this technique is that it gives an accurate reproduction, provided, however, that the formation of air bubbles is avoided by an appropriate operating technique. On the other hand, its major drawback is the time it takes to obtain a second imprint and, above all, the time it takes to harden.

C. Two-Dimensional Profilometry

Two-dimensional profilometry represents the section of the skin on a plane perpendicular to the mean plane of the skin surface. The detecting organ is very often a mechanical detector whose measuring point (round peak of a diamond pyramid with a 90° or 60° angle at the peak) follows the local altitude variations in the relief and transforms them into an analog signal $v = f(\text{time})$, the stylus being displaced in the measuring direction at a regular speed.

Three basic principles can be used to transform the local relief variations into an electrical signal:

1. Mechanical stylus and inductive detector
2. Mechanical stylus and optical detector
3. Optical sensor with or without interferometer

1. Inductive Mechanical Detectors

This is the oldest method and, excluding the new optical detector with interferometers, the most accurate. Its principle consists of transforming the vertical movements of the diamond tip (Fig. 6) into an electrical signal. This conversion takes place thanks to a bobbin-nucleus system mounted on the pivoting arm of the detector. An electrical amplification system makes it possible, thanks to an adjustable window, to select a part of the feeler's course and to magnify it to discern relief variations with a very low amplitude.

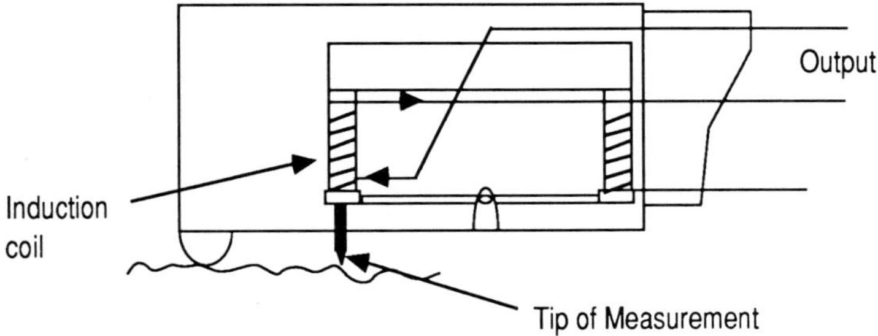

Figure 6   Mechanical profilometer with induction system.

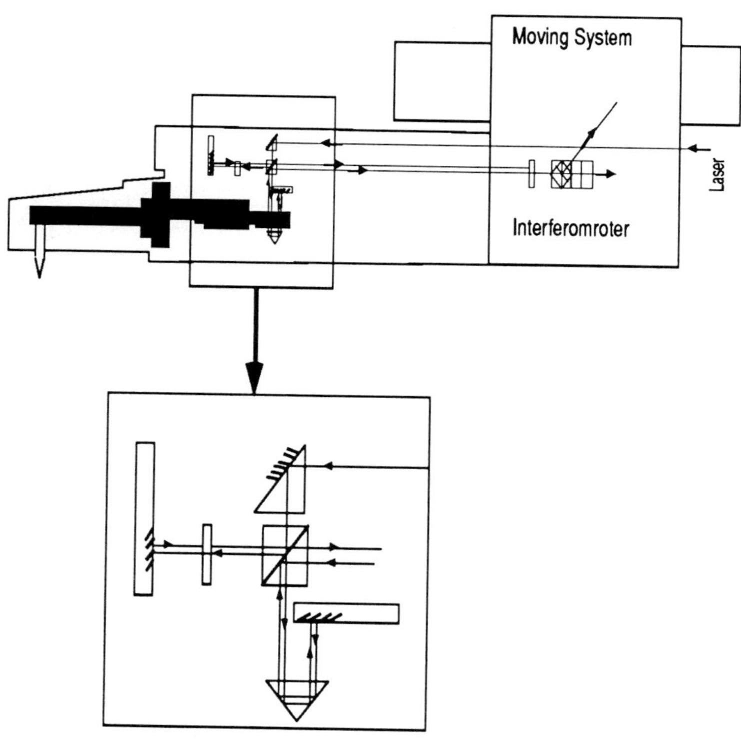

Figure 7   Mechanical sensor and optical measurement.

2. Mechanical Sensor and Optical Measurement

Such a system was created a few years ago, and the improved version is due to Rank Precision Industries with the Form Talysurf system (Fig. 7). The principle uses the vertical shifting of a mechanical stylus transformed in an optical interferometer. This interferometer analyzes the difference between a vertical reference position and the actual position. A second interferometer measures the exact horizontal (x) position of the stylus.

Such a system has two advantages:

1. The coordinates x and y are known with very good accuracy.
2. The vertical range of the system is very wide and can reach 4 mm with very good precision. Such a system is very useful in the study of surfaces that present a very important defect of form.

3. Optical Sensor

A recently manufactured optical sensors is the laser RM 600 Rodenstock stylus (Fig. 8). It uses a 1 μm diameter focus obtained from a laser diode and analyzes the size of this focus by means of a detector that generates lens

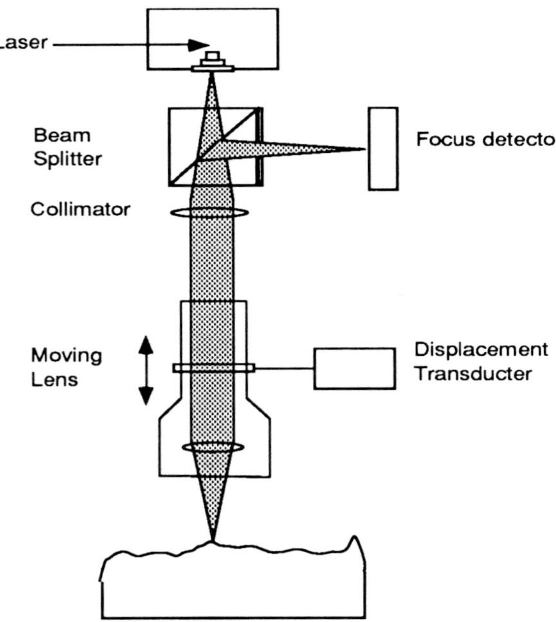

Figure 8   Optical profilometer.

movement to obtain a perfect point. The movement of the objective lenses is a measure of the roughness of the surface.

D. Elimination of Form Defects and Waviness

For any zone to be analyzed, the surface subjected to the making of a replica is about 2–8 cm^2. The general form of the surface of this area is never a perfect plane, but it corresponds to any equation $z = f(x, y)$. Under such conditions, the skin relief represents only the higher frequencies of the entire surface spectrum.

The lower frequency components are characteristic of the form defect of the studied zone. Figure 9 compares the spectrum of the profile obtained on a same surface before (Fig. 9A) and after (Fig. 9B) correction of the shape defect.

The study of skin relief necessitates filtering the lower frequencies in the spectrum before any calculating processes. This can be done through generally used methods.

1. Electrical Filtering

This well-known method consists of using a resistance-capacity (RC) circuit with one or various levels. Should such a circuit be used, the signal entering the filter, which is the signal yielded by the transducer, has a sinusoidal form

$$V_E = V_0 \sin\left(2\pi \frac{x}{L}\right)$$

where L is the spatial period.

The output of such an RC filter yields a signal whose altitude is

$$V_S = \frac{V_0}{1 + L^2/4\pi^2 R^2 C^2}$$

and the phase

$$\phi = \arctan \frac{L}{2\pi RC}$$

If we define the filter in accordance with the manufacturers, a wavelength with a L_c cut representing the value of the input signal wavelength, for which the amplitude of the output signal is 0.50 that of the input signal, the signal is

$$V_S(x) = \frac{V_0}{[1 + K(L/L_c)^2]} \sin(2\pi x/L + \phi)$$

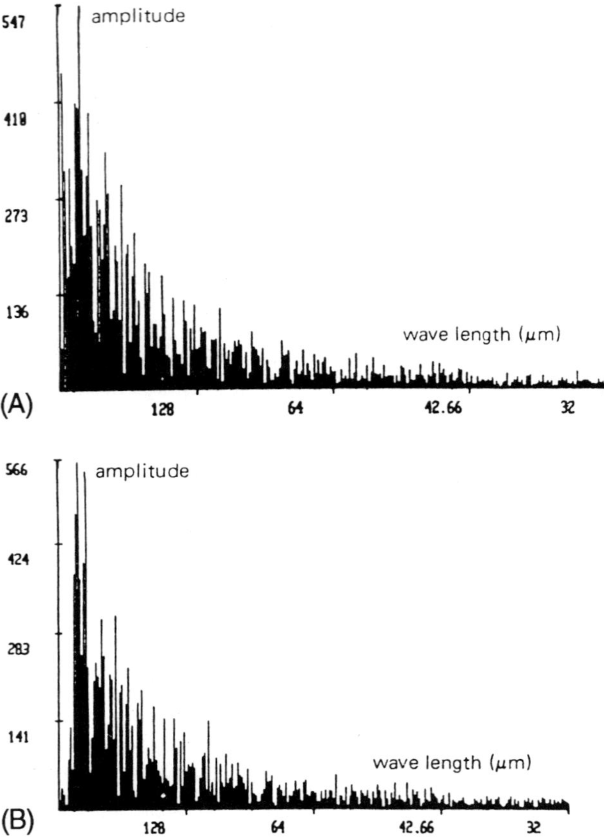

Figure 9 Frequency spectrum of a surface: (A) actual surface; (B) after filtering of the form defect.

Currently, profilometers have five filtering values: 80, 250, 800, 2500, and 8000 μm. Note that when studying numeric filters, such a restriction can be avoided. The expression of $V_S(x)$ makes it possible to anticipate the response of the filter in relation to the different wavelengths L the input signal can contain. An example is given (Fig. 10) for different filter values characterized by their cutoff ($L_c = 800$ and 2500 μm).

The advantage of the RC filter is that it is easy to make. However, it has three disadvantages:

1. The law $V_s = F(L)$ varies as $1/L$; therefore, with a slow variation, the filter is not very selective.

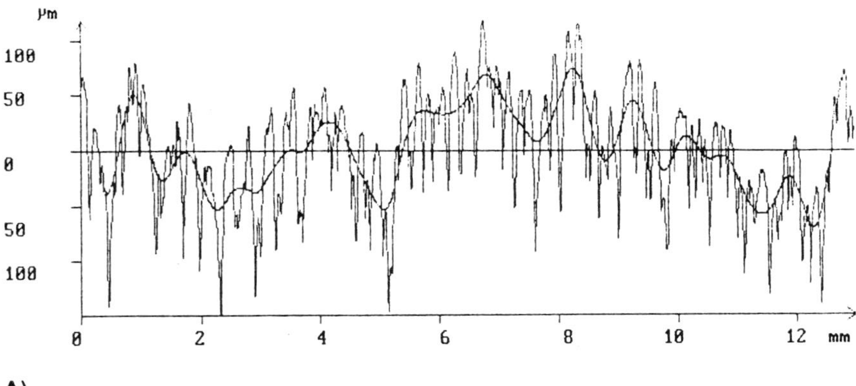

A)

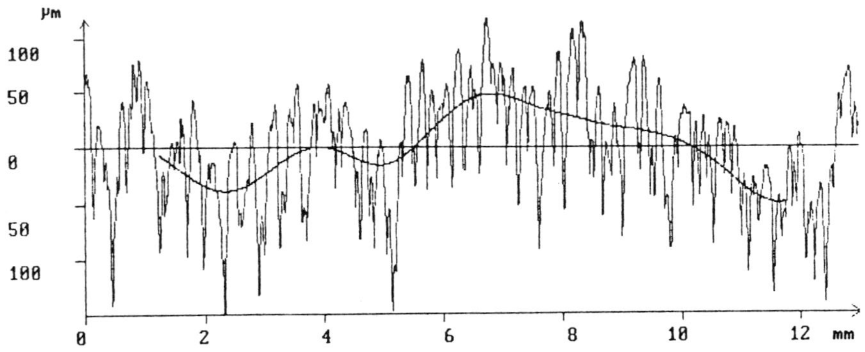

B)

Figure 10 Electrical filtering with different filter values: (A) $L_c = 0.8$ mm; (B) $L_c = 2.50$ mm.

2. It requires as many different filters as there are L_c values. In practice, manufacturers have limited the number to five.
3. Its most important defect is to present a difference in phase between the real profile and the filtered profile.

2. Numeric Filtering

Numeric filtering has numerous possibilities. Introduced recently to the study of surface profiles, it was limited to its simplest achievements.

Two methods are commonly used:

1. Filtering by decomposition of the profile in straight segments
2. Filtering by calculation of the actual average line of the profile

a. Filtering by Decomposition into Straight Segments.   This method, invented for the study of industrial surfaces, is accepted according to international standards. It is based on the following principle.

Over a length chosen from the five values of L_c given by manufacturers, one can realize straightening of part of the profile. This operation is made by using the mean square line evaluated over this part (Fig. 11).

This operation is repeated along the entire profile. Roughness parameters are deduced from the analysis of each of these parts of the profile. This form of filtering is good for profiles showing slowly varying defects of shape but can introduce erroneous roughness when the shape of the replica presents fast variations.

Figure 11 shows some examples of filtering by using the standard method with usual filtering lengths 0.80 and 2.5 mm.

b. Numeric Filtering by Means of a Rectangular Window.   The following principle is used. If the profile is defined by equidistant N points separated by a distance h, the filtering is done by means of a rectangular window. This method calculates at each point of the profile the average value obtained over $2k + 1$ points symmetrically distributed around the point with the abscissa x.

$$g(x) = \frac{1}{a} \operatorname{rect} \frac{x}{a}$$

where $g(x) = 0$ for $|x| > \dfrac{a}{2}$

$\quad\quad\, g(x) = 1$ for $|x| \leq \dfrac{a}{2}$

If $V_0(x)$ is the skin profile, the filtered profile is given by

$$V_s(x) = g(x) * V_0(x) = \frac{1}{a} \int V_0(t) \operatorname{rect}\left(x - \frac{t}{a}\right) dt$$

$$= \frac{1}{a} \int V_0 \, dt = \overline{V_0(t)}$$

If the choice of the number k has been judicious, this value may correspond to the form defect of the analyzed profile. The amplitude therefore depends on the number of $2k + 1$ points that have undergone smoothing. The choice of the number k of smoothing points used is related to that of the L_c wavelength of the cut.

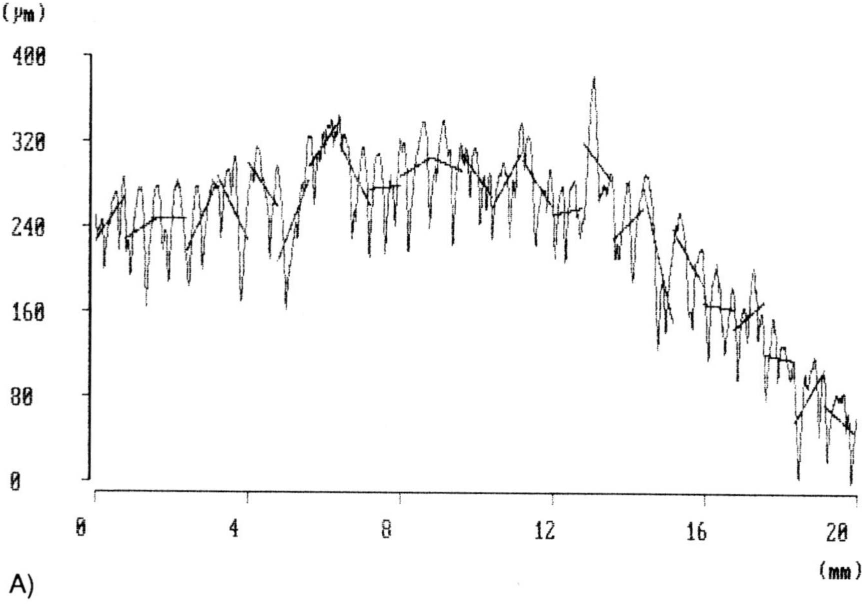

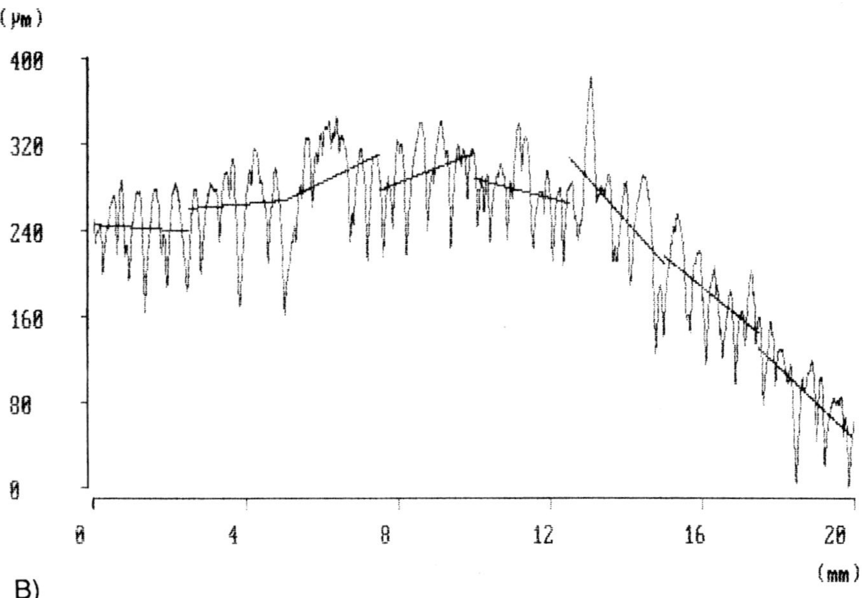

Figure 11 Filtering by standard method: (A)L_c = 0.8 mm; (B)L_c = 2.50 mm.

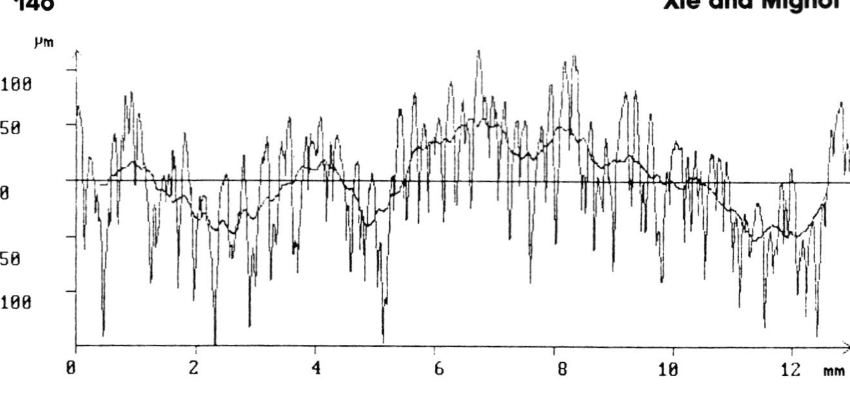

A)

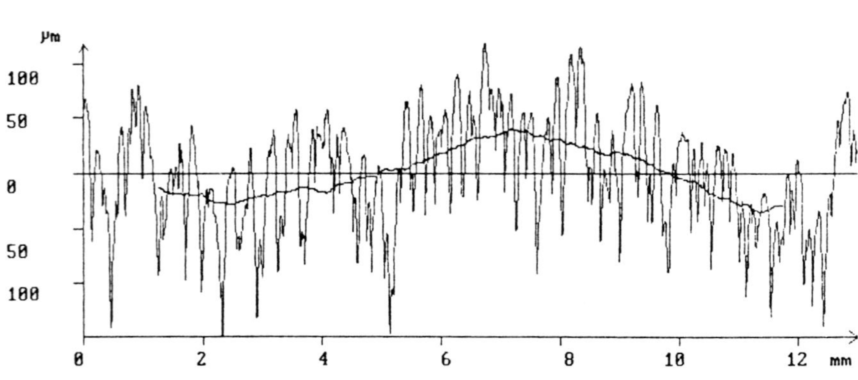

B)

Figure 12 Numeric filtering using a rectangular window: (A) $L_c = 0.8$ mm; (B) $L_c = 2.50$ mm.

Figure 12 shows the result of numeric filtering carried out on the same profile using successive values of k (or a).

3. Extension of Numeric Filtering

Many filtering methods can be used in surface topography measurement. Each of these numeric filters uses a window whose shape answers to a weighting function. The well-known laws have triangular, parabolic, Gaussian, or Hamming shape. The future standardized numeric filter will be of Gaussian shape, which is defined as

$$g(x) = e^{-x^2/\sigma^2}$$

The advantage of such a law is not to introduce any difference in phase between the $V_0(x)$ input signal and the $V_s(x)$ filtered signal. Another advantage is the possibility to avoid calculation of its Fourier transform, which has the same Gaussian form. The use of such a filter gives a $V_s(x)$ profile closer to the ideal filtered profile than those given by the numeric rectangular window or by electrical filtering. An example of such an application is given in Figure 13.

The use of one of the filtering processes described in this chapter now provides us with a filtered profile of the form that represents the microrelief of the skin surface. The next step consists of exploiting such a filtered profile to deduce the characteristic dimensions of the relief.

E. Data Processing

The results of a study of mechanical surfaces have been used to analyze the profiles of the skin surface. It is only recently that it appears necessary to add to these specific methods, which correspond better to the characteristic relief of the skin. In this section we successively look into classic methods processing and new, more specific methods.

1. Using Standardized Parameters

For almost 40 years, the mechanical industries have taken an interest in surface topography (9–11). During this period, standards have been developed that fulfill the requirements of the industrial sectors, but it is not possible to give a detailed description of all the standards described in standard ISO in a few pages. We can, however, classify the classic parameters into first, *amplitude parameters*, which describe the vertical distribution of the points that constitute the profile. The primary parameters used by numerous authors to study skin profiles are

Extreme parameters, such as R_t, the maximum distance detected between the highest peak and the bottom of the lowest valley, $R_{\max}$, equivalent to R_t but for the points situated inside one of the five or more parts of the profile, and R_p, the height, evaluated from the mean line of the highest peak encountered along the total length.

Average parameters: R_a, the arithmetic average of the profile into five equal parts, and R_z the average difference between the altitude of the five highest peaks and the five lowest valleys.

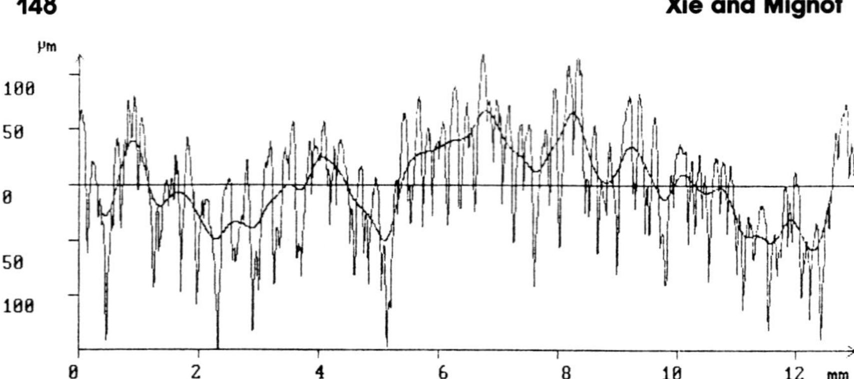

A)

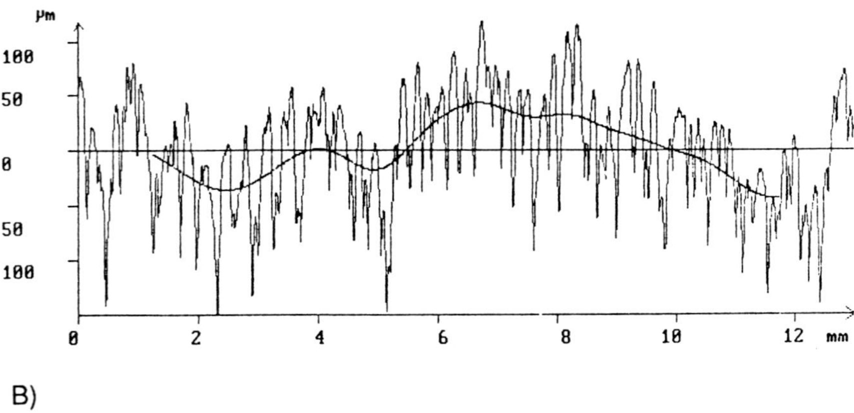

B)

Figure 13 Numeric filtering using a Gaussian window: (A) L_c = 0.8 mm; (B) L_c = 2.50 mm.

Skin relief is characterized by a succession of plateaus separated by furrows of variable depth. *Spacing parameters* make it possible to study the horizontal distribution of the relief. Among the different parameters that can be used, HSC, the high spot count, is the number of peaks situated above the average line or above a line parallel with this mean line. S_m is average spacing between measured furrows at the mean line level.

Hybrid parameters use both height and spacing parameters. The principal parameters are Δs, the quadratic average of the slopes at each point (the arithmetic average being zero), and Δq, the ratio between the quadratic average of the heights and slopes.

Over the few years these different classic parameters have been used by many authors to define skin relief. Figure 14 shows the use of two parameters depending on aging.

It is clear that the use of these classic parameters requires the prior elimination of any profile form defect, either by electrical filtering or by a numeric method.

2. Need to Develop Specific Parameters

The classic parameters invented to study mechanical surfaces have for many years made it possible to give a satisfactory quantification of skin relief, but the specificity of skin relief required the development of particular parameters with two different aims.

First the number of available parameters among which the user must choose should be reduced. Since these parameters are not all independent, the choice is very difficult.

Figure 15 shows the correlation between classic parameters and proves the unnecessary use of a great number of parameters.

Second, the particular nature of skin relief formed of plateaus separated by furrows should be taken into account.

Recently, two interesting trials have been carried out with a view to fulfilling these requirements.

Cook et al. (10) used decomposition of skin relief in a succession of peaks separated by deep furrows.

Mignot et al. (12) used a decomposition that resembles both that of Cook et al. and that used in the automotive industry to characterize functional surfaces (13,14). This method uses the following process.

The initial profile given by the detector is straightened according to a method of least squares. The correction is sufficient because the average value of the profile is of no consequence in the parameters that will be developed. This characteristic is one of the advantages of this method since the errors due to either electrical or numeric filtering are eliminated. In this way, only the highest points (summits of plateaus) and the bottom of the furrows of the profile, thus straightened, are retained. If the h_i are the depths of successive furrows measured from the peak of neighboring plateaus (Fig. 16A), only those that surpass a minimum value linked to the distribution of the depths of all the furrows retained.

In practice, only those furrows with an h_i depth are taken into account. For example,

$$h_i \geq 0.05\sigma$$

                                                      Xie and Mignot

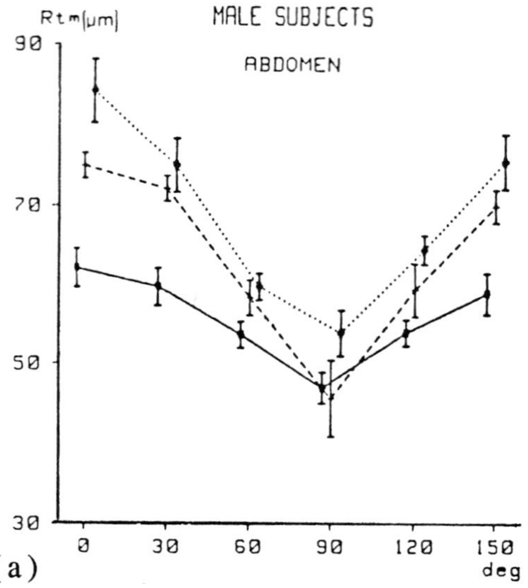

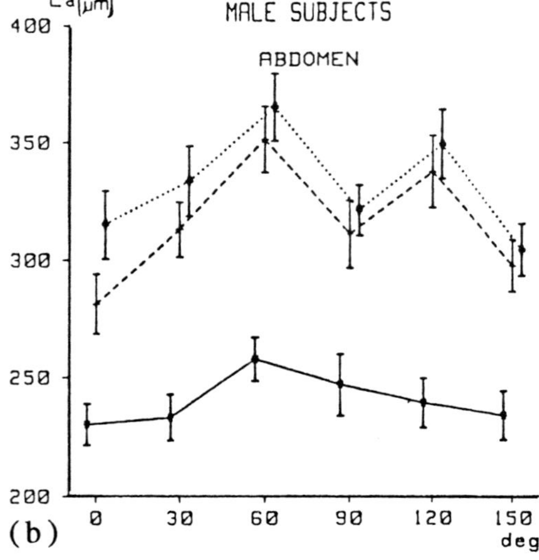

Figure 14 Use of classic parameters: (a) R_{tm} ISO parameter; (b) λ_a parameter (mean spacing between peaks and valleys); solid line, 5 years; dashed line, 25 years; dotted line, 55 years.

	Ra	Rp	Rv	Ry	Sm
Ra	1	0,93	0,91	0,97	0,47
Rp	0,93	1	0,81	0,95	
Rv	0,91	0,81	1	0,95	
Ry	0,97	0,95	0,95	1	
Sm	0,47				1

Figure 15 ISO parameters.

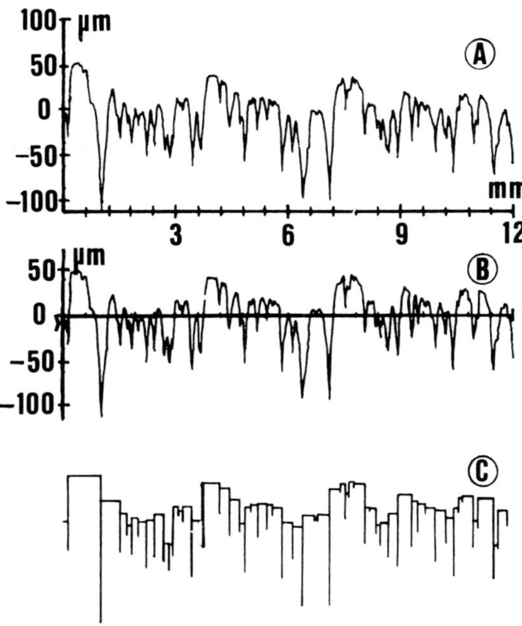

Figure 16 Decomposition of the skin surface into characteristic motifs: (A) initial profile; (B) straightened profile; (C) decomposition into elementary profiles.

This arbitrary value was chosen because, in the hypothetical Gaussian distribution of furrows, 5% of the values corresponding to a depth lower than $h = 1.65\sigma$, where σ is the root-mean-square (rms) of the distribution, are eliminated. Cook et al. (10) use a fixed value for this threshold.

The p distribution made it possible to obtain

The average value $\bar{z}$ of all the furrows
The skewness $R_{Sk} = \mu(3)/\mu(2)^{3/2}$
The kurtosis $R_{Ek} = \mu(4)/\mu(2)^{4/2}$

where the $\mu(j)$ represent the centered moments of the distribution of the h_i, such as

$$\mu(j) = \int h^j p(h)\, dh$$

and $\sigma^2 = \mu(2)$, the variance of the distribution. The coefficients R_{Sk} and R_{Ek} characterize the symmetry and the peakiness of the distribution.

By using the same statistical parameters the distribution of the width w of the plateaus around the average value w can be studied. Note, moreover, the resemblance between this parameter w, which is specific to study of the skin, and the more general S_m. However, with the help of the parameter S_m, which measures the spacing on the average line, we can verify (Fig. 16B) that many plateaus escaped this parameter, which explains the greater sensitivity observed when width w is used. Like the classic R_a and R_{tm} parameters, $\bar{z}$ is a parameter expressing an average.

Another interesting aspect of this method of analysis resides in the possibility of automatically distinguishing the primary from the secondary furrows; the separating principle can be based on the following criteria:

1. A primary furrow is characterized by its depth. Any depth exceeding a given threshold taken from the histogram of the repartition of the depth of the furrows is classified as a primary furrow. For example, we can choose z limit $= z + 1.65\sigma$, where σ is the rms of the distribution of the depth z.

2. Proximity: two important neighboring furrows do not fall into the same category of primary furrows. In fact, in a profile representing a surface cut on a plane perpendicular to the former, two primary furrows can represent a neighboring intersection. In this case, the distance separating the primary furrows measured along the recorded profile should not be taken into account since it minimizes the actual average width separating the primary furrows.

3. If the first two conditions are fulfilled, other primary furrows have locally become less deep. This decrease in depth may exist inside the plateaus, either because of the presence of neighboring furrows or because of the crossing of one or several primary furrows (each is edged with a primary furrow but can be crossed by different furrows). Therefore, all plateaus presenting an important width are examined to detect the eventual presence of other primary furrows. If in particular a succession of furrows of respective altitude z_i

$$z_{i-2} > z_{i-1} > z_i < z_{i+1} < z_{i+2}$$

should meet inside such a plateau, the furrow with altitude z_i is classified as primary even though it is not very deep.

Thus, so that two interesting furrows are not counted as one, the following condition is applied to the width of a newly detected plateau: a minimum width $>= 0.9w$.

Many of our fellow workers are concerned about aging of the skin, which is also the preoccupation of numerous laboratories. Skin relief is sensitive to the aging mechanism and can be used as a means of evaluating aging of the skin. Even though two-dimensional measurements are subject to errors due to

Localization of the measuring zone
Anisotropy of the relief
Nonhomogeneity of the surface

Nevertheless the results give interesting indications. A few interesting examples related to measuring classic profilometer R_{tm} and morphologic parameter $\overline{w}$ are given (Fig. 17). Note that the use of morphologic parameters leads to a less important dispersion of results (notably for $\overline{w}$).

Figure 18 gives an example of decomposition into elementary patterns (motifs) for two men (25 and 83 years old) and shows the interest of such a method of measurement of the depth of furrows and width of plateaus.

3. Wrinkles and Surfaces of Any Shape

In both two-dimensional profilometers, the use of a specific amplification is linked to the maximum range that the profilometer can offer. For example, with an amplification of 1000, the sensitivity given by the minimum variation that can be detected by the analog-digital conversion chart (12 bits) is 0.07 μm, and the maximum range is 50 μm (linearity zone given by the constructor). Thus, any difference in level surpassing this maximum range cannot be measured with the industrial system. On some surfaces deep wrinkles can present differences in height amounting to several millimeters.

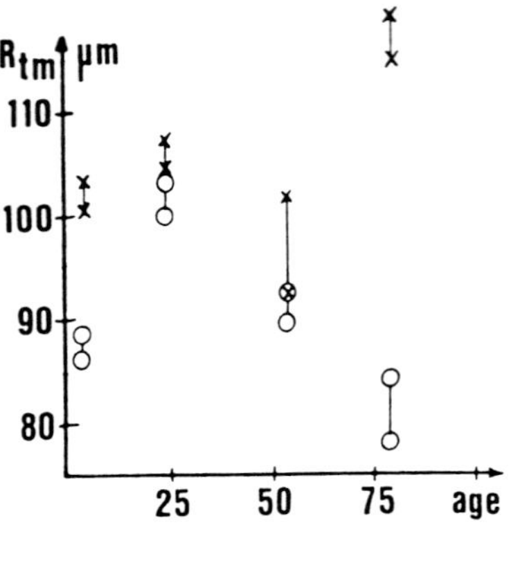

A)

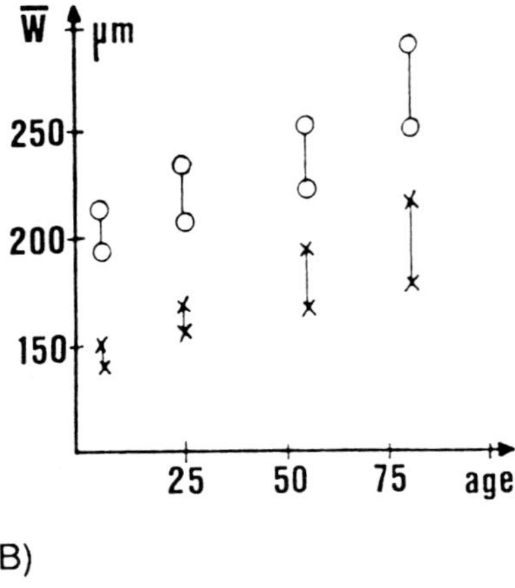

B)

Figure 17   Classic parameter R_{tm} (A) and mean depth $\overline{w}$ of furrows (B).

To explore very important differences (in height), two different solutions are currently possible:

1. Use optical interferometers, which can combine great sensitivity and a greater range of measuring scale (5 mm).
2. Use classic profilometers modified to eliminate the previous limitations.

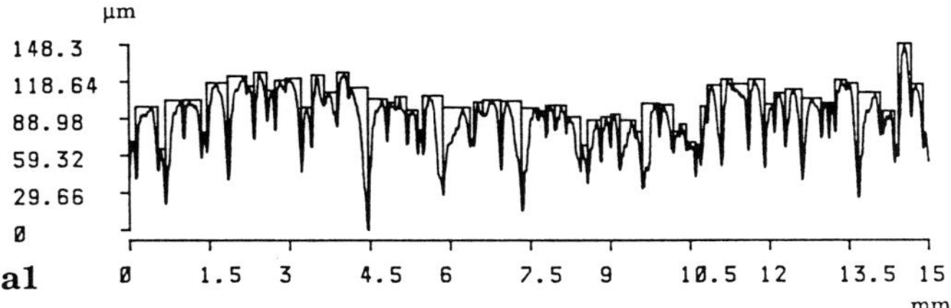

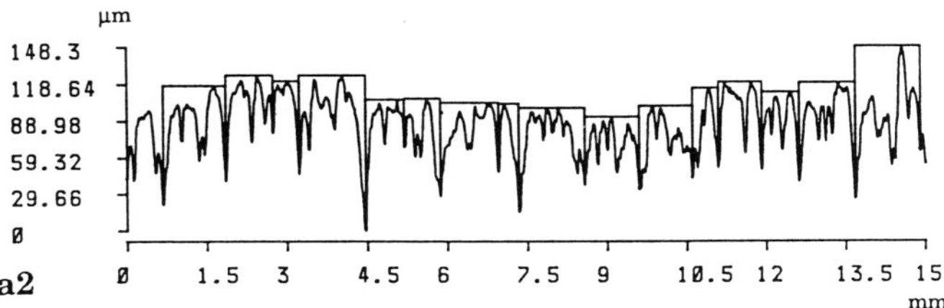

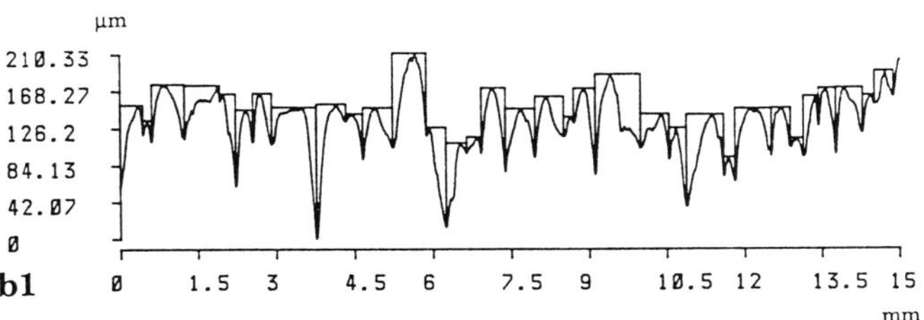

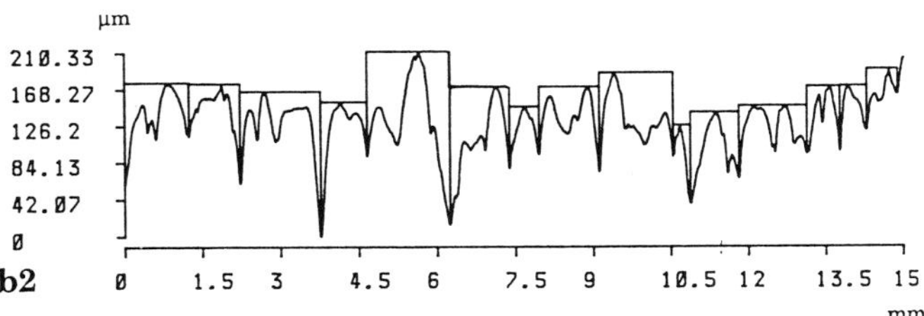

Figure 18 Decomposition into elementary patterns: (1) all significant patterns; (2) detection of principal furrows. (A) A 25-year-old man. (B) An 83-year-old man.

Optical interferometers arrived on the market only a few years ago. The measuring instrument can be either a mechanical sensor ensuring direct contact with the surface to be analyzed or an optical sensor. Such an example is shown in Figure 7 for mechanical and optical system realization.

Transformation of a classic profilometer into a wide-range system is based on the vertical displacement of the stylus relative to the sample when the signal produced by the sensor approaches the limits of the system. This displacement is carried out by a step-by-step motor. Generally, the signal produced by the appliance varies between -5 and 5 V, and can be converted into a numeric signal over 12 bits (0–4095). This range of variation can be separated into five parts (Fig. 19).

From (minsat $+ \delta$) to α: when the measuring point reaches this zone, it leaves the central zone and must be brought back by the movement of the motor. This extreme zone must consist of at least one linear part of the signal $i = f(z)$; α is a value dependent on the scale that is used.

From α to β is the normal measuring zone in which a classic profilometer operates. The linear relationship is $i = f(z)$. As long as the signal produced remains in this zone, the sample is shifted step by step under the sensor and the profile is stored.

From β to (maxsat $- \delta$): Like the second zone, this high zone is a prohibited zone: Any point that reaches it brings about a stop to the horizontal transfer of the sample. A vertical displacement is made to return the signal to the linearity zone.

These vertical displacements are carried out by a stepping motor with a 1 μm step. The mechanical error that inevitably accompanies these displacements is eliminated given that it is not necessary to know its precise position. This is done by adopting the following principle.

When the numerical signal reaches the limit α or β, its value is exact, known, and store. A vertical displacement transfers the stylus so that the signal returns to about the average value (2048) of the measuring scale. After such a vertical transfer, the new signal represents the height of the same point of the surface before displacement, the difference being equal to a quantity named offset. Thus the real height of the experimental point after the $i + 1$ vertical displacement is

$$Z_{i+1} \text{ real} = Z_{i+1} + \text{offset}_i$$

where offset is the sum of all the previous vertical displacements.

$$Z_j \text{ real} = Z_j \text{ measured} + \text{offset}_i$$

The reference of the heights is given by the altitude of the first measuring point. Thus, the exact position of the vertical motor is irrelevant since the

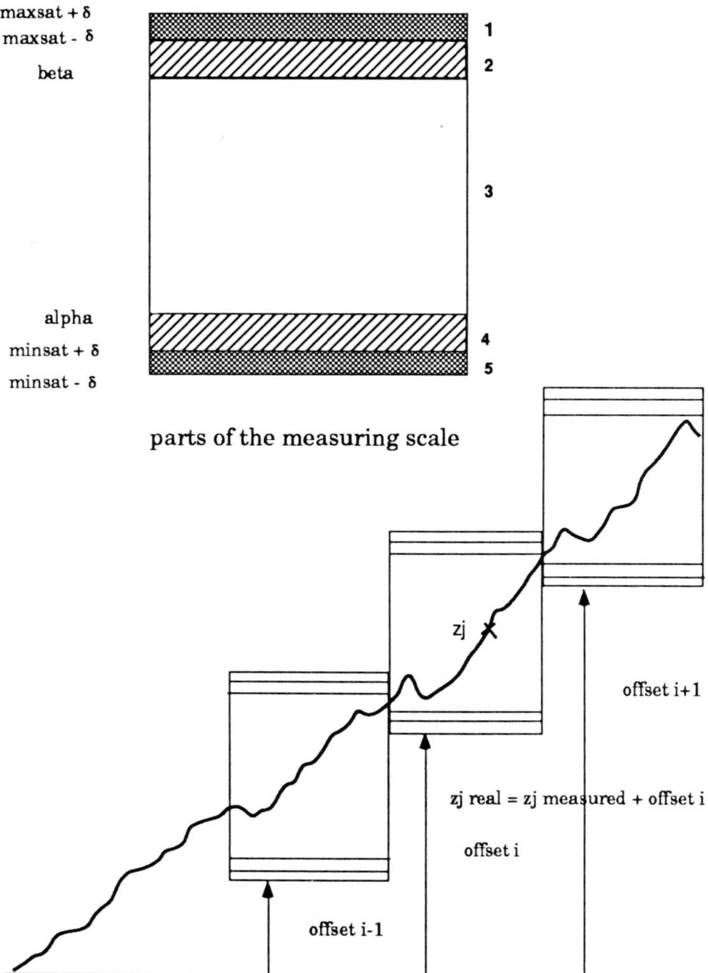

Figure 19 Principle of the wide-range system.

exact value of the position of the point is the value it had before the vertical displacement. The only problem is therefore linking by way of software of the signal before and after displacement, the precision of which depends only on the precision of the analogic digital convertor. Although the previously mentioned principle appears simple (a simple transfer of the scale), this procedure is accompanied by two possible causes of error, the first due to the accuracy of the convertor and the second related to the slight displacement of the stylus.

F. Three-Dimensional Surface Analysis

Although it is possible to use image analyses to solve such a problem, this procedure entails a very powerful computer, which explains why it is rarely used industrially. The only method currently used consists of a profilometer that describes a series of parallel profiles of which the entire group constitutes a scanning of the surface (16,17).

1. Principle

The principle is given in Figure 20, and the measuring system consists of a profilometer (mechanical or optical) whose signal is processed by a personal computer. A system comprising two step-by-step motors ensures the horizontal displacement of the sample under the stylus, which is kept in a fixed position on the horizontal plane. A third vertical motor can ensure displacement

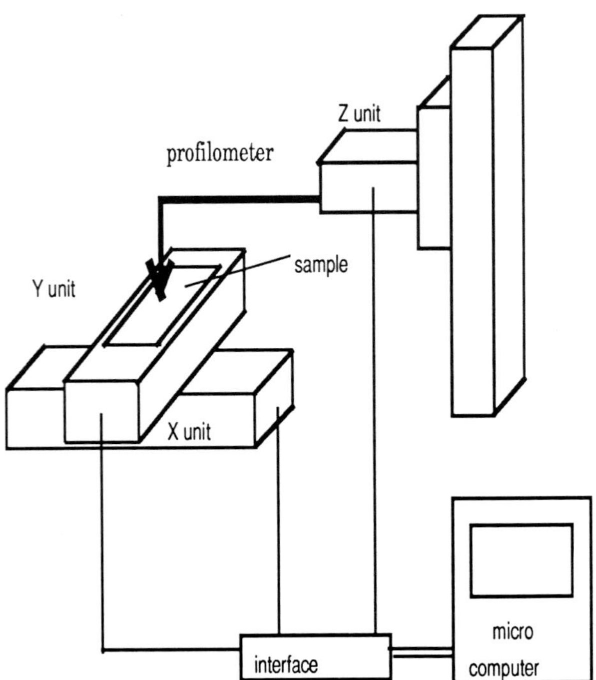

Figure 20   Principle of the three-dimensional system.

of the stylus relative to the samples to extend the measuring range of the system. Contact between the motor and the computer can be made according to the IEEE standard or by means of other systems. However, scanning of a surface, according to a 256-line matrix comprising 256 points (65,536 points), requires about 1.5 h under these conditions. Such a long duration is not feasible for an industrial process. Furthermore, the solution uses the scanning motor, not step by step, but in an almost continuous rotation by picking up the data in midstream. This can be done by using an auxiliary microprocessor that manages the motors and reads the signal instead of the computer. The data are stored in the memory and transferred to the computer at the end of the line or at the end of the matrix. With such a method the time needed to obtain a 65,536-point matrix can be reduced to 15 m.

2. Separation for Waviness and Defects of Form

As in two-dimensional measurement, undulation and defect of form are always present in a skin surface replica. There are two possible ways of eliminating the form defect or undulation from the altitude z of each experimental point:

1. The analyzed surface $z = f(x, y)$ representing any orientation relating to the defined horizontal plane can be rectified by calculation of the plane $z(x, y) = a + bx + cy$ passing through the experimental points.
2. Numeric filtering by gliding is a two-dimensional extension of the method used in profilometry. It consists of displacing a surface element of known dimensions and form on the surface and finding an average that can be weighted by any function chosen beforehand by the user.

Figure 21 shows an example of the size and the form allocated to the filters that are used. Mask 15 × 15 uses 177 experimental points, and it is possible to weight each point according to its distance from the center. Since deformation of the image should be avoided, symmetrical masks are used.

A low-pass filter is used to give prominence to the furrows of the skin while eliminating low-amplitude, high-frequency defects.

If x and y are the coordinates of the current point of the surface, the mask extends from

$$x - mx < x < x + mx$$
$$y - my < y < y + my$$

An example of such skin surface filtering is given in Figure 22.

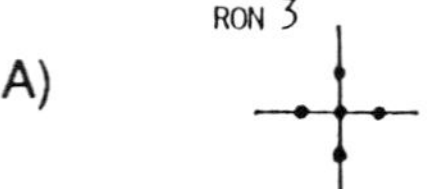

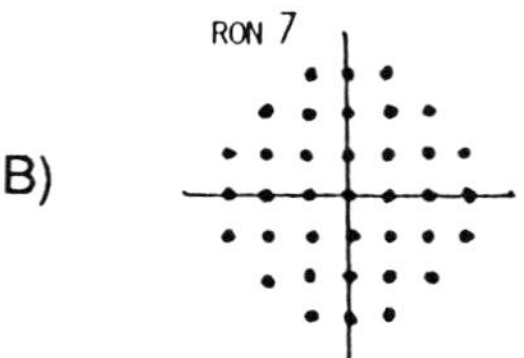

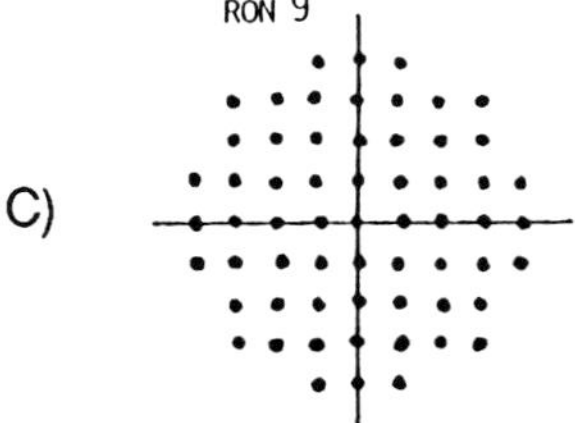

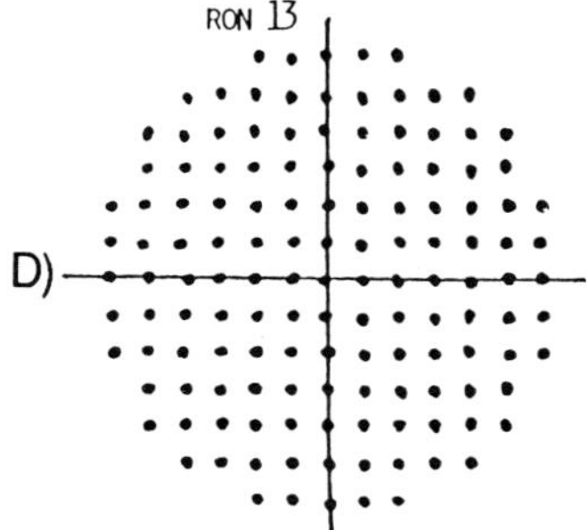

Figure 21   Shape and size of the surface element used in two-dimensional filtering: (A) size = 3 (5 points); (B) size = 7 (37); (C) size = 9 (61); (D) size = 13 (137).

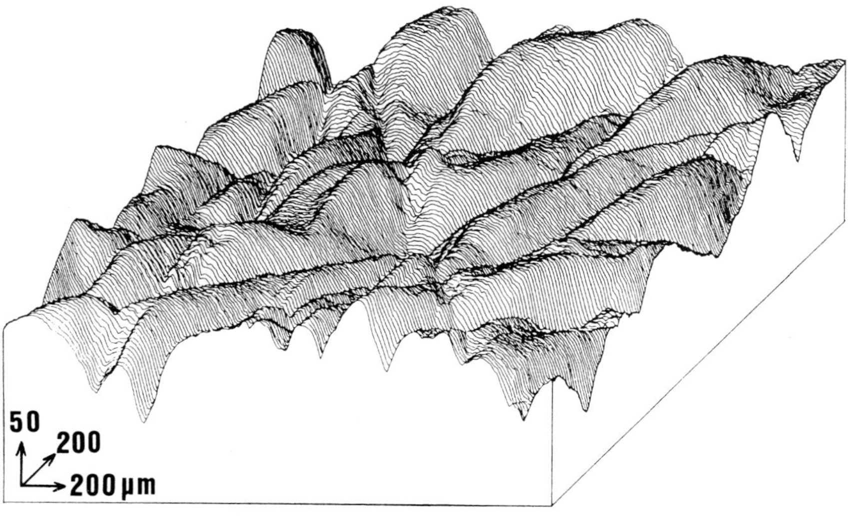

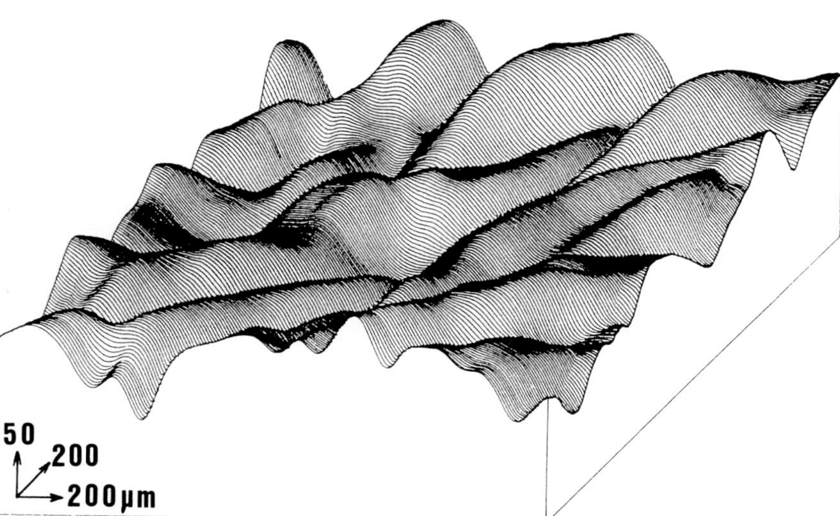

Figure 22   Example of skin surface filtering: (A) initial surface; (B) after low-pass filtering.

A high-pass filter is rarely used for the skin, except perhaps to give prominence to minor, low-amplitude defects with a pathologic cause.

Peuker and Douglas developed an interesting method to study the relief of the earth (18). This method can be easily extended to microrelief, especially that of the skin. Characterization of the nature of any point on the surface is deduced from study of the local variations of the relief around the point along a closed circuit that surrounds it. In the same way, we successively study points, such as peaks, hollows, and valleys. Other points, such as passes and crests, could be studied using the same method, but these are of secondary importance for skin relief. If n experimental points with a height z_i are found along a closed contour, Z_c is the height of the central point.

N is the number of sign changes along the closed circuit (Fig. 23), Δ^+ is the sum of all positive differences, Δ^- is the sum of negative differences $(Z_c - Z_i)$. If T_p is the threshold beyond which the difference Δ^+ or Δ^- becomes significant, then

The central point is a peak if $\Delta^+ = 0$, $|\Delta^-| > T_p$, $N = 0$.
The central point is situated in a valley if $\Delta^+ - \Delta^- > T_p$, $N = 2$.
The central point is a hollow if $\Delta^- = 0$, $\Delta^+ > T_p$, $N = 0$.

The accuracy of the analysis depends on the neighborhood. The shorter the distance of each point from the center, the more insignificant differences are considered. An example of the application of these methods to the skin surface is given in Figure 24. Figure 24 shows the horizontal representation of a family of particular points (valleys).

The interest of this method surpasses the vertical distribution of a single family of points. In fact, if the analyzed surface is characterized by 256×256 points, the total number of points are not sensitive to the influence of an external agent (hydration, sun filter, or moisturizing cream) in the same way. It is also interesting to remember those experimental points that may be sensitive to the effect of an agent.

Since skin relief is determined mainly by the presence of furrows, the distribution of furrow depth compared to the average height of the surface can supply additional interesting information.

Knowing the probability $p(z)$ so that the depth of a furrow can be situated between the values z and $z + dz$ results in the histograms of Figure 25, which make it possible to statistically follow, with the help of successive, centered moments of distribution, even the lesser variations in relief.

4. Three-Dimensional Quantification of Microrelief

The aim of all the different methods examined thus far is not merely to give a graphic representation of surface topography. In addition, quantitative data are required even though officially recognized three-dimensional parameters,

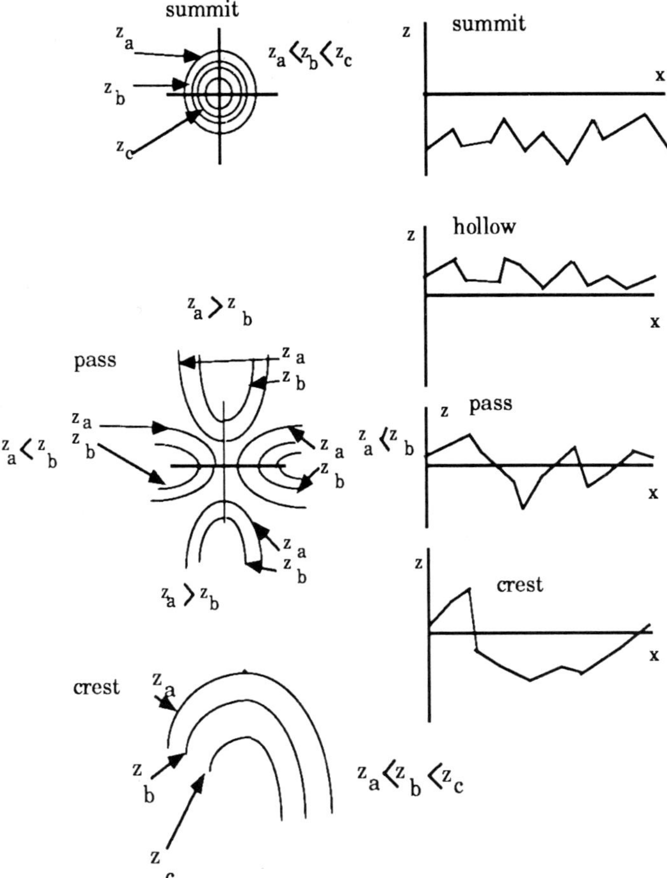

Figure 23 Definition of particular points on the skin surface.

as in two-dimensional studies, do not exist. This field is still new as far as its applications to quantification of microrelief are concerned, but specific parameters in two directions can already be foreseen.

Roughness parameters represent the three-dimensional extension of parameters established in two dimensions. Since in two-dimensional measurement (profilometry) such roughness parameters as R_a, R_{tm}, and R_{pm} are defined over a basic length, one can extend these definitions three dimensions.

If the skin surface is filtered by the method previously described, the connected surface is divided into a given number of elementary surfaces (for example in square forms with sides equal to one basic length). Over each of

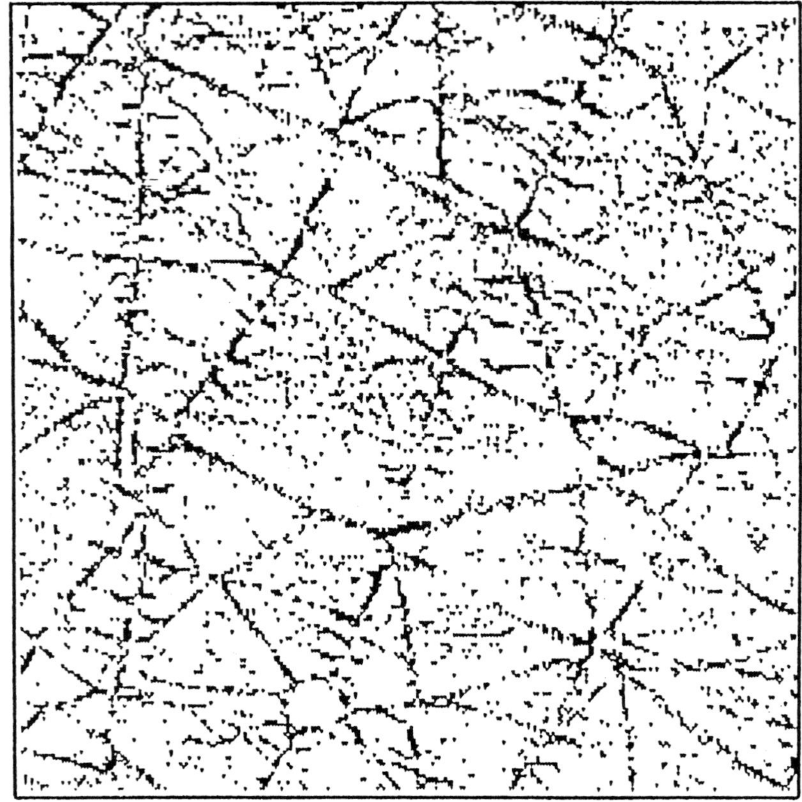

Figure 24 Detection of particular points on the skin surface: example of furrows.

these elementary elements parameters are evaluated by a definition based on two-dimensional analysis. For example,

$$R_a = \frac{1}{N} \sum R_a \qquad \text{with} \qquad R_a = \frac{1}{n} \sum_i \sum_j |z_{ij} - \bar{z}|$$

where n is the number of points over this element of the surface, z the mean value of the surface obtained after filtering at the point (i, j), and N the number of elementary areas.

Statistical parameters result from the distribution of the heights $p(z)$ of all the points on the surface after study of the successive, centered moments.

Additional characteristics of the condition of the surface can be obtained from the same function $p(z)$:

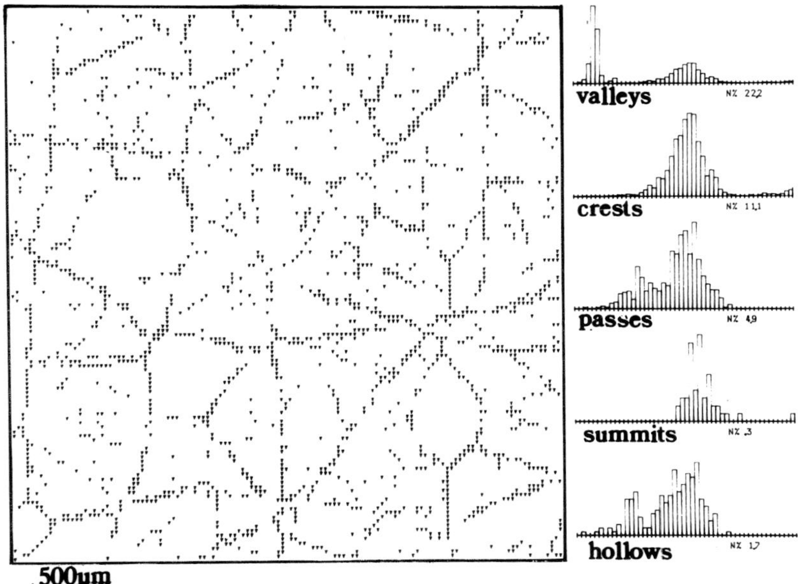

Figure 25 Particular points on the skin surface: example of furrow distribution and probability densities.

Longuet-Higgins (19,20) showed that if the $p(z)$ distribution is known, it is possible to evaluate the successive moments of the surface M_{00}; M_{02}, M_{04}, and M_{22} from which the density of the peaks, the average curve of the peaks, the anisotropic coefficient of the surface, the wavelength according to x and y, and the densities of zero or of extrema can be derived. Such a statistical three-dimensional study provides a new way of characterizing skin topography.

5. Relation Between Two-Dimensional and Three-Dimensional Analysis

Although three-dimensional analysis is more complete, it is sometimes difficult to use it to study local detail. It is also interesting to extract, from data representing a surface, the actual profile that exists between two points of this surface irrespective of the disposition of the two points (Fig. 26).

Knowing the function $z(x, y)$ at any point and storing all these values in the computer's memory make it possible to have rapid access to all the points (or the intermediate points obtained through interpolation) between any two points on the surface represented by its intersection with a vertical

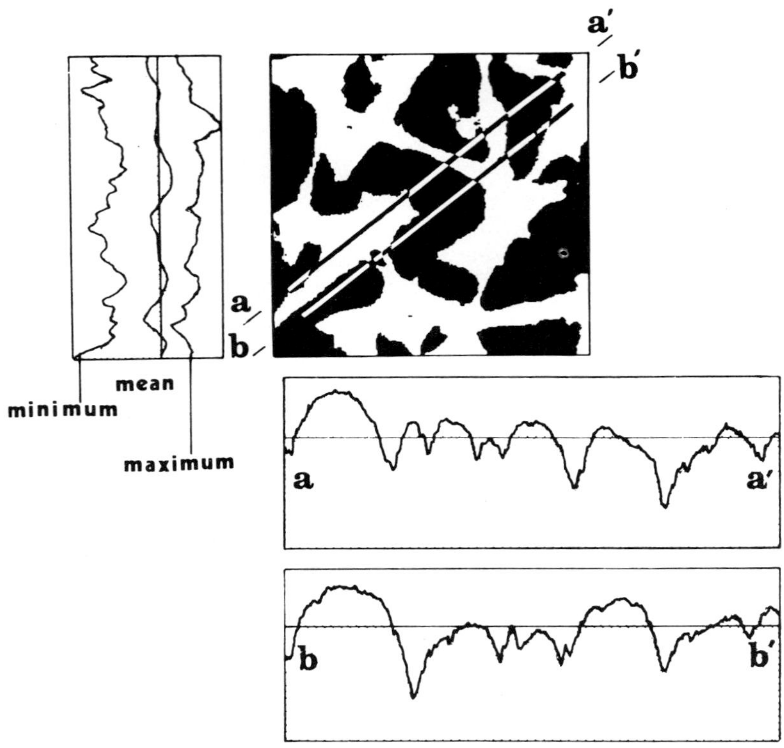

Figure 26 Two-dimensional analysis deduced from the surface: extraction of two parallel profiles.

plane. Thus, any two-dimensional roughness parameters can be extracted and used to quantify the local properties of the skin surface in the direction of the profile.

6. Study of Skin Relief by Methods Used in Image Analysis

The distribution of furrows on the skin surface or of the form and size of plateaus demarcated by the furrows are dimensions made accessible through image analysis.

Detection of characteristic elements of the surface requires developing specialized software to make it possible to detect, count, and characterize these elements. Such techniques are developed in image analysis and can be applied to the "image" from a three-dimensional profilometer. We obtain the proposed results by carrying out the following successive operations:

Filtration of the image to reduce noise and increase contrast while reinforcing linear forms

Detection of the points of the image that belong to the lines using contextual information and local, statistical analysis

Detection of the segments of the straight line of the image and from these segments construction of linear forms

Suppression of discontinuities

a. Preparation of Data for Furrow Quantification by Smoothing Operator. The application of a classic smoothing operator, which consists of replacing the altitude at a point of the image with the average value in the neighborhood of this point (Fig. 27B), is not well suited to images of the skin (21–23). In fact, it lessens the contrast, which consequently makes it more difficult to detect the lines and the appearance of discontinuities.

A specific algorithm based on the principle designed by Nagao and Matsugama (21) must therefore be developed and schematized (Fig. 27C). Each of the M_k masks measuring 5×5 pixels is applied to the neighborhood of a point (i, i) of the image and supplies an average value M_k and a variance T_k. The altitude in (i, j) after application of the filter is replaced by the average value m_1.

This algorithm chooses the most significant direction and the minimum variance and makes it possible to eliminate noise by smoothing while reinforcing the contrast. Figure 27D shows an example of application of the Nagao filter to the same skin surface.

Earlier algorithms do not give complete satisfaction, particularly regarding secondary furrows whose initial contrast is very insignificant. To prevent furrows from disappearing after filtering, a new method by Paton (24) uses directional masks (straight segments measuring 5 pixels). Figure 28 shows the shape of the masks that were applied (eight possible directions).

b. Thresholding the image. After filtration and reinforcement of the furrows, their quantification is facilitated on an image reduced to two levels. In fact, the initial image can consist of 4096 gray levels, which makes calculating longer and drawn out on a microcomputer. The smoothed image must be transformed into a two-level image representing the lines and the background. This thresholding must use local statistical properties. If $I(i, j)$ is the gray level of the image at one point and m the average value of the gray levels in a given neighborhood (5×5 or 7×7) and if

$$m - I(i, j) > S \qquad \text{then} \qquad I(i, j) = 1$$

If not, $I(i, j) = 0$ and the point (i, j) does not belong to a furrow. Figure 29 illustrates the results obtained from this operator by applying the same initial image using two different values of threshold S.

c. Analysis of Plateaus. Since the image is binary (white = 0, plateau; black = 1, furrow), detection of the size and direction of the plateaus is

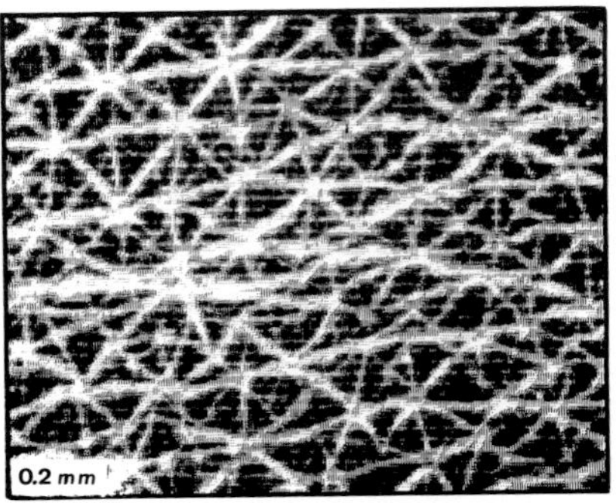

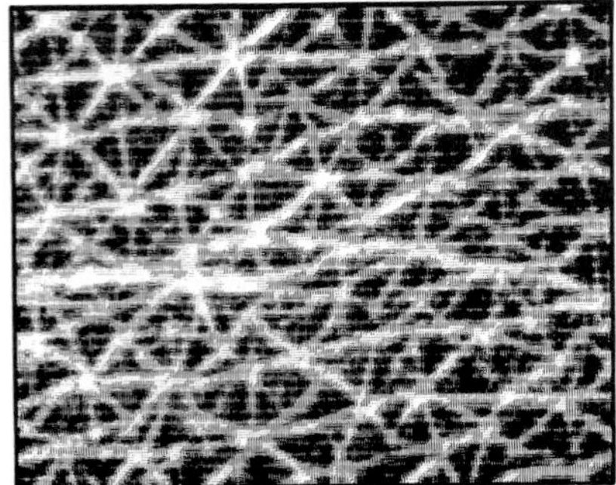

a

b

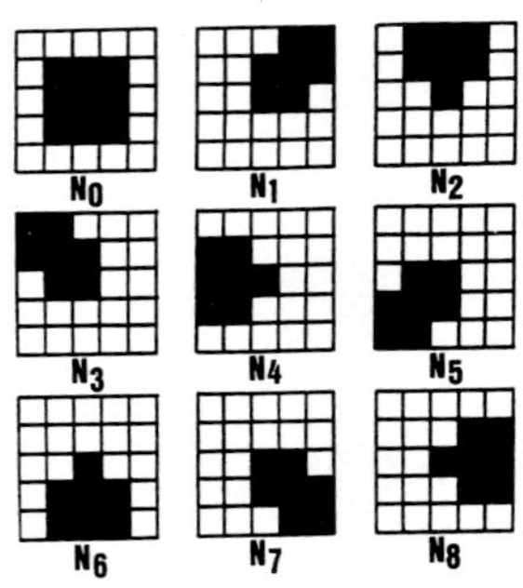

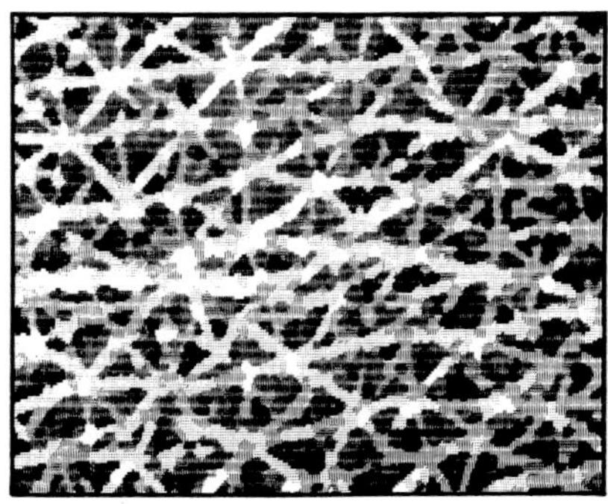

c

d

Figure 27 Detection of furrows and plateaus: smoothing operator. (A) Initial skin surface; (B) classic smoothing operator effect; (C) Nagao masks; (D) Nagao smoothing operator.

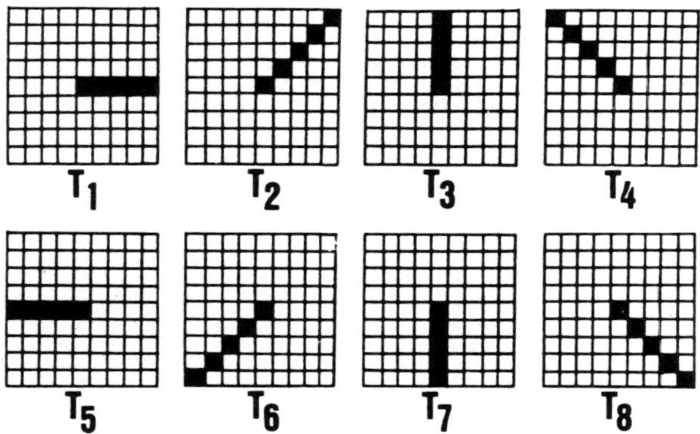

Figure 28 Directional reinforcement masks.

made possible by scanning the image line by line. The intersection of a plateau and a line of the image creates a straight segment made up of pixels whose value is 0. Each segment that is detected is defined by three parameters Y, X_1, and X_2, with Y = line number and X_1 and X_2 the abscissas of the two extremities of the segment. Two segments (Y_1, X_{11}, X_{21}) and (Y_2, X_{12}, X_{22}) overlap if:

$$(Y_1 - Y_2) = 1$$
$$X_{22} > X_{11}$$
$$X_{21} > X_{12}$$

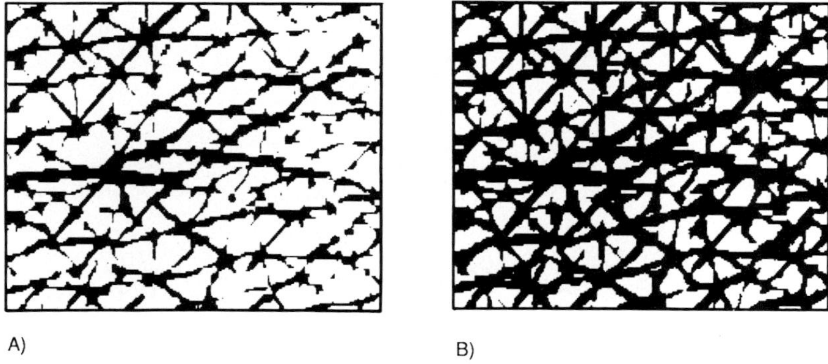

Figure 29 Detection of furrows: thresholding the image. (A) Level = 20; (B) level = 30.

  Xie and Mignot

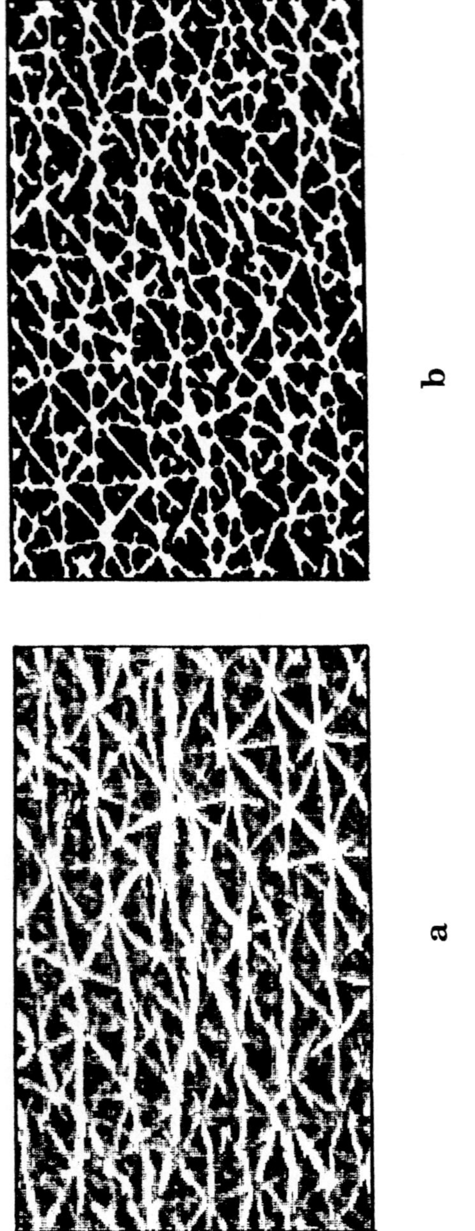

Figure 30 (A) Initial surface; (B) determination of the plateau.

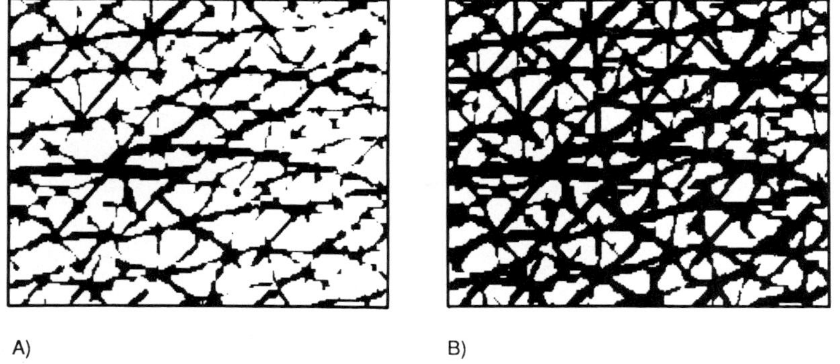

Figure 31 Detection of furrows: thresholding the image. (A) Level = 20; (B) level = 30.

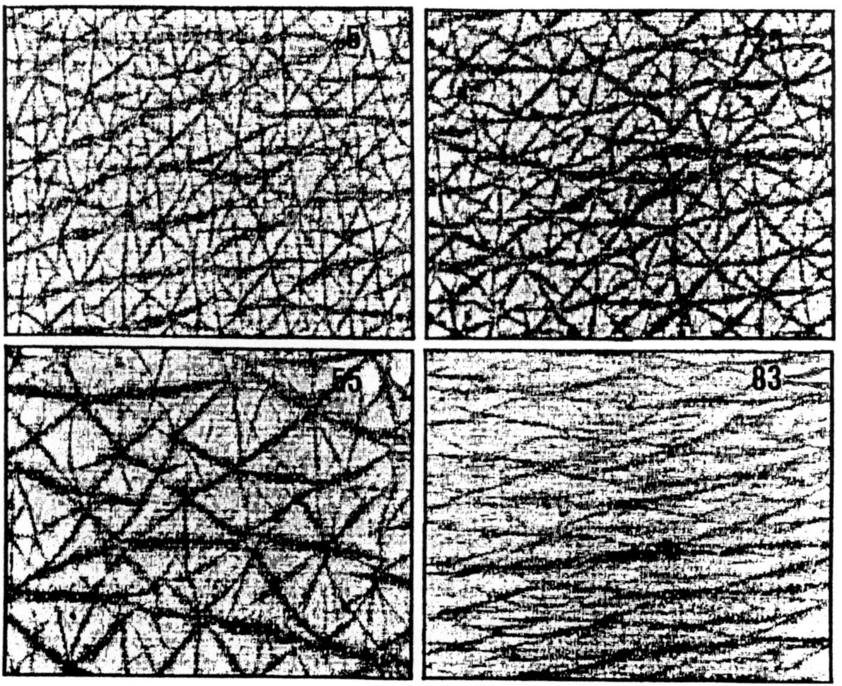

Figure 32 Initial skin surfaces: male subjects 5, 25, 55, and 83 years old.

When an entire group of segments overlap, they form a plateau whose area or dimensions can be calculated easily. Figure 30b shows an example of the initial image and the contours of the plateaus determined from it.

d. Furrow Processing.   The lines obtained after thresholding do not have a consistent width (Fig. 31). Skeletonization aimed at obtaining lines of unit-width is required to calculate the densities. Different skeletonization algorithms can be applied (25–27).

Figures 32 and 33 are examples of the skeletonization of initial images of skin replicas. They illustrate the accuracy of the results. Figure 32 shows the initial skin surfaces (subjects 5, 25, 55, and 83 years old).

e. Detection of Straight Segments of the Image. Search for Furrows.   The straight segments of imposed minimum length (5 points) are detected by specific masks locating these segments in eight characteristic directions. An example of these masks is shown (Fig. 34.) At each point on the masks a coefficient $S(l, m)$ representing the importance related to point (l, m) of the configuration k is affected. The application of configuration k in the neighborhood of point (i, j) of the image gives a value E_k calculated as follows.

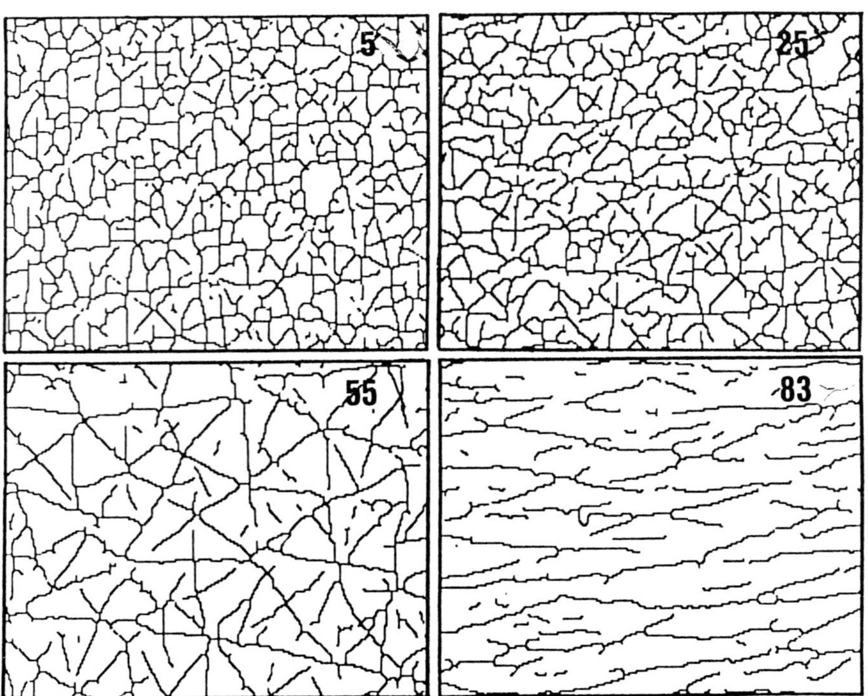

Figure 33   Skeletonization of the furrows (same areas as in Fig. 32).

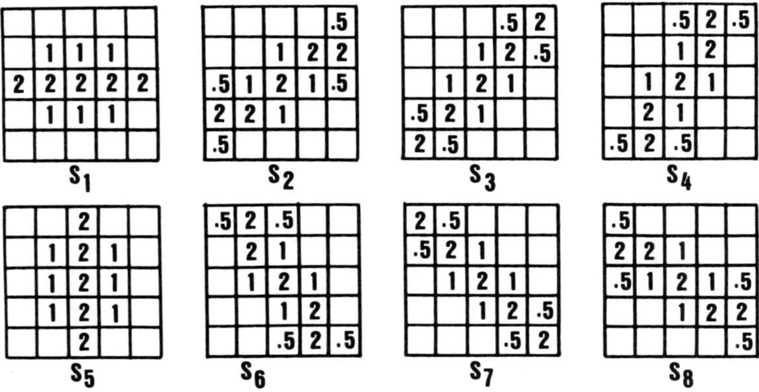

Figure 34 Masks used in furrow orientation detection.

$$E_k = \frac{1}{16} \sum_{p=1} \sum_{q=1} S_k(p, q)\, I(i + p - 3, j + q - 3)$$

The possible presence of a k-type segment is given by

$$E_L = (E(k))$$

and the detected segment is conserved in (i, j) of the image. This same point is then a point of intersection. It is now possible to obtain quantitative information from the skin plateaus and furrows.

Figure 35 illustrates the density and orientation variations obtained according to the aging of male subjects between 5 and 83 years old. From such figures one can obtain the values of the densities (in number of segments and percentage in the eight measuring directions), as well as the overall density of furrows in families around 5, 25, 55, and 83 years old. These results connect with those of profilometry.

G. Effect of Aging on Skin Relief

Table 1 relates the evolution of classic parameters R_a, R_{tm}, R_{ek}, S_m and thus also the morphologic $\bar{z}$ and $\bar{w}$ parameters with age (5, 25, 55, and 80 years). In this example (abdomen and volar forearm), the relief does not vary the same way in two different sites and shows that important variations occur after 25 years.

With the use of classic parameters, such as R_a and R_{tm}, the height of the relief decreases continuously in the forearm site after 25 years, whereas a minimum value is obtained at 55 years in the abdomen site. An important increase occurs during the last studied period at both sites.

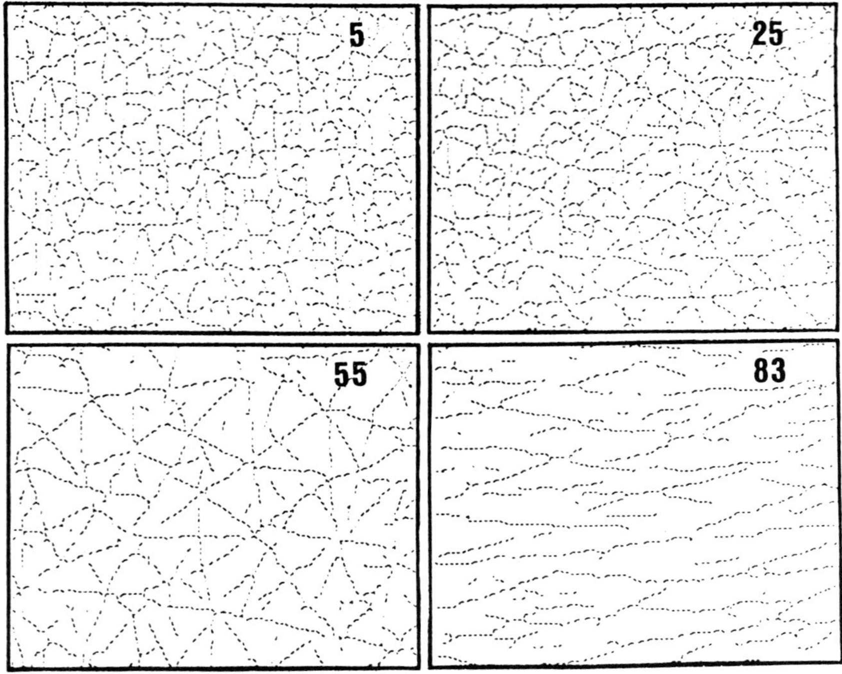

Figure 35 Detection of furrow direction (same areas as in Fig. 32). Use of straight segment decomposition.

In contrast, the variation in the space parameter S_m shows a more uniform variation with aging. A continuous increase in this mean distance between furrows (measured at the mean level) confirms the visual aspect of the skin surface. At both sites, an increase in the value of S_m is obtained with aging. Nevertheless, such a result shows only the evolution of this mean distance between principal furrows. More information is obtained from morphologic parameter $\overline{w}$. The S_m parameter cannot take into account all secondary furrows located at the top of plateaus, whereas all furrows are counted when using parameter $\overline{w}$. This difference in parameter definition explains the difference in results: $\overline{w}$ is approximately 50% of S_m. In a complementary fashion, three-dimensional analysis of the skin surface allows the detection of furrow directions and measurement of the corresponding density of distribution.

Table 2 gives an example of the evolution with aging of the density of furrows of the volar forearm in four arbitrary directions relative to the arm axis.

Table 1 Evolution of Roughness Parameters with Aging

Parameter	Age (years)				
	5	25	55	80	
R_a	16 ± 0.8	17 ± 1	16.3 ± 1.2	24 ± 3	Abdomen
	11 ± 1	15.5 ± 1.5	10.3 ± 2	9 ± 2.5	Forearm
R_{tm}	102 ± 6	105 ± 6	97 ± 7	117 ± 6	Abdomen
	87 ± 2	102 ± 5	92 ± 4	80 ± 5	Forearm
E_k	3.1 ± 0.2	2.95 ± 0.2	3.25 ± 0.3	2.90 ± 0.2	Abdomen
					Forearm
S_m	305 ± 22	352 ± 15	386 ± 41	502 ± 49	Abdomen
	312 ± 21	305 ± 28	392 ± 33	472 ± 51	Forearm
$\overline{Z}$	32 ± 2	31.8 ± 2.3	35.2 ± 3	43 ± 2.7	Abdomen
	28.5 ± 1.8	31.2 ± 2.7	29.9 ± 1.9	27.1 ± 3.4	Forearm
$\overline{w}$	146 ± 9	164 ± 11	172 ± 18	184 ± 30	Abdomen
	203 ± 15	215 ± 18	233 ± 20	256 ± 28	Forearm

The decrease in furrow density and the number of characteristic directions is in good agreement with the results by Corcuff et al. (28,29) using an image analysis method.

IV. CONCLUSION

Skin relief has interested dermatologists for about 20 years, but it was only a few years ago that specific means of quantification were developed. The development of personal computers has made it possible to elaborate chains of portable measurements and does not require considerable investment in equipment. However, future development of these techniques will require the

Table 2 Evolution of Furrow Density (%) with Aging in Four Main Directions

Age (years)	Main direction (degrees)				Density of all furrows (%)
	0	45	90	135	
5	45.1	26.0	19.9	9.0	19.5
25	45.1	31.1	13.0	10.8	18.6
55	34	33.8	14.2	18.0	14.9
75	38.8	33.3	16.7	11.2	9.7

evolution of two extremities of the measuring chain: the sensor and the software for processing.

Sensors are oriented in an optical direction, since only they can assure great accuracy and the large measuring scale required to study the skin. Although they were only recently used to measure mechanical surfaces, their use has confirmed their validity. The passage from two-dimensional to three-dimensional studies opens up a new domaine. The skin surface is not isotropic and is sometimes nonhomogeneous. However, this brings up the notion of measuring time, still acceptable with regard to two-dimensional measurements when the analyzed surfaces do not present any important form defects. Three-dimensional measurements require developing rapid systems to displace the sample and store and treat the data.

Three-dimensional measurements have thus far contributed only to graphic information—visualization of pseudoperspectives and contour curves, cuts at different levels, and histograms of distribution, for example—but a truly quantitative study based on the distribution of heights and local slopes of the surface has yet to be developed. There are interesting mathematical theories, however, even though they were developed for other disciplines.

Sensors and the analysis of signs developed to study skin relief are amenable to development, either in dermatology—the study of skin transplants and the healing of wounds—or in other disciplines— the role of the condition of the surface in certain joint afflictions (arthritis) or in the tribologic behavior of prostheses. The recent elaboration of some of the methods presented here proves their interest and shows that considerable progress has yet to be made. A much greater field of application exists than that explored thus far.

REFERENCES

1. Cummins H, Midlo C. Fingerprints, palms and soles. New York: Blakiston, 1961.
2. Lin WC, Dubes RC. A review of ridges counting in dermatoglyphics. Pattern Recognition 1983, 16 (n1): 1–8.
3. Alter M. Dermatoglyphics analysis as a diagnostic tool. Medicine (Baltimore) 1966; 16:35–56.
4. Moayer B, Fu KS. A syntactic approach to fingerprint pattern recognition. Pattern Recognition 1975; 7:1–23.
5. Peklenik J. Investigation of the surface topography. Ann CIRP 1967 XV:381–5
6. Sarkamy L. A method for studying the microtopography of the skin. Br J Dermatol (1962), 74:254–258.

7. Hayer MD. A detail duplication test for dental materials. NY State Dent J (1959); 25:154–7.

8. Facq JM. New pressure less replicas technique for the study of human skin. Toilet Goods Association. Proceedings of Scientific Section (1967); 47 (16):16.

9. Cook TH. Profilometry of skin. A useful tool for the substantiation of cosmetic efficacy. J Soc Cosmet Chem (1980); 31:339–51.

10. Cook TH, Craft TJ, Brunell RL. Quantification of the skin topography by skin profilometry. Int J Cosmet Sci (1982); 4:195–205.

11. Makki S, Agache P, Mignot J, Zahouani H. Statistical analysis and three dimensional representation of the human skin surface. J Soc Cosmet Chem (1984); 35:311–25.

12. Mignot J, Zahouani H, Rondot D, Nardin PH. Morphological study of the human skin relief. Bioengin Skin. (1987); 3:177–96.

13. Boulanger J. Nouvelles méthodes de calcul des critères d'état de surfaces. Rev Prat Controle Ind (1975); 117:205–33.

14. Fahl CF. Motif combination. A new approach to surface profile analysis. Wear (1982); 83:165–79.

15. Chuard M, Nardin PH, Rondot D, Mignot J. Range expansion and automation of a classical profilometer. J Manufact Systems (1987); 6 (3):223–31.

16. Williamson JBP. Topography of solid surfaces. Proceedings NASA Symposium on Interdisciplinary Approaches to Friction and Wear. San Antonio. P.M. Ku edit. (November 1967) (NASA SP-181), 85–142.

17. Thomas TR. Recent advances in measurement and analysis of surface microgeometry. Wear (1975); 33:205–33.

18. Peuker TK, Douglas DH. Detection of surfaces specific points by local parallel processing of discrete terrain elevation data. Comp Graph Im Process (1975); 4:375–87.

19. Longuet-Higgins MS. Statistical properties of an isotropic random surface Philos Trans Soc (1957); 250A:157–74.

20. Longuet-Higgins MS. The statistical geometry of random surfaces. Hydrodynamic stability, Proceedings 13th Symposium on applied math. Am Math Society Boston 1962:105.

21. Nagao M, Matsuyama T. Edge preserving smoothing. Comput Graph Im Process (1979); 9:394–407.

22. Coquerez JP, Devars J. Detection des contours dans les images aefiennes; nouveaux opefateurs. Traitement Signal (1985); 1:45–65.

23. Grant G, Reig AF. An efficient algorithm for boundary tracing and featuring extraction. Comput Graph Im Process (1981); 17:225–37.

24. Paton K. Line detection by local methods. Comput Graph Im Process (1979); 9:316–32.

25. Shapiro B, Pisa J, Sklansky J. Skeleton generation from x, y boundary sequences. Comput Graph Im Process (1981); 15:136–53.

26. Stefanelli R, Rosenfeld A. Some parallel thinning algorithms for digital pictures J Assoc Comput Mach (1971); 18:255–64.

27. Montanari V. Continuous skeletons from digitized images. J Assoc Comput Mach (1969); 16:534–49.
28. Corcuff P, de Rigal J, Lévêque J-L. Skin relief and aging. J Soc Cosmet Chem (1983); 34:177–90.
29. Corcuff P, de Rigal J, and Lévêque J-L. Image analysis of the cutaneous micro-relief. Bioengin Skin (1982); 4(1):16.

13

Age-Related Changes in Skin Microrelief Measured by Image Analysis

PIERRE CORCUFF and JEAN-LUC LÉVÊQUE

L'Oréal
Aulnay-sous-Bois, France

I. INTRODUCTION

The considerable physiologic importance of the skin surface as the interface between the individual and the environment explains the intensive research efforts made in this field over the past decade. The geometric organization of the skin surface is remarkable and reflects the subjacent structures. This organization is responsible for the ''appearance'' of each individual, which has a scientifically recognized social impact (1).

However, the intensity of these investigations has contributed to the extreme confusion surrounding the subject. Indeed, the vocabulary is confused, with such terms as skin surface patterns, microtopography, microrelief, texture, microdepressionary network, furrows, crests, lines, and plateaus. Similarly, there is a profusion of investigative methods, including visual scoring, profilometric measurements, densitometric methods, and image analysis. Finally, it is far from clear exactly how the descriptive parameters used (distance, height, orientation, anisotropy, texture, structure, density, roughness, and periodicity) correspond to topography. Our aim is to contribute to the clarification of this area by giving a brief description of microrelief and the methods used for its measurement, before going on to discuss the published results and what they tell us about chronologic and actinic aging and their impact on the mechanical properties of the skin.

179

II. DESCRIPTION OF SKIN MICRORELIEF

The skin surface presents a number of depressions that are roughly rectilinear and can be classified according to depth and the magnification required to describe them. The most visible features are wrinkles, which vary in depth from 100 μm to several millimeters according to age and environmental factors.

Wrinkles are situated in particular sites, for example the expression lines of the face and folds around the joints. Under low magnification ($\times 10$), the skin presents a network of features: parallel furrows criss-cross, forming rectangles, squares, lozenges, trapezoids, and triangles. Hashimoto (2) proposed a simple classification into four groups of lines.

Primary lines are wide and 20–100 μm deep according to site and age. They cross to form parallelograms, rectangles, or squares. Secondary lines are narrower (depth 5–40 μm); they are branches of primary lines and form diagonals within the shapes made by the latter. Primary and secondary lines

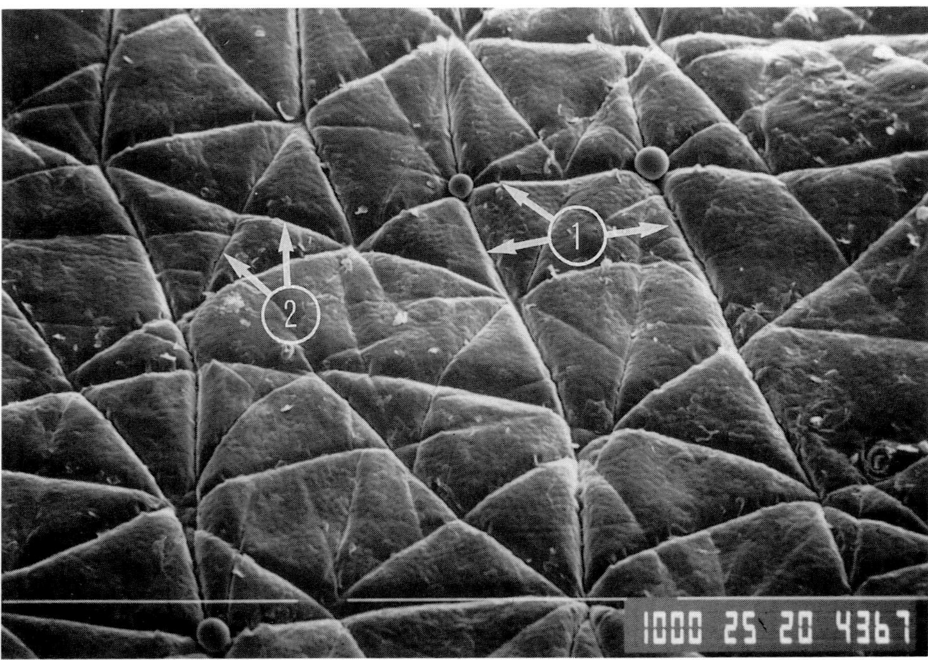

Figure 1 Scanning electron micrograph of skin surface showing typical drawings of microrelief: (1) primary lines, and (2) secondary lines.

generally intersect at the points where sweat ducts and hair shafts emerge (Fig. 1).

At higher magnification ($\times 100$), precluding study with the naked eye, tertiary lines form the boundaries of the corneocytes and quaternary lines traverse individual corneocytes.

Only primary and occasionally secondary lines are assessed by image analysis; these features form the microrelief.

III. INVESTIGATIVE METHODS

As soon as a skin biopsy specimen is removed it retracts, showing that the skin is under permanent tension: this is what creates the typical drawings. The topography of the skin can therefore only be observed in vivo. For practical reasons (mainly the delayed ease of the observation and the presence of a translucent horny layer that creates optical disturbances—reflection and diffraction), nearly all studies are based on replicas. Silicon dental resins give an accurate negative reproduction of the skin surface (Fig. 2).

Observations can be made directly on the negative or on a positive replica made using Araldite, which enables the use of a conventional microscope or scanning electron microscopy after gold coating. These visual methods are widely used and provide qualitative results.

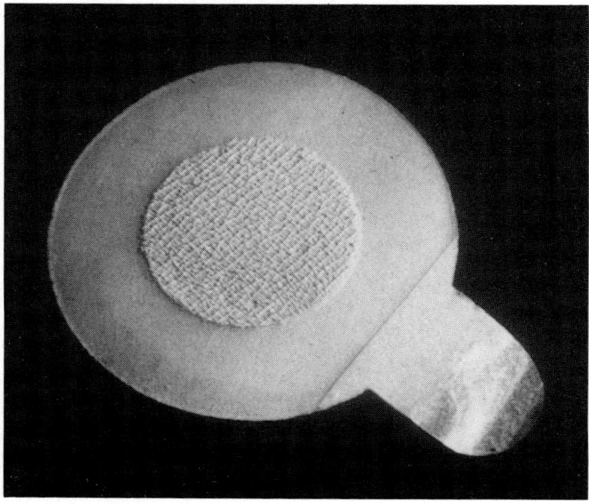

Figure 2 Negative Silflo replica of the surface of the forearm inserted in an adhesive paper ring.

The most widely known quantitative method, profilometry, was first used in the early 1970s (3,4). An apparatus designed for measuring the roughness of metal surfaces was adapted to the skin. Basically, the method consists of moving a stylus linearly across the skin surface and obtaining a trace. A series of scans is necessary to obtain a mean profile representative of the area studied. The profiles give rise to more than 10 quantitative parameters, which are then analyzed using a computer. The parameters were originally defined for use in metallurgy and are often difficult to interpret in terms of skin microrelief. The method is lengthy and delicate and gives only two-dimensional readings. The results must be interpreted with care, since the skin surface is strongly anisotropic. The choice of the direction of the scan must therefore be taken into account when analyzing the results. Makki et al. (5), aware of this difficulty, further developed the method to obtain three-dimensional images; however, the time required to reproduce the relief of 1 cm^2 skin was prohibitive (>1 hr) for routine studies. The clearest review of this methodology remains that done by Cook (6).

An alternative approach, first described in 1981 (7), is based on the shadow principle, a method used by NASA to study lunar topography. When

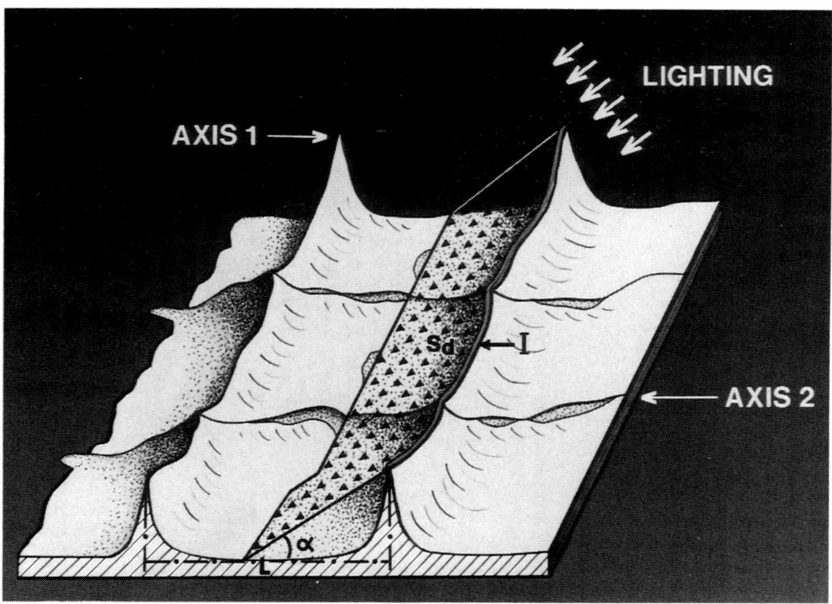

Figure 3 The shadowing principle used in image analysis: α incident lighting angle; *Sd*, surface area of shadows; *I*, intercept length.

applied to the topography of negative imprints, it gives a three-dimensional analysis of 1 cm^2 in less than 5 minutes (Fig. 3). Under oblique lighting, the shadows created behind the crests (negative furrows) can be selected and measured (Fig. 4).

The main orientations of the skin furrows are then determined, together with the density and mean depth of lines oriented in a given direction. A mathematical model is used to calculate the total skin surface area within 1 cm^2 of projected surface. This value is known as the coefficient of developed skin surface (CDSS) and expresses the reserve of tissue or "deformation reservoir."

These stereologic parameters fall within the concept of fractality (8). The skin surface is very irregular, and as a result, measurements depend on the degree of magnification and the angle of lighting. This angle can be used as a filter: with an angle of 26°, for example, depressions of less than 15 μm are not recognized, whereas at 38°, it is not possible to measure wrinkles and

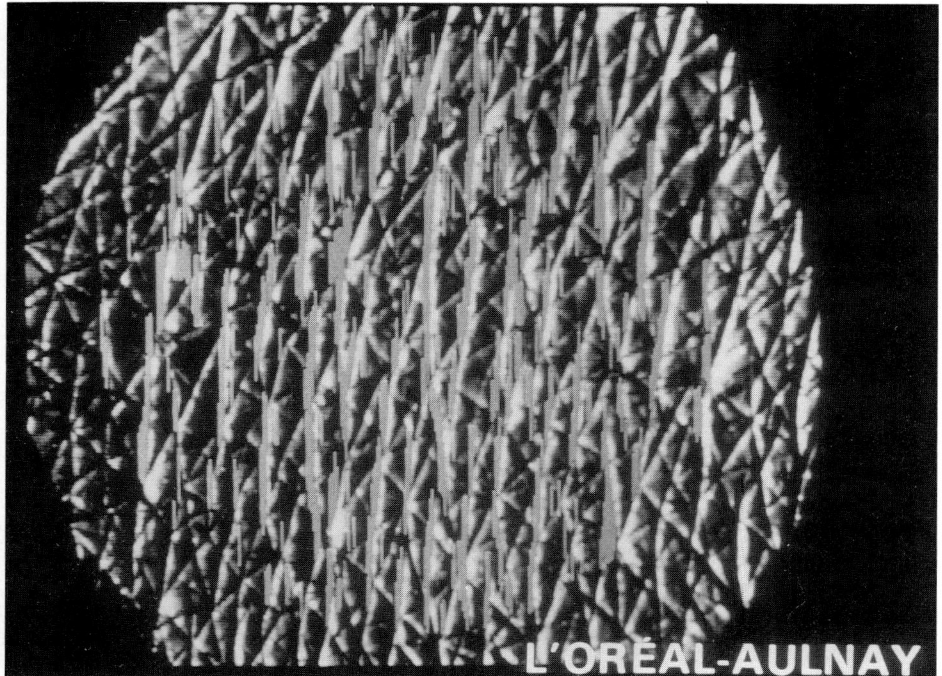

Figure 4 Image analysis of negative replica: the binary (gray) overlay corresponds to selected shadows for automatic measurements.

primary lines simultaneously (9). This configuration selects only primary lines, as defined earlier, with a lighting angle of 26°. However, these limitations should not make us forget the richness of the data obtained for a large surface area in a short period of time, allowing routine studies of a large number of samples with the inherent advantages of better statistical validity.

Since 1985, numerous variants of image analysis have been advanced (10–15). The image is recorded by means of a video camera, a mechanical profilometer (16), or, more recently, a scanning laser (17). Acquisition using a camera is performed either under diffuse lighting conditions (18), which limit the study to two dimensions, or under oblique lighting at an angle of 25° (19), which preserves the three-dimensional information. The latter option demands a multidirectional study, given the anisotropy of the structure. Some authors have taken this factor into account (20); others have not (21).

Acquisition by profilometry allows three-dimensional reconstruction of the skin surface point by point. Progress in computerized data handling has reduced the acquisition time with a laser probe to acceptable proportions (less than 5 minutes).

These novel methods of image analysis preserve the three-dimensional information for both primary and secondary lines (22).

IV. PARAMETERS OF MEASUREMENT

At the observed scale, the skin cannot be considered a finite object, but rather a structure. As a result, only global or statistical approaches can be envisaged. The global approach demands little computing power, being based on probabilistic geometry and stereologic parameters (23). Basically, stereology can only be applied to isotropic structures (24). A multidirectional study is therefore necessary, ignoring the periodicity of the events. The tools that imply a statistical approach require more computing power. Profilometric parameters are only suitable for isotropic structures. Here again, a multidirectional study is obligatory, and this was previously limited by a lack of computing power and speed.

Since 1985, these limits have been receding and parameters of structure and texture are beginning to emerge; such parameters are far better for describing the skin surface than the classic Euclidian parameters of distance and height. Such tools as convolution (25), Fourier spectrum (26), and covariance (27) allow the description of parameters of structure, orientation, and periodicity, and fractal geometry gives access to parameters of texture (28).

Research teams involved in this area are still seeking data capture systems and measurement parameters adapted to quantifying microrelief. As a result, most publications are entitled ''A new method for. . .'' rather than ''Changes in skin texture with aging,'' for example.

V. AGE AND SKIN MICRORELIEF

Image analysis is too recent to have contributed entirely to the study of changes in skin microrelief with aging. Agache et al. (29) recently conducted an exhaustive review of the data acquired by means of profilometry and image analysis. It emerges that a certain number of similar findings have been reported by various teams studying different sites. Among these findings are the absence of sex-related differences and an increase in anisotropy with age, together with the lack of secondary lines and an increase in the distance between the primary lines plus their reorientation (Fig. 5). Opinion is divided with regard to the changes in the depth of skin furrows. Some profilometric studies have concluded that there is a decrease with age (30). In our opinion,

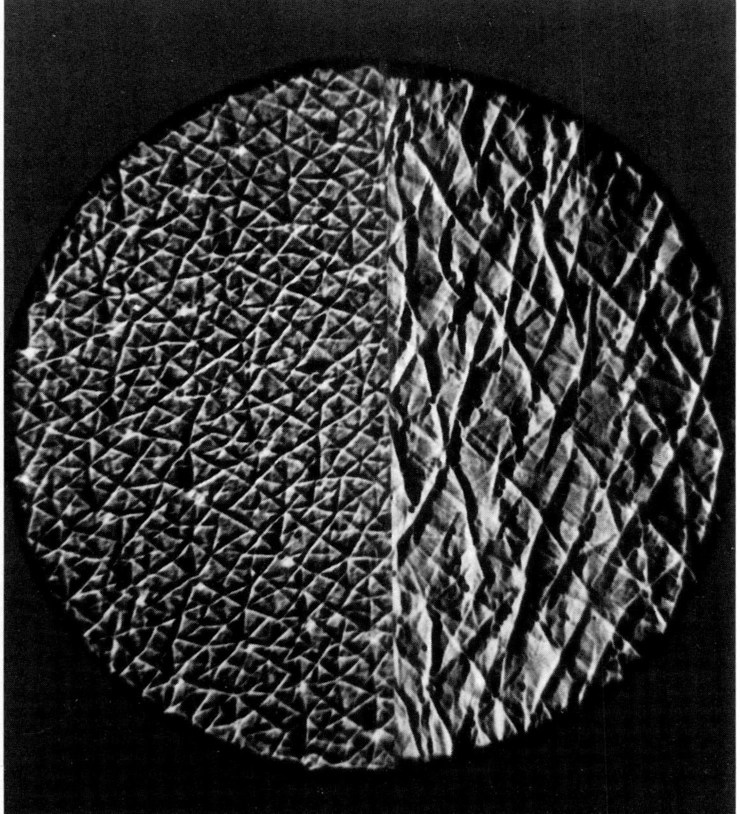

Figure 5 Montage of negative replicas from the volar forearm: left; star-shaped pattern of a 10-year-old child; right, irregular pattern of a 69-year-old woman.

this results from a bias introduced by the principle of the directional trace, since the authors did not take into account the reorientation of the primary lines with age.

The study on the cheek performed by Hayashi et al. (31) also provided complementary and contradictory data. Indeed, they reported a decrease in the roughness parameter that may correspond to a decrease in the depth of the primary lines. In contrast, they confirmed that the distance between the lines increases, that the anisotropy increases, and that there is a loss of periodicity of surface features with age. Finally, it is noteworthy that Nakayama et al. (21) reported ethnicity-related differences.

Each skin site adapts and deforms according to local tensions, which repeated throughout life, give rise to remodeling of skin texture (32). Experimentally, the best documented sites are the arm, the ventral face of the forearm, the leg, the abdomen, and the face.

As a result of the complexity of this remodeling, only studies based on image analysis have thus far been able to measure overall events. We now look at three examples in detail.

The volar forearm (33) can be considered a site that is relatively protected from sunlight and is therefore interesting for the study of the effects of aging per se. It is nonetheless exposed to frequent and extensive mechanical deformation, that is, flexion-extension and rotation. This probably explains why the deformation reservoir is high in children (CDSS = 1.16). Several phenomena are involved in the kinetics of aging: a progressive loss of the second

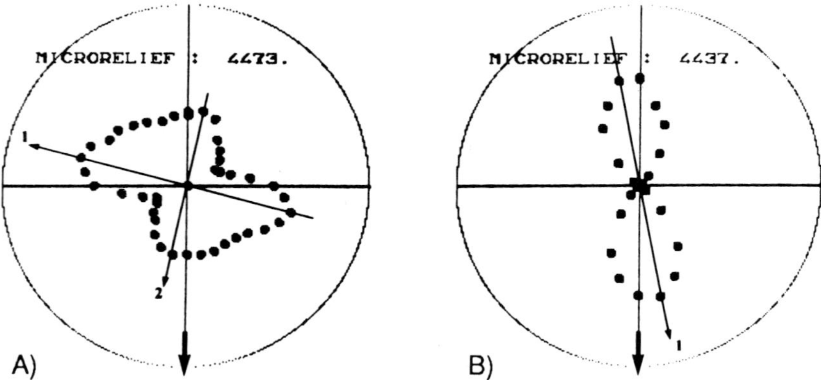

Figure 6 Typical roses of directions on the volar forearm. The vertical arrows indicate the long arm axis. (A) Young skin showing two perpendicular directions of furrows (butterfly image). (B) Aged skin with a single direction of furrows (helical aspect).

axis of skin furrows and a rotation of the first axis, which, from being approximately perpendicular to the axis of the arm in children, becomes almost parallel to it in the elderly (Fig. 6). Meanwhile, the furrows of the first axis deepen and, from the sixth decade of life onward, become more widely spaced. Despite the spacing of one axis and the disappearance of the other, the deformation reservoir increases progressively up to 1.22 in the elderly subject. This increase in the tissue reserve is a phenomenon generally observed during aging (Fig. 7).

The external face of the leg (34) is also a zone that is exposed little to the sun. In addition, it undergoes mechanical deformations of lower amplitude than the forearm. It is a site that ages slowly; indeed, the elderly retain furrows perpendicular to the axis of the limb. In contrast, as for the forearm, the other axis rotates to become parallel to the axis of the leg, that is, in the direction of the strongest constraints. The deformation requirements being low, the reservoir is small in children (CDSS = 1.02) and increases only moderately in the elderly (1.08).

The site that suffers most from the rigors of time and weather is the *face*. Here, things change very quickly. At the age of 25 years, crow's-foot wrinkles around the eye are permanently in place (Fig. 8). The site of the crow's-foot has been extensively studied for several reasons. An epidemiologic study by Daniell (35) concluded that this feature was reinforced in smokers. Measurements by Grove et al. (20) are noteworthy for two reasons: the study was multidirectional, and correlations between the morphometric parameters and

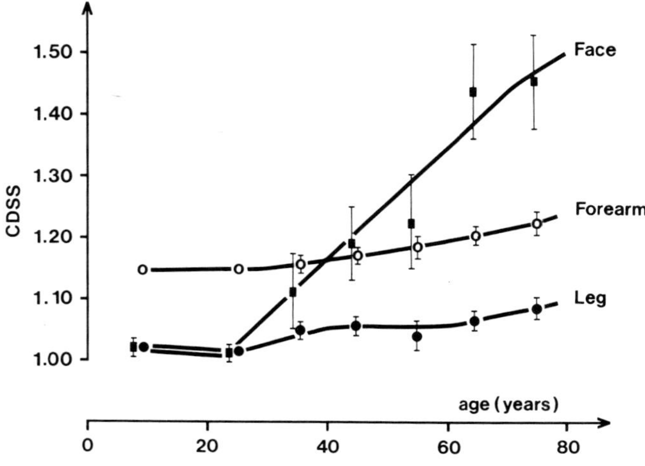

Figure 7 Evolution of the CDSS during aging at various body sites.

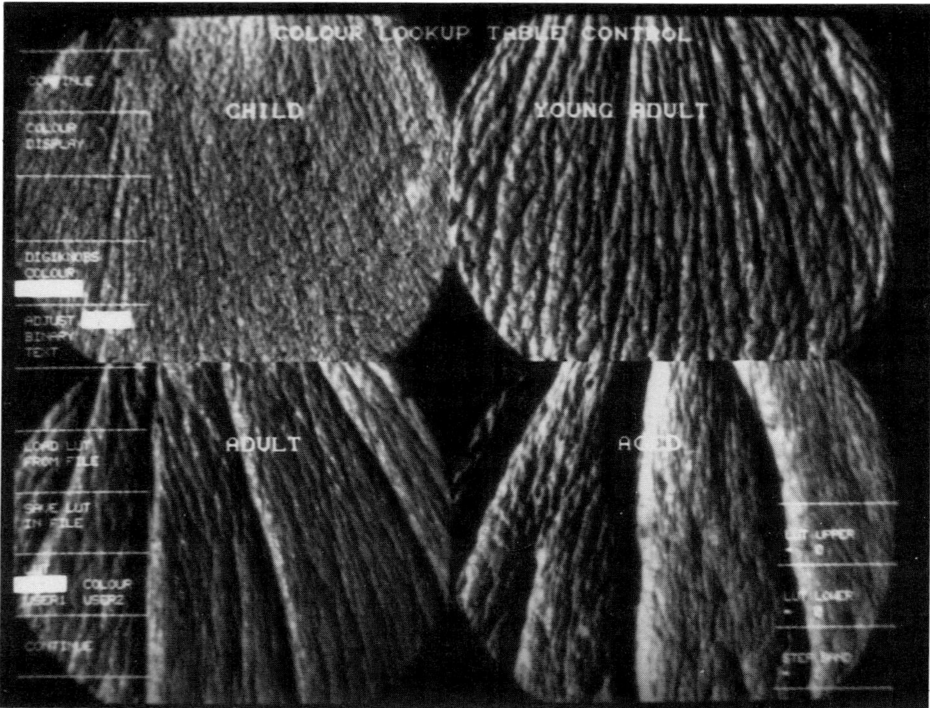

Figure 8   Crow's-foot area of the eye. Montage of stored images with the image analyzer.

Daniell's classification were attempted. Numerous extrinsic factors act synergistically in the aging of the face. There are very wide interindividual differences, as shown by the study of the depth of the furrows of the forearm and the crow's-foot wrinkles (Fig. 9). The corresponding anatomic features appear to be more deeply situated than those associated with microrelief (36). The crow's-foot of the eye presents characteristics that, overall, create an ex ceptional site. Indeed, it is not affected by joint movements, it is subject only to the actions of the facial muscles, at the point where the lower part of the face meets the forehead, and, unusually, is subject only to compression (in

Figure 9   Individual plots of furrow depth versus age: (A) on the volar forearm, the increase in depth starts in the fifties; (B) crow's-foot wrinkles increase in depth from 25 years of age. Notice the large individual variations.

100
80
Depth (µm)
60
r = 0·710
40
20
0   20   40   60   80   100
Age (years)

(A)

600
500
400
300
200
Depth (µm)
150
r = 0·394
100
75
50
25
0   20   40   60   80   100
Age (years)

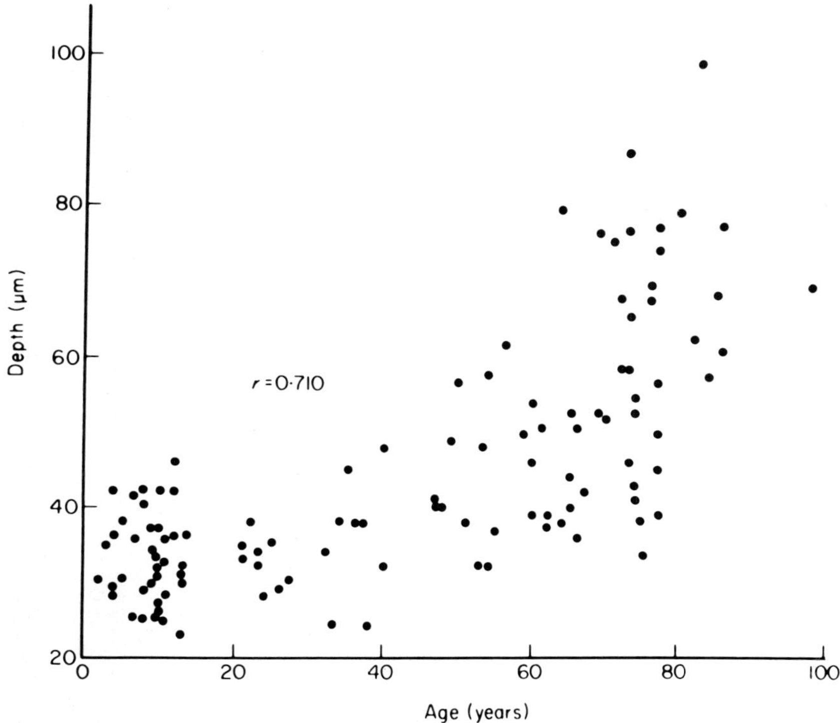

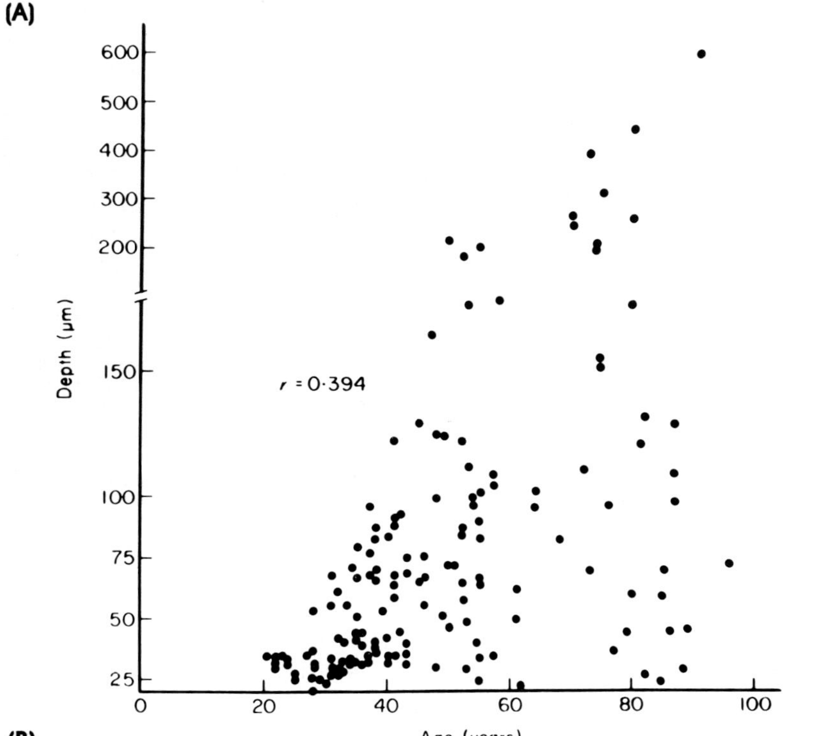

(B)

opposition to extension). This is perhaps why the deformation reservoir is small in children (CDSS = 1.02). This reservoir, which reaches 1.45 in an elderly population living in a temperate region, can easily exceed 2 in subjects who have been greatly exposed to the sun: the depth of the lines in these subjects can be measured in millimeters. At this level, one can speak of sunlight-accelerated aging, or *actinic aging*.

VI. EFFECTS OF ULTRAVIOLET LIGHT

The effects of ultraviolet (UV) light on the skin are well documented. This subject can be approached in several ways. Epidemiologic studies conducted by Australian researchers (37) on immigrant Anglo-Saxon populations in Australia, New Zealand, and South Africa are rich in information.

For obvious ethical reasons and to reduce the experimental time scale, most laboratory work on the effects of UV light on the skin have been done

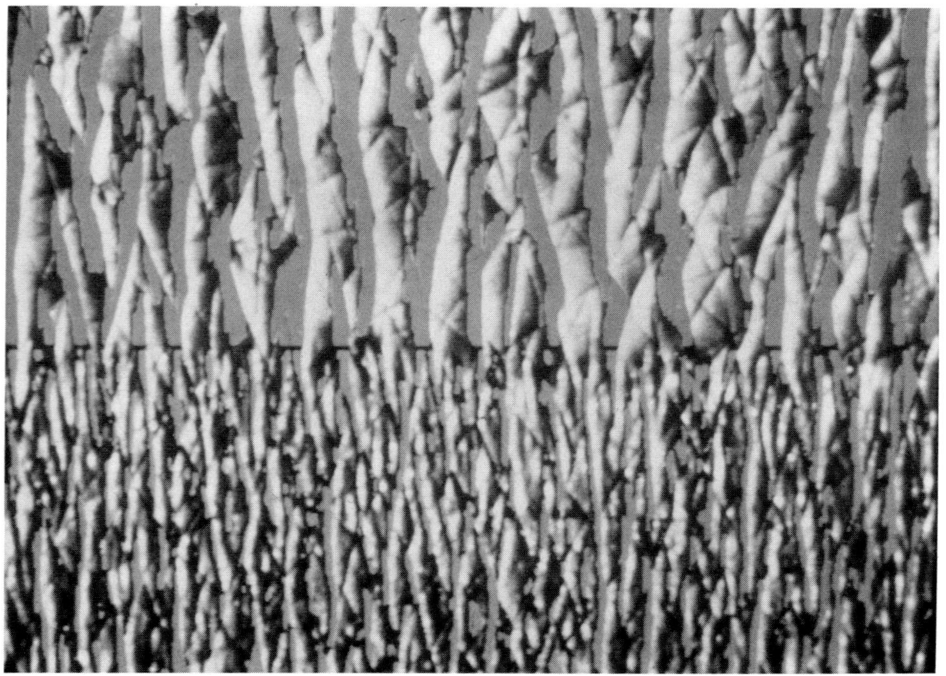

Figure 10 Automatic measurement of primary lines of the back of a volunteer who received a single UV irradiation of 2 MED: Lower binary overlay, shadows from the protected area; upper binary overlay, shadows from the irradiated area.

on animals. Standardized protocols exist for the study of microrelief in human by means of "noninvasive" methods (38): solar simulators can be used to deliver a known dose of UV of certain wavelengths. It has been shown that the application of single doses above the minimal erythemal dose (MED) leads to extensive changes a few days later in skin microrelief. This phenomenon resembles, in certain respects, that occurring during aging (Fig. 10). Indeed, there is an increase in the distance between the lines and their depth. However, there is no increase in the CDSS, contrary to the situation in aging.

Mathematic modeling of the skin surface based on the cyclöid arch (7) illustrates the differences between chronologic aging and the response to this type of stress (Fig. 11). These modifications are maximal between days 5 and 7 after exposure and thereafter decrease gradually. They represent the response of the skin to an acute UV aggression and probably reflect the cutaneous edema that follows the inflammatory reaction.

With regard to the effect of prolonged exposure to the sun, there are fewer experimental data. However, one recent study (39) also showed that furrow

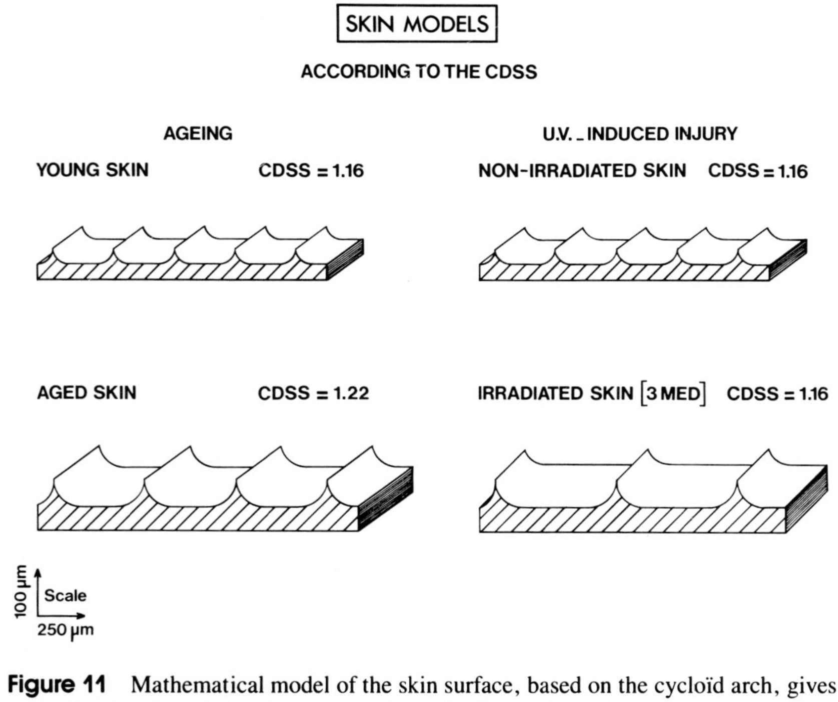

Figure 11 Mathematical model of the skin surface, based on the cyclöid arch, gives easy visualization of the changes in microrelief in evolving phenomena.

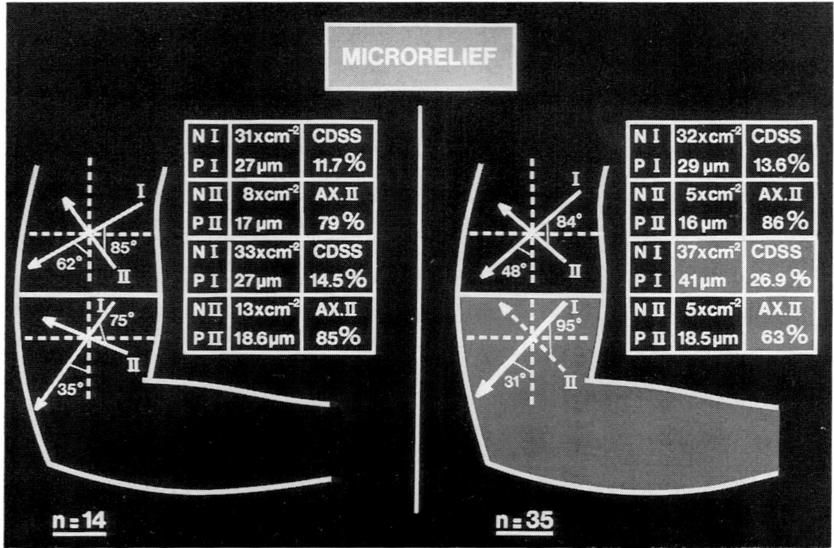

Figure 12 Comparative study of the arm of 14 sedentary subjects (left) and sun-exposed skin of 35 professional cyclists. N = line density; P = depth of furrows; I = first axis of furrows; II = second axis of furrows; AX.II = percentage of presence of the second axis of furrows in the population.

depth increases with an increase in line density. Under the particular experimental conditions of this study, the CDSS was greatly increased (Fig. 12).

VII. AGING, MECHANICAL PROPERTIES, AND MICRORELIEF

In fact, remodeling of the microrelief is an ongoing phenomenon that depends on the forces exerted by the subjacent dermis. This strict dependence has been studied by Ferguson and Barbenel (40), as well as by Takahashi and Marks (41) and ourselves (42). Dynamic tests of monoaxial tension show that simultaneous reorganization or reorientation takes place throughout the thickness of the skin, involving bundles of collagen fibers, Langer's lines, and the primary lines of the microrelief. When repeated throughout the life of an individual, these constraints eventually leave a permanent imprint on the surface pattern (Fig. 13). The deformation reservoir is called upon differently according to whether the skin is young or old (Fig. 14). It appears that the surface pattern, drawn according to the organization of the collagen bundles, in fact reflects the mechanical state of the elastic network responsible for holding the collagen fibers together (43). In our most recent study (44), con-

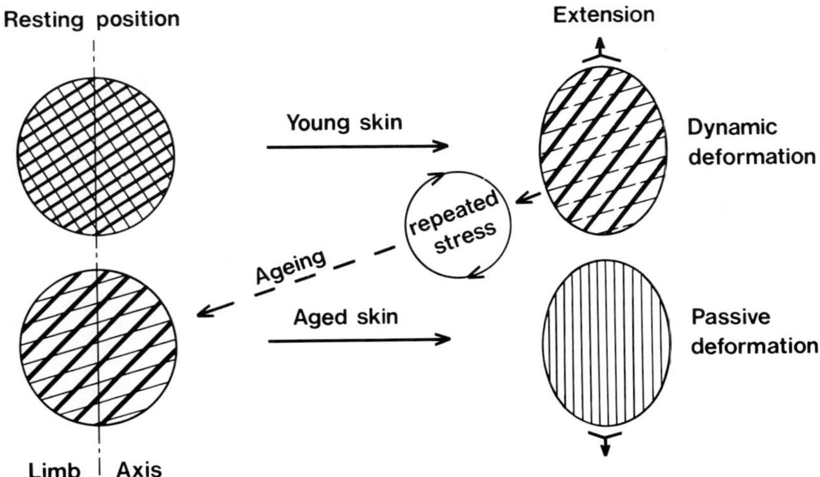

Figure 13 Hypothetical explanation of the evolution of microrelief during aging in relation to mechanical constraints.

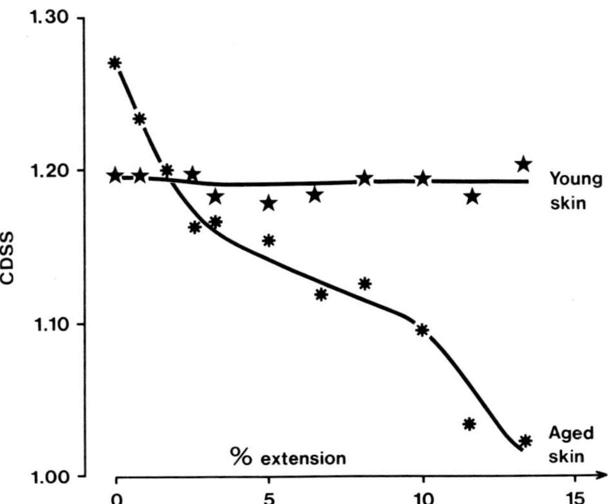

Figure 14 Role of the reservoir of deformation (CDSS) in young and aged skin when considering uniaxial stretching of the skin (volar forearm).

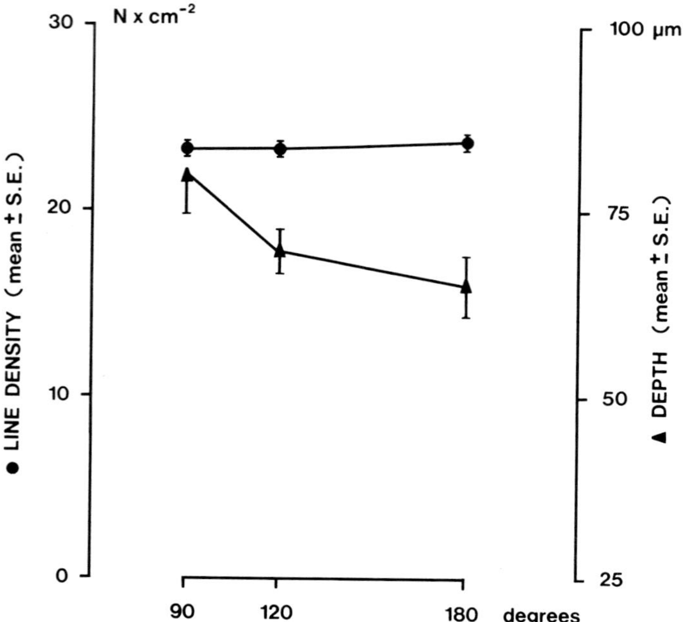

Figure 15 Evolution of microrelief parameters of the volar forearm in aged subjects (over 70 years old) according to the angle of the elbow joint. Notice the constancy in line density (24 cm^{-2}) associated with a weak standard error. A line density of 24 cm^{-2} equals an average distance of 400 μm between parallel furrows.

cerning the primary lines of the forearm of young adults and elderly subjects according to position, we found what appeared to be an "end point" in the aging process. This final image would correspond to the primary lines oriented parallel to the axis of the limb, with an average spacing of the order of 400 μm (Fig. 15); there is a very large tissue reserve (about 40%) that forms a "redundance," compensating for the loss of elasticity of the skin.

VIII. CONCLUSION

Since the beginning of the 1980s, image analysis has provided objective information on the development of lines and changes in the microrelief during aging. Unfortunately, the diversity of the techniques used makes it difficult to compare the results obtained by different teams: further standardization is therefore required. The advantages of this noninvasive method for studying the skin surface result from the strict relationships between the microrelief and the organization of the dermis.

However, the precise nature of these relationships remains mostly a matter of speculation. Dynamic tests reflect the mechanical properties of the skin and provide important clues. Our knowledge of this area is important for the objective evaluation of the antiaging treatments that today inundate the market. According to this recent technology, the evolution of dermal disorders, such as scleroderma, striae distensae, and those induced by corticotherapy, can be conveniently and precisely assessed, leading to follow-up of their eventual regression by therapy. The rapid improvement of image analyzers (higher performance and lower costs) will allow a great democratization of such investigations in the next few years.

REFERENCES

1. Graham JA, Kligman AM. Physical attractiveness cosmetic use and self perception in the elderly. Int J Cosmet Sci 1985; 7(2):85–98.
2. Hashimoto K. New methods for surface ultrastructure. Comparative studies of scanning electron microscopy, transmission electron microscopy and replica method. Int J Dermatol 1974; 13:357–81.
3. Marks R, Pearse AD. Surfometry: a method for evaluating the internal structure of the stratum corneum. Br J Dermatol 1971; 84:117.
4. Kadner H, Biesold C. Zur technik der Ranhigkeits messung der Hantoberflache mit derm Perth-O-Meter. Dermatol Monatsschr 1971; 157:758–9.
5. Makki S, Mignot J, Zahouani H, et al. Statistical analysis and three dimensional representation of human skin surface. J Soc Cosmet Chem 1984; 35:311–25.
6. Cook TH. Profilometry of skin. A useful tool for the substantation of cosmetic efficacy. J Soc Cosmet Chem 1980; 31:339–59.
7. Corcuff P, de Rigal J, Lévêque JL. Image analysis of the cutaneous microrelief. Bioeng Skin Newslett 1982; 4(1):16–31.
8. Mandelbrot B. The fractal geometry of nature. New York: W. H. Freeman, 1983.
9. Corcuff P, Chatenay F, Lévêque JL. A fully automated system to study skin surface patterns. Int J Cosmet Sci 1984; 6:167–76.
10. Tankosic P, Burlet C. Morphometric analysis of anisotropic and multioriented structure by use of an electronic image analyzer (Quantimet 720): application to the study of the human cutaneous microrelief. Acta Stereol 1986; 5(1):87–92.
11. Gormley DE. Computer models and images of the cutaneous surface. Dermatol Clin 1986; 4(4):641–9.
12. Nomine JP, Vincent L, Meyer F, Serra J, Escande JP, Arnaud-Battandier J. Cutaneous aging and mathematical morphology. Acta Stereol 1987; 6(3):895–900.
13. Kahn E, Roussel J, Gavoille A, Robert C, Robert A. Use of texture parameters in image analysis of human cutaneous microrelief. Acta Stereol 1987; 6(3): 889–94.
14. Miller DL. A simple, low cost image analysis system for evaluation of skin surface. Bioeng Skin 1987; 3(3):243.

15. Barton SP, Marshall RJ, Marks R. A novel method for assessing skin surface topography. Bioeng Skin 1987; 3:93–107.
16. Hoppe U, Sauermann G. Quantitative analysis of the skin surface by means of digital signal processing. J Soc Cosmet Chem 1985; 36:105–23.
17. Zahouani H. Quantification de la topographie des surfaces. Thesis 115, Besançon, France, 1989.
18. Awajan A, Rondot D, Mignot J. Quick method of measuring the furrows distribution on skin surface replicas. Med Biol Eng Comput 1989; 27(4):379–89.
19. Barton SP, Marks R. Image analysis as a tool for measuring biological phenomena of the skin. Int J Cosmet Sci 1988; 10:137–44.
20. Grove GL, Grove MJ, Leyden JJ. Optical profilometry: an objective method for quantification of facial wrinkles. J Am Acad Dermatol 1989; 21:631–7.
21. Nakayama Y, Kawasaki K, Kumagai H, Kaneko O, Mitsui T. Application of image analysis to the study of skin surface microtopography in relation to aging. J Appl Cosmet 1986; 4:97–110.
22. Awajan A, Rondot D, Mignot J, Agache P. Detection et quantification des plis principaux et secondaires de la peau par traitement et analyse d'images vidéo. Innov Tech Biol Med 1989; 10(1):53–67.
23. Corcuff P. A 3D approach of unflat surfaces by automatic image analysis: the skin microrelief. Acta Stereol 1987; 6(3):901–6.
24. Weibel E. Stereological methods (1 and 2). New York: Academic Press, 1989.
25. Rosenfeld A, Kak AC. Digital picture processing (1 and 2). New York: Academic Press, 1982.
26. Russ JC. Computer assisted microscopy. Raleigh: North Carolina State University, 1988.
27. Serra J. Image analysis and mathematical morphology. London: Academic Press, 1984.
28. Flook AG. A comparison of quantitative methods of shape representation. Acta Stereol 1984; 3(2):159–64.
29. Agache PG, Mignot J, Makki S. Microtopography of the skin and aging. In: Kligman AM, Takase Y, eds. Cutaneous Aging. Tokyo: University of Tokyo Press, 1988.
30. Mignot J, Zahouani H, Rondot D, Nardin PH. Morphological study of human skin relief Bioeng Skin 1987; 3:177–96.
31. Hayashi S, Mimura K, Nishijima Y. Changes in surface configuration of the skin caused by aging and application of cosmetics: three-dimensional analysis according to a new system based on image analysis and Fourier transform. Int J Cosmet Sci 1989; 11:67–85.
32. Lapiere CM. The aging dermis: the main cause for the appearance of "old" skin. Br J Dermatol 1990; 122(35):5–12.
33. Corcuff P, de Rigal J, Makki S, Lévêque JL, Agache P. Skin relief and aging. J Soc Cosmet Chem 1983; 34:177–90.
34. Corcuff P, Lévêque JL, Grove GL, Kligman AM. The impact of aging on the microrelief of peri-orbital and leg skin. J Soc Cosmet Chem 1987; 82:145–52.

35. Daniell HW. Smoker's wrinkle. A study in the epidemiology of "crow's feet." Ann Intern Med 1971; 75:873–80.
36. Pierard G, Lapiere CM. The microanatomical basis of facial frown lines. Arch Dermatol 1989; 125:1090–2.
37. Holman CDJ, Armstrong BK, Evans PR, et al. Relationship of solar keratosis and history of skin cancer to objective measures of actinic skin damage. Br J Dermatol 1984; 110:129–38.
38. Corcuff P. Stereology of the skin surface: a comparison between aging and UV-induced damages. In: Morganti P, Montagna W, eds. Cosmetic dermatology. Roma: International Ediemme, 1986; 157–63.
39. Corcuff P, Francois AM, Lévêque JL, Porte G. Microrelief changes in chronically sun-exposed human skin. Photodermatology 1988; 5:92–5.
40. Ferguson J, Barbenel JC. Skin surface patterns and the directional mechanical properties of the dermis. In: Marks R, Payne PA, eds. Bioengineering and the skin. London: MTP Press, 1981; 83–92.
41. Takahashi M, Marks R. Conformational and functional changes in the stratum corneum after forced extension. Bioeng Skin 1986; 2:39–48.
42. Corcuff P, Gracia AM, de Lacharrière O, Lévêque JL. Image analysis of the skin microrelief as a non-invasive method to approach the dermal architecture. In: Pierard GE, Pierard-Franchimont C, eds. The dermis. Liege, Belgium: Monographies dermatologiques liégeoises, 1989; 102–13.
43. Imayama S, Braverman M. A hypothetical explanation for the aging of skin. Am J Pathol 1989; 134(5):1019–25.
44. Corcuff P, de Lacharrière O, Lévêque JL. Extension induced changes in the microrelief of the human volar forearm: variation with age. J Gerontol Med Sci 1991, 46(6):223–27.

14

Size and Shape of Corneocytes at Various Body Sites: Influence of Age

PIERRE CORCUFF and JEAN-LUC LÉVÊQUE

L'Oréal
Aulnay-sous-Bois, France

I. INTRODUCTION

Our knowledge of the size of horny cells in the stratum corneum has greatly improved over the last two decades with the development of technical methods, leading to a better understanding of their biologic and physiologic roles. Obtaining corneocyte samples from the skin surface, first performed by Wolf in 1939 (1), has now become one of the simplest noninvasive techniques. With regard to the biologic significance of these dead cells, if we can decipher the "mummified" messages they contain, we shall obtain precious information on the physiology of the deep epidermis. An important step forward was made by Grove and Kligman (2), who showed that a relationship existed between the projected area of corneocytes and the rate of epidermal turnover.

The physiologic function of corneocytes is related to their peculiar shape, which is adapted to the construction of a barrier against environmental aggression. Several teams have shown the relationship between the projected area of corneocytes and the penetration of various substances, on the one hand (3–5), and transepidermal water loss, on the other (6, 7).

However, the intense series of measurements started by Plewig at the beginning of the 1970s (8, 9), leading to the publication of the textbook *Stratum*

199

Corneum in 1983 (10), was not founded on Wolf's technique but on the McGinley group's adaptation (11) of Williamson's method for sampling cutaneous bacterial flora (12). This technique permits the observation of isolated corneocytes, essential for accurate measurements and morphologic studies.

II. CORNEOCYTE SAMPLING METHODS

Among the various corneocyte sampling methods proposed in the literature, only two have stood the test of time: the detergent scrub technique and the stripping technique.

A. Detergent Scrub Technique

This is the method that has engendered the most important advances in the field of cutaneous desquamation and corneocyte morphology. The skin is wet with phosphate buffer containing 0.1% Triton X-100, a nonionic detergent, and gently scraped; the suspension obtained contains a majority of isolated

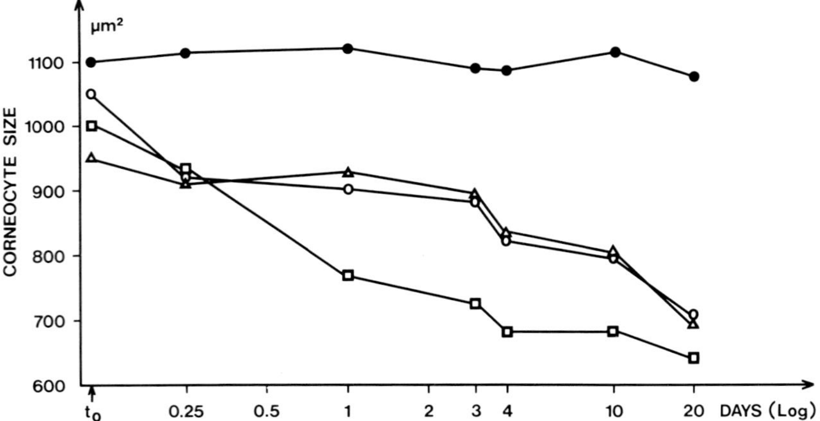

Figure 1 Evolution of the mean projected area of corneocytes with time, according to sampling procedures and relative humidity (RH): corneocytes in phosphate buffer and Triton X-100 (scrub method; solid circles); corneocytes on Corneodisc, RH = 50% (open circles); corneocytes on Corneodisc, RH = 10% (triangles); corneocytes on Corneodisc, RH = 90% (squares). Samples were obtained from adjacent areas of the volar forearm of a male subject aged 45 and kept at room temperature. Corneocyte size was determined from measurement of 500 cells by automatic image analysis (Quantimet 970).

corneocytes. A preliminary study (13) showed that such suspensions typically contain 70% individual corneocytes, 10% cell debris, 20% corneocyte aggregates, and less than 1% artefacts. Further developments of the method with a view to standardizing the number of cells obtained in no way affect the morphology of the corneocytes obtained. Certain authors have proposed motorized appliances with or without scraping of the skin surface (14, 15). These automatic procedures have influenced not the size but the number of cells obtained per unit area of skin.

One advantage of the detergent scrub method is that the cells are in osmotic equilibrium in the sampling solution. The samples can be stored for lengthy periods without modifying the projected area of the corneocytes, as shown in Figure 1. The use of a preservative (NaN_3) is recommended for long storage periods.

B. Stripping Method

Although it was developed before the detergent scrub technique, few studies have been published concerning corneocytes isolated by the stripping method. There are several reasons for this: in particular, contrary to the detergent scrub method, the population of single (i.e., measurable) cells is relatively small. Other problems involve the reproducibility of the harvesting technique, the choice of adhesive, and the optical quality of the sample. Nonetheless, most teams have used the technique, and Plewig (8) reported that the results obtained did not differ from those of the detergent scrub technique, stating that ''the effect of moisture, air drying, with or without a coating film of immersion oil, can be neglected.''

Because attempts to revive corneocytes by dissolving the adhesive have given unsatisfactory results, we designed a new sampler, the Corneodisc. Its main advantages are that the support is semirigid, the adhesive is adapted to the task, and the adhesive and support are perfectly transparent and homogeneous. The use of the corneodisc facilitates the sampling procedure and increases the number of individual corneocytes available for measurement. If the sample contains an excessive number of cells, it can be reduced by counterstripping. The optical quality of the sample is such that the corneocytes can be measured by means of automated techniques with no prior staining. Figure 2 shows the quality of the images obtained.

In contrast, Plewig's statement must be reexamined. As shown in Figure 1, the projected area of the corneocytes decreases rapidly with time, particularly under conditions of high relative humidity. Indeed, under these conditions the cell contour becomes rounded and the cells themselves become more transparent, probably as a result of ''ballooning.''

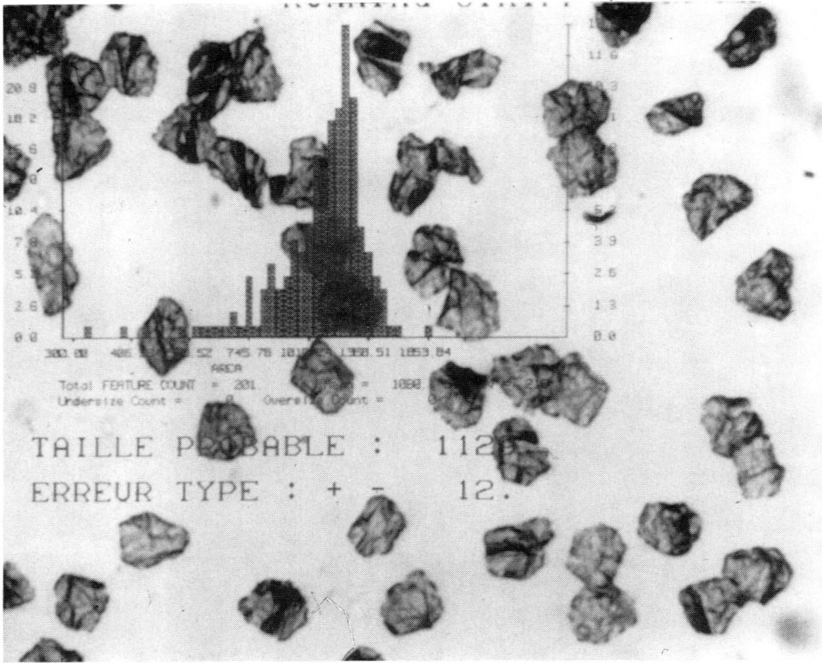

Figure 2 Corneocytes on Corneodisc as seen on the television display of the Quantimet 970. Note the good contrast of unstained features. Histogram and results are overlaid at the end of the automatic measuring procedure.

In addition, the projected area immediately after stripping is almost always smaller than that of suspended corneocytes of the same origin (Table 1). Finally, as shown in figure 3, there is a weak linear correlation between the results obtained by the two methods. Our interpretation is that measurements recorded immediately after stripping are representative of the state of the corneocytes in situ (humidity conditions in the stratum corneum), whereas suspended cells are in a state of equilibrium with the reference buffer.

The large changes in corneocyte size with time (-15% in 24 h) mean that measurements must be performed immediately.

III. MORPHOLOGIC FEATURES OF CORNEOCYTES

The peculiar ''disklike'' geometry of corneocytes means that a minimum of only two measurements are required to describe them: the projected area and the thickness.

Table 1 Comparison of the Projected Surface Area of Corneocytes Harvested by Two Different Methods.[a]

Sample	Stripping	Detergent
1	992	1061
2	1023	1110
3	837	1023
4	800	965
5	769	1022
6	996	940
7	1019	1210
8	906	1060
9	960	1025
10	810	945
11	964	992
12	964	1000
13	837	966
14	837	979
15	1074	1243
16	842	862
17	882	991
18	728	800
19	878	938

[a]Samples come from two adjacent areas of the volar forearm of 19 adults. Results are expressed in $\mu m2$.

A. Projected Area

This parameter is evaluated using an optical microscope, since the corneocyte has a diameter of approximately 50 μm. Different teams use manual methods (16) based on planimetry, semiautomatic methods (17) based on microspectrophotometry, or automated methods (18) based on image analyzers. None of these methods introduce a significant technical bias, so that results can be compared from one team to another.

Whether manual or automated, measurements performed on corneocyte suspensions containing 70% representative elements lead to "robust" statistical estimations. Most authors agree on the small variations in corneocyte size within a given sample.

It is generally considered that 50 manual measurements give the mean projected area to within 3%; 500 automated measurements give 1% accuracy. In contrast, the projected area of corneocytes is affected by various intrinsic and environmental factors. Some intrinsic factors appear to have little influence,

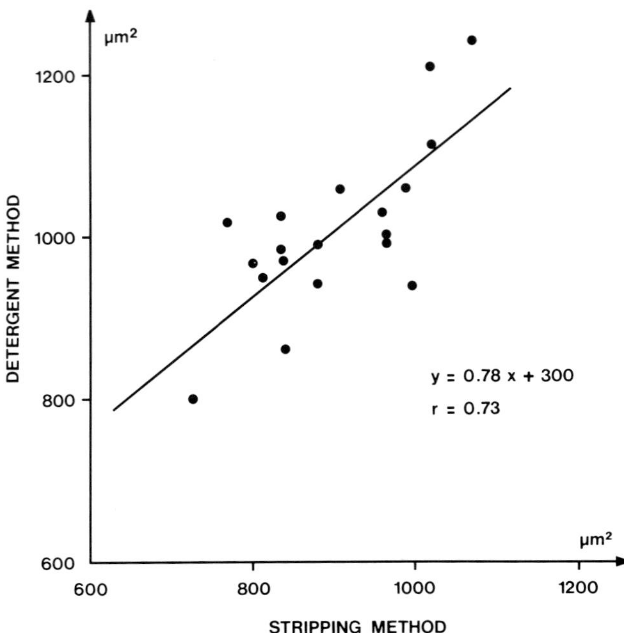

Figure 3   Linear correlation between the sizes of corneocytes reported in Table 1.

such as ethnicity (9, 18–21) and sex (9, 19, 20), whereas site (8) and age—
which we shall consider later—are more important. Disease states clearly
play an important role (22, 23), as does skin dryness (24).

Extrinsic factors include the seasons (25), sunlight (26), mechanical friction (27), chemical irritants (28), cosmetic agents (29), and medical treatment (30). With one or two exceptions (31), these factors induce concomitant
modifications of epidermal activity.

Most workers in this field agree that there is an inverse relationship between epidermal turnover and the projected area of corneocytes. In other
words, an increase in epidermal turnover due to an aggression (UV light or
irritation, for example) is reflected by a reduction in corneocyte size; slowing
of epidermal turnover (e.g., during aging) leads to an increase in size (32).

B. Thickness

Whereas corneocyte diameter is measured using optical instruments, their
thickness (less than 1 μm) is close to the limit of resolution of the classic light
microscope (0.6 μm). This makes it difficult to measure diameter and thickness at the same time. In an early work, Marks et al. (7) compared the modal

volume of a corneocyte population, measured using a Coulter counter, with its mean projected area determined by planimetry. Although the thickness value obtained by this method is a rough approximation, the results suggested that no corneocyte flattening occurred with aging, contrary to general opinion.

The interferometric method used by Plewig et al. (33) is better adapted to this type of measurement, since the resolution is of the order of 10 nm. Unfortunately, it has not been widely used because it is a delicate procedure and permits only simple statistical analysis. Although this method has shown variations in corneocyte thickness according to anatomic site, it has provided no information concerning age-related changes.

Confocal microscopy (34), a novel technology, gives three-dimensional images and may provide a new approach to this problem, although the resolution is only 0.15 μm in the Z axis. Figure 4 shows that the diameter and

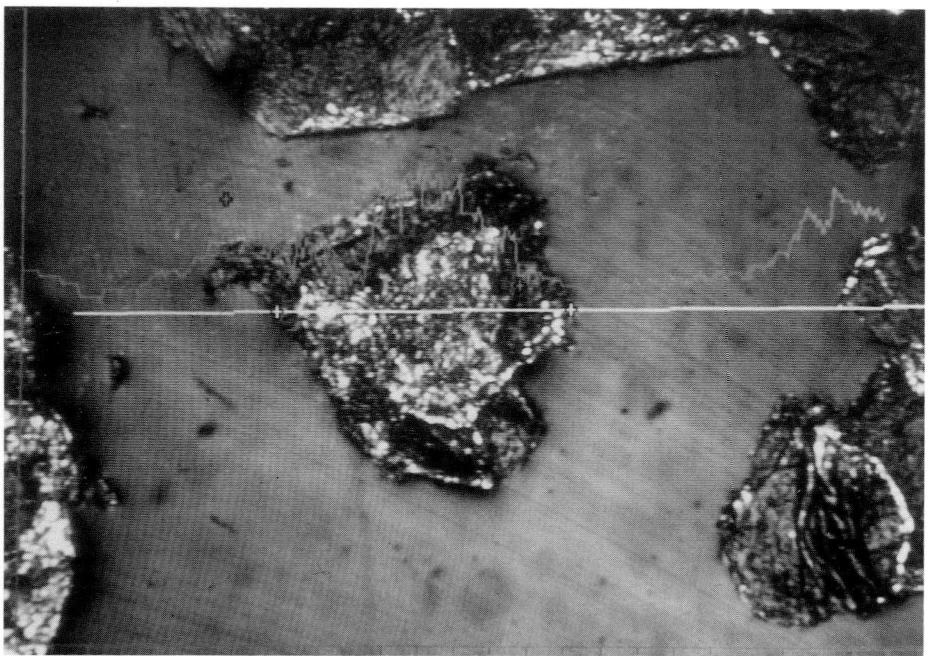

Figure 4 Confocal image of a single corneocyte obtained with the tandem scanning reflected light microscope (TSM, Tracor). This image is the three-dimensional reconstruction from 50 optical sections 0.1 μm in depth performed by Misis Image (St. Etienne, France). The altitude profile corresponds to the line crossing the corneocyte. Measurements are recorded using two pointers: diameter 40 μm and mean thickness approximately 0.55 μm.

thickness of corneocytes can be measured simultaneously. The altitude profile shows that thickness is variable and must therefore be determined using a statistical method.

The first results obtained give a corneocyte thickness of between 0.3 and 0.5 µm, compared with 0.2–0.4 µm according to Plewig et al. and 0.6–1.0 µm according to Marks et al. Whatever the true value, the influence of aging on this parameter remains to be studied.

C. Corneocyte Morphology

The qualitative description of corneocyte morphology is made at two levels. In the first, light microscopy is used to describe the overall shape (hexagonal, pentagonal, or elliptical) and the presence or absence of nuclear debris (35) (phantoms and remnants) and trabeculae. In the second, scanning electron microscopy is used to describe the surface aspect of the corneocyte envelope, the presence or absence of microvilli, and the density and depth of folds (Fig.

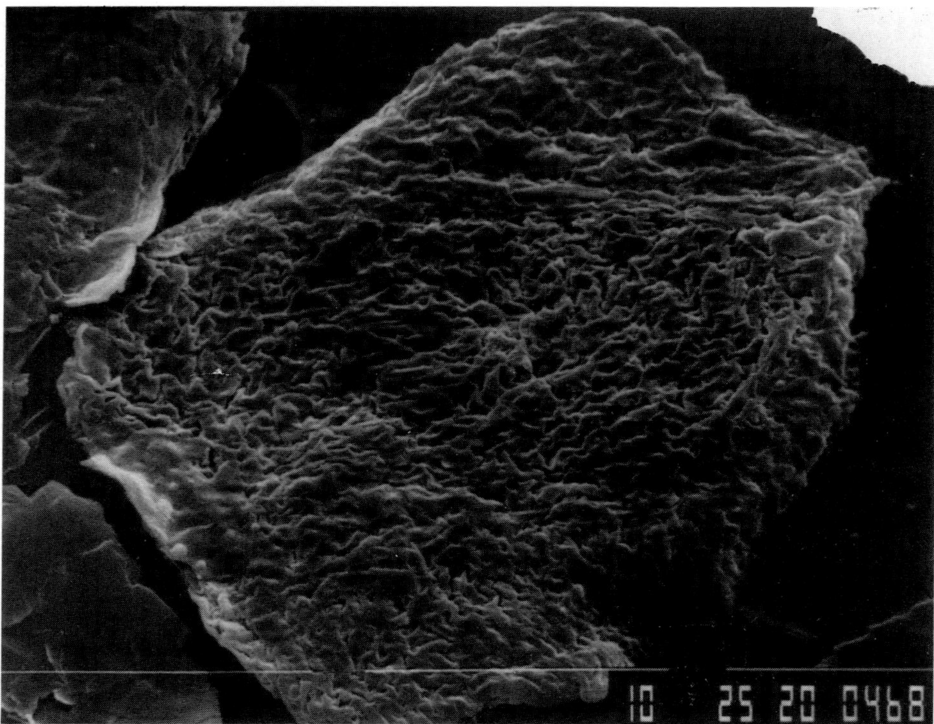

Figure 5   Surface aspect of a corneocyte by scanning electron microscopy.

5). Corneocytes are not dealt with in the following section because they do not appear to change with age (36).

The "healthy" corneocyte, in both young and aged subjects, has an essential function, that is, protecting the skin and limiting exchanges. The hexagonal shape is in no way a chance occurrence: it is a good compromise between the circle (minimal projected area) and a geometric form that avoids the existence of "chinks in the armor" (leaks and penetration) and excessive thickness, since each edge interlocks with the neighboring corneocyte. It is therefore the most economical and effective protective shape. Nature does not respect mathematic models. Thus, the corneocyte often takes a pentagonal shape (Fig. 6).

The recent purification of cornified envelopes (40) has revealed the existence of two morphologically different classes: a polygonal form with a rigid texture and an irregular shape with a fragile appearance. The fragile envelopes are found in the stratum compactum, whereas the stratum disjunction contains almost rigid envelopes. Each class could represent a different step in maturation of the corneocyte. We see later how to interpret the various proportions of these forms in relation to aging.

IV. INFLUENCE OF AGE

As we have just seen, most of the information available in the literature concerns measurements of the projected area of corneocytes obtained by the detergent scrub method. Although Plewig (9) initially found a sex-related difference in corneocyte size (generally larger in female subjects), this was not borne out in later studies by Plewig himself (25) or by other teams (19, 20, 37). Because no ethnicity-related difference has been found, either (8, 18, 19, 21), one might expect the results obtained by the various workers in this field to concur. However, seasonal variations and the presence of uncontrolled inflammatory conditions can engender significant differences.

The most important source of variation is the anatomic site studied. Most workers have studied the arm, either the forearm (volar and dorsal) or the upper arm (inner and outer). Figure 7 shows the values obtained for the forearm by various teams (7, 9, 20, 38). As can be seen, there is relative agreement between the teams, and there is a clear linear relationship between age and corneocyte size, with changes starting at birth.

Figure 8 shows corresponding data obtained for the upper arm. Although there are stronger disagreements between the results of the various teams, the general pattern of change is the same. These two sites can be considered relatively protected (by clothing) from external aggression and mechanical insult. Studies concerning sites that are better protected, such as the chest (39)

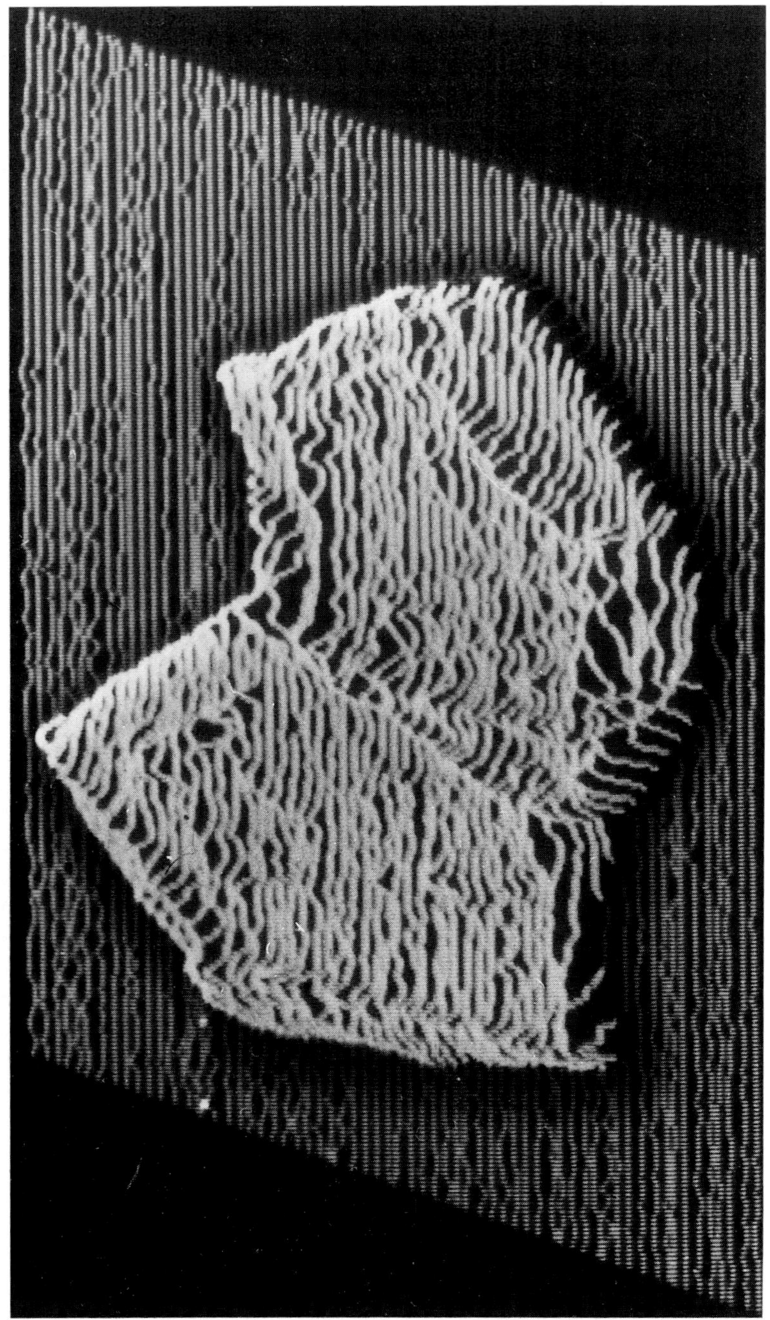

Figure 6 Confocal image of corneocytes showing a pentagonal contour. Trabeculae are clearly drawn. (From Zeiss.)

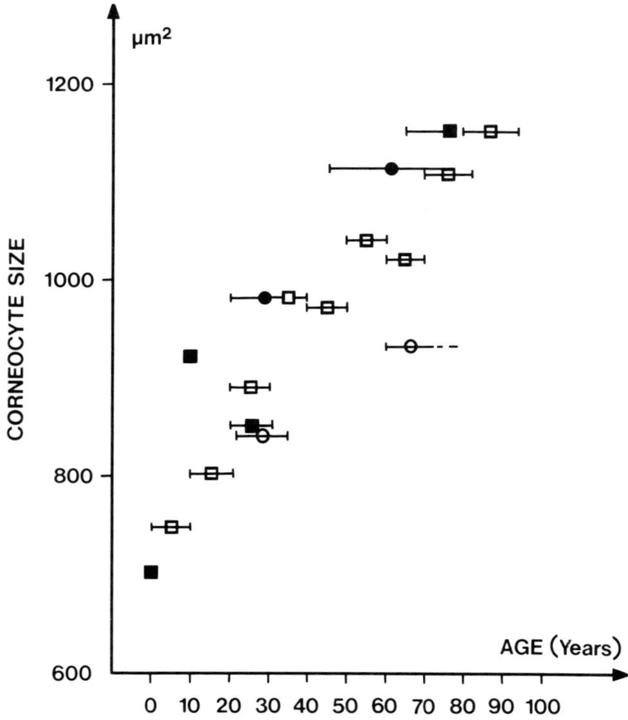

Figure 7 Evolution of the corneocyte size versus age on the forearm. Data from Plewig (9) (solid squares); Marks et al. (7) (solid circles); Grove et al. (20) (open circles); Lévêque et al. (38) (open squares).

and the abdomen (9, 19), fully confirm the linear relationship between corneocyte size and age.

However, this rule does not apply to all body sites. Indeed, the changes in the corneocytes of the forehead are rather anomalous. As shown in Figure 9, the data obtained by various teams are widely divergent. A projected area of 555 μm^2 in subjects of the 20–30 year age group has even been reported (4). In addition, it appears that the projected area is larger in newborn and pre-pubertal children than in adults below the age of 50 years. This raises the possible role of hormonal interactions (sebaceous function).

Comparison of age-related changes in the size of corneocytes from ''protected'' and ''exposed'' sites provides additional information. Figure 10 summarizes the changes reported for two protected sites (leg and forearm) and

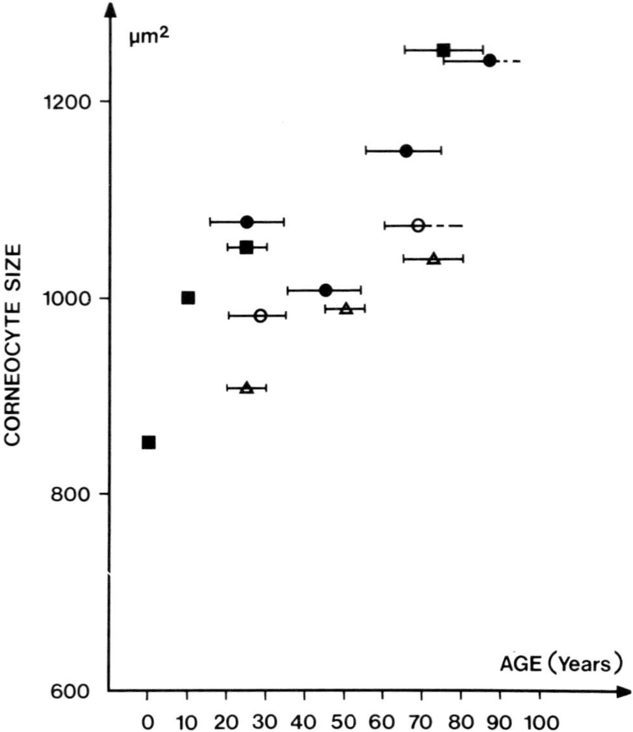

Figure 8 Evolution of corneocyte size versus age on the upper arm. Data from Rougier et al. (4) (open triangles). All other data as listed in Figure 7.

two exposed sites (back of the hand and cheek). The protected sites show similar linear changes with age; the exposed sites also show parallel changes, but these are not linear with age. Corneocyte size remains stable between the ages of 25 and 55 years; thereafter, the curves rapidly join those of the protected sites.

Overall, these results suggest that from the earliest age all sites change at the same rate (identical slopes) but with different starting points. As a result, the projected area of corneocytes may be predetermined (genetically) according to the aggression each site will undergo during life, the smallest cells being in the most exposed areas. The plateau that occurs during adulthood is in accordance with the observation (26) that, in the presence of aggression (e.g., UV radiation), epidermal turnover remains high, giving rise to smaller

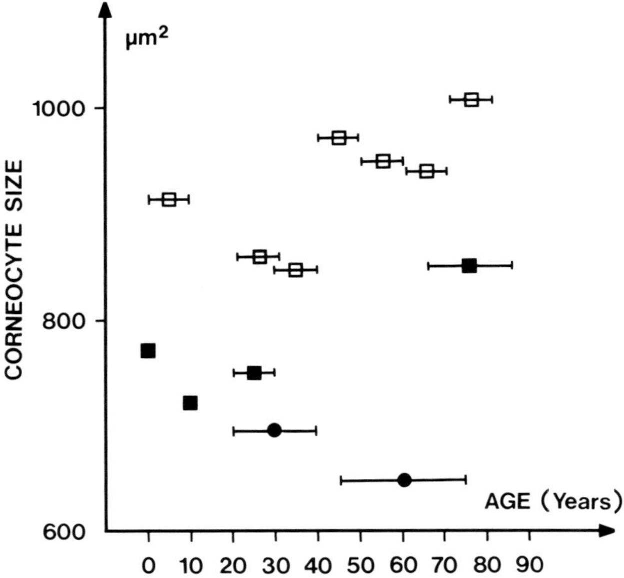

Figure 9 Evolution of the corneocyte size versus age on the forehead. Data from Corcuff (unpublished results; open squares). All other data as listed in Figure 7.

corneocytes. The sharp increase in size observed around the age of 60 years might correspond to both a more sedentary life-style (reduced aggression) and exhaustion of the capital of epidermal cells (reduced turnover).

A recent study concerning changes in morphology of cornified envelopes with age confirms the increase in corneocyte size (R. Aubert, E. Picard, R. Bazin, and E. Soudant, personal communication). It gives additional information on the degree of maturation of horny cells: the proportion of rigid envelopes increases with age. This means a higher ratio of mature corneocytes in the stratum corneum of aged people. Such evolution could be related to important changes in cutaneous barrier function as recorded in aged people from penetration measurements.

V. ACTINIC AGING

The various changes according to the degree of exposure of the anatomic site to the environment raise the question of the impact of photoaging on corneocyte size. Among the extrinsic factors that may influence this parameter,

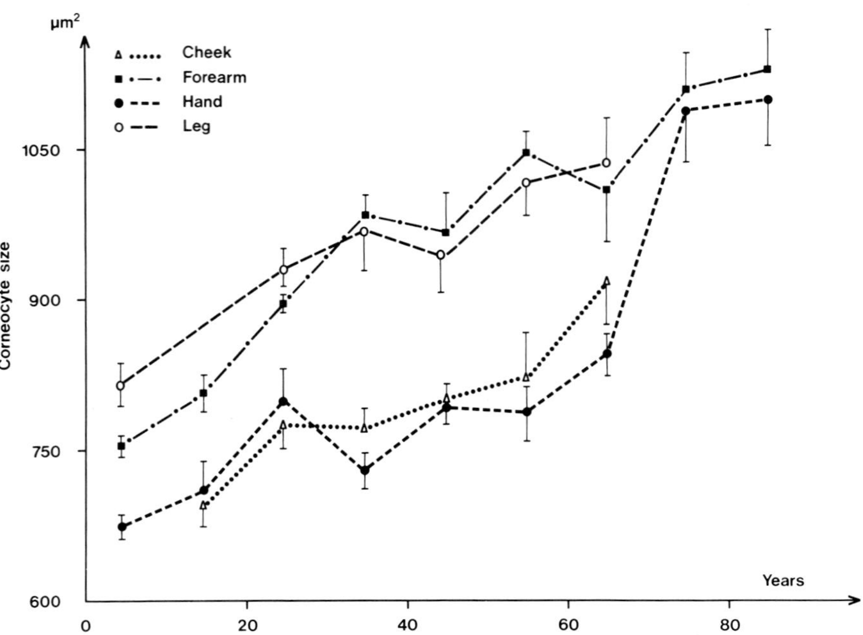

Figure 10 Comparative evolution of the corneocyte size (mean ± standard error of the mean) versus age at various body sites.

ultraviolet radiation (i.e., sunlight) appears to play the principal role, for the following reasons. First, it was shown by Mackenzie (31) that mechanical friction does not alter the projected area of corneocytes. Second, Herrman et al. (25) found that corneocytes are smaller in summer than in winter. Finally, we showed that this reduction in size during summer is more marked in populations particularly exposed to the sun (26).

In skin subject to inflammation of pathologic, mechanical, clinical, or therapeutic origin, the acceleration of epidermal turnover is associated with a decrease in corneocyte size. UV-induced erythema does not escape this rule, as shown in Figure 11, with a maximal reduction in size 20 days after exposure.

This time lag is approximately that taken for the keratinocytes to transit to the skin surface (41,42), assuming that desquamation has not been strongly disturbed. The duration of this size reduction is short when the irradiation is virtually instantaneous. In contrast, if exposure is chronic (sunlight), the corneocytes remain reduced in size as long as the aggression persists. In a study of professional cyclists (43), we found that the size of corneocytes from the

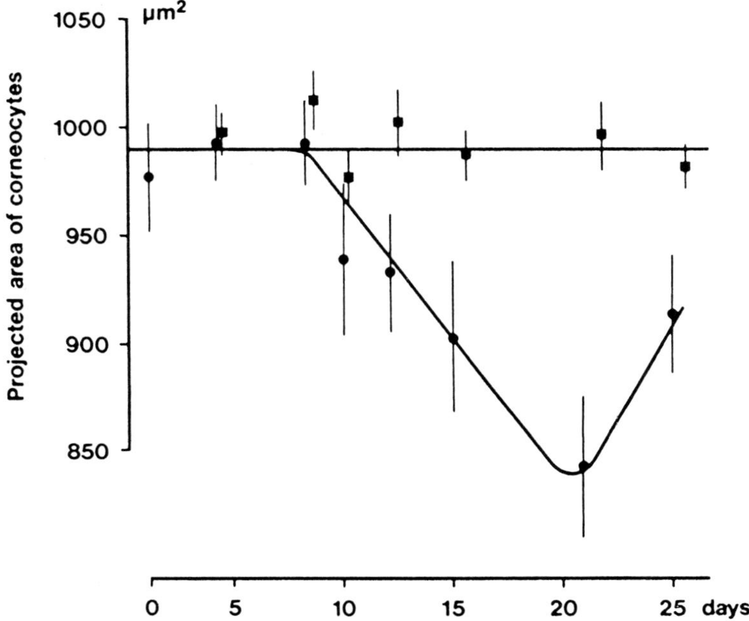

Figure 11 Changes in corneocyte size on the back of volunteers following a single UV irradiation of 2 MED: protected area (squares); irradiated area (circles).

area of the arm protected by the shirt was "normal" (936 μm^2), but in the adjacent, exposed area the projected area was smaller (810 μm^2).

If corneocyte size is reduced permanently by exposure, this parameter might serve as a marker of photoaging. Unfortunately, as seen earlier, size changes continue the normal course when the aggressive factor disappears. Although this does not mean that corneocytes do not bear the hallmarks of photoaging, these remain to be discovered.

VI. CONCLUSION

The main advantages of studying corneocyte size are the simplicity and rapidity of sample collection and measurement. The noninvasive technique provides immediate information concerning the living layers of the epidermis. This rapid diagnostic tool can be applied to all anatomic sites. Furthermore, corneocyte size can be used as a marker of inflammation or biologic aging but does not reflect permanent actinic aging. Doubtless the corneocyte contains other messages so—back to work!

REFERENCES

1. Wolf J. Die innere Struktur der Zellen des Stratum desquamans der menschlichen Epidermis. Z Mikrosk Anat Forsch 1939; 46:170–202.
2. Grove GL, Kligman AM. Corneocyte size as an indirect measure of epidermal poliferative activity. In: Marks R, Plewig G. eds. Stratum corneum. Berlin: Springer Verlag, 1983; 191–5.
3. Zesch A, Schaefer H, Hoffman W. Barriere und reservoir funktion der einzelnen Hornschichtlagen der menschlichen haut fur lokal aufgetragene Arzneimittel. Arch Dermatol Res 1973; 246:103–7.
4. Rougier A, Lotte C, Corcuff P, Maibach HI. Relationship between skin permeability and corneocyte size according to anatomic site, age and sex in man. J Soc Cosmet Chem 1988; 39:15–26.
5. Elias PM, Cooper ER, Korc A, Brown BE. Percutaneous transport in relation to stratum corneum structure and lipid composition. J Invest Dermatol 1980; 76:297–301.
6. Wilson DR, Maibach HI. A review of transepidermal water loss: physical aspects and measurements as related to infants and adults. In: Ed: Maibach HI, Boisits EK, eds. Neonatal skin. New York: Marcel Dekker, 1982; 83–100.
7. Marks R, Nicholls S, King CS. Studies on isolated corneocytes. Int J Cosmet Sci 1981; 3:251–8.
8. Plewig G, Marples RR. Regional differences of cell sizes in the human stratum corneum. I. J Invest Dermatol 1970: 54:13–8.
9. Plewig G. Regional differences of cell sizes in the human stratum corneum. II. Effects of sex and age. J Invest Dermatol 1970; 54:19–23.
10. Marks R, Plewig G, eds. Stratum Corneum. Berlin: Springer Verlag, 1983.
11. McGinley KJ, Marples RR, Plewig G. A method for visualizing and quantitating the desquamating portion of the human stratum corneum. J Invest Dermatol 1969; 53:107–11.
12. Williamson P, Kligman AM. A new method for the quantitative investigation of cutaneous bacteria. J Invest Dermatol 1965; 45:498–503.
13. Corcuff P, Delesalle G, Schaefer H. Quantitative aspect of corneocytes. J Soc Cosmet Chem 1982; 33:1–7.
14. Marks R. Quantification of desquamation and stratum corneum cohesivity. In: ed. Lévêque JL, Cutaneous investigation in health and disease. New York: Marcel Dekker, 1989; 33–47.
15. Corcuff P, Chatenay F, Saint-Léger D. Hair skin relationships: a new approach to desquamation. Bioeng Skin 1985; 1:133–9.
16. Marks R, Barton SP. The significance of the size and shape of corneocytes. In: Marks R, Plewig G, eds. Stratum corneum. Berlin: Springer Verlag, 1983; 161–70.
17. Grove GL, Lavker RM, Kligman AM. Use of microspectrophotometry in dermatological investigation. J Soc Cosmet Chem 1978; 29:537–44.
18. Corcuff P, Lotte C, Rougier A, Maibach HI. Racial differences in corneocytes: a comparison between black, white and oriental skin. Acta Derm Venereol (Stockh) 1991; 71:146–48.

19. Marks R. Measurement of biological aging in human epidermis. Br J Dermatol, 1981; 104:627–33.
20. Grove GL, Lavker RM, Hoelzle E, Kligman AM. Use of non intrusive tests to monitor age associated changes in human skin. J Soc Cosmet Chem 1981; 32:15–26.
21. Takahashi M, Watanabe H, Kumagai H, Nakayamay Y. Physiological and morphological changes in facial skin with aging. 2-. A study on racial differences. J Soc Cosmet Chem Jpn 1989; 23(1):22–30.
22. Hölzle E, Plewig G. Effects of dermatitis, stripping and steroids on the morphology of corneocytes. A new bio assay. J Invest Dermatol 1977; 68:350–6.
23. Goldschmidt H. Surface area measurements of psoriatic corneocytes: effects of intralesional steroid therapy. J Invest Dermatol 1979; 73:558–60.
24. Lévêque JL, Grove G, de Rigal J, Corcuff P, Kligman AM, Saint-Léger D. Biophysical characterization of dry facial skin. J Soc Cosmet Chem 1987; 82:171–7.
25. Herrmann S, Scheuber E, Plewig G. Exfoliative cytology: effects of the seasons. In: Marks R, Plewig G, eds. Stratum corneum. Berlin: Springer Verlag, 1983; 181–5.
26. Corcuff P, Lévêque JL. Corneocyte changes after acute UV irradiation and chronic solar exposure. Photodermatology 1988; 5:110–5.
27. Lee S, Park YK, Kim YK, Kang JS. an experimental study on corneocytes of acutely and chronically irritated skin. Arch Dermatol Res 1983; 275:49–52.
28. Hamami I, Marks R. Structural determinants of the response of the skin to chemical irritants. Contact Dermatitis 1988; 18(2):71–5.
29. Nicholls S, Lawson A, Barton SP, Marks R. Changes in corneocyte size after application of topical corticosteroids and vehicles to normal skin. In: Marks R, Plewig G, eds. Stratum corneum. Berlin: Springer Verlag, 1983; 242–7.
30. Breiner W, Scheuber E, Plewig G. Effects of 13-cis retinoic acid therapy on the qualitative and quantitative exfoliative cytology of the human stratum corneum. Arch Dermatol Res 1982; 273:191–2.
31. Mackenzie IC. Effects of frictional stimulation on the structure of the stratum corneum. In: Marks R, Plewig G, eds. Stratum corneum. Berlin: Springer Verlag, 1983; 153–60.
32. Marks R. Epidermal and corneocyte size changes with age. Br J Dermatol 1980; 102:738–9.
33. Plewig G, Scheuber E, Reuter B, Waidelich W. Thickness of corneocytes. In: Marks R, Plewig G, eds. Stratum corneum. Berlin: Springer Verlag, 1983; 171–4.
34. Boyde A. Applications of tandem scanning reflected light microscopy and three dimensional imaging. Ann N Y Acad Sci 1986; 483:428–39.
35. Tring FC. A rapid method for identifying nucleated horn cells. Br J Dermatol 1976; 94:339–40.
36. Marks R, Lawson A, Nicholls S. Age-related changes in stratum corneum, structure and function. In: Marks R, Plewig G, eds. Stratum corneum. Berlin: Springer Verlag, 1983; 175–80.
37. Sauermann G, Hoppe U. Bestimmung des Zellvolumens humaner Hornepithelzellen. J Soc Cosmet Chem 1981; 32:355–70.

38. Lévêque JL, Corcuff P, de Rigal J, Agache P. In vivo studies of the evolution of physical properties of the human skin with age. Int J Dermatol 1984; 23(5): 322–9.
39. Holzle E, Plewig G, Ledolter A. Corneocyte exfoliative cytology: a model to study normal and diseased stratum corneum. In: Marks R, Plewig G, eds. Skin models. Berlin: Springer Verlag, 1986; 183–93.
40. Michel S, Schmidt R, Shroot B, Reichert U. Morphological and biochemical characterization of the cornified envelopes from human epidermal keratinocytes of different origin. J Invest Dermatol 1988; 91(1):11–5.
41. Epstein WL, Maibach HI. Cell renewal in human epidermis. Arch Dermatol 1965; 92:462–8.
42. Baker H, Kligman AM. Technique for estimating turnover time of human stratum corneum. Arch Dermatol 1967; 95:408–10.
43. Lévêque JL, Porte G, de Rigal J, Corcuff P, Francois AM, Saint-Léger D. Influence of chronic sun exposure on some biophysical parameters of the human skin; an in vivo study. J Cutan Aging Cosmet Dermatol 1988; 1(2):123–7.

15

Influence of Age on Stratum Corneum Cohesion, Desquamation, and Epidermal Turnover

R. MARKS

University of Wales College of Medicine
Cardiff, Wales

I. INTRODUCTION

Most aspects of epidermal structure and function change as a function of the aging process. It is therefore not surprising that quite striking alterations take place in stratum corneum cohesion, desquamation, and turnover during intrinsic aging. Note that discussion on this topic is mainly confined to intrinsic aging: the effects of cumulative environmental injury (mostly what has come to be known as photoaging) are much more unpredictable and dependent on the degree of damage sustained.

II. STRATUM CORNEUM COHESION

Stratum corneum cohesion refers to the binding forces within the stratum corneum that unite corneocyte to corneocyte. It is on these forces that the stratum corneum depends for its structural integrity, and it is the gradual release of these intracorneal binding forces that allows desquamation to occur. Corneocytes are lost to the exterior when the forces that bind them to the neighboring horn cells are exceeded by an external shearing force.

It is not entirely clear what is responsible for the corneocyte-corneocyte bond. It is clear that desmosomal junctions are retained to an extent. Desmosomal structures are present ultrastructurally within the stratum corneum

(1), although not as clearly lamellated as in the epidermis. Desmosomal protein is certainly present within the stratum corneum although its components are in different proportions in the horny layer compared to the epidermis (2). Apart from desmosomal contacts, the corneocyte cell wall is thrown into folds that interdigitate one cell into the adjoining cells, and the disklike shape ensures that this arrangement is strongly resistant to shearing forces.

The intercellular space contains substances that must also be of importance in modulating intracorneal cohesion and the process of desquamation. Some of these materials are complex sphingolipids, and according to the "bricks and mortar" concept of the Elias school (3), these are important in the binding together of corneocytes. This group points to the disorder of X-linked ichthyosis, in which there is an inherited deficiency of steroid sulfatase (4), as strong evidence for this concept. They propose that it is the ratio of cholesterol sulfate to free cholesterol under the control of steroid sulfatase that is all important to desquamation.

However, not all workers accept that lipid substances have an all-important role in the process. Dissolution of the stratum corneum is dependent on trypsin in callus (5), and at least at this site protein bonds must be important in corneocyte binding. Work by the Cardiff group has shown that organic solvents are not successful in removing corneocytes from the skin surface, whereas many corneocytes can be dislodged by the nonionic detergent Triton X-100 (6). When analysis of the nonionic detergent-soluble substance was performed, glycoproteins were identified to which antibodies were raised, which it was suggested might be of importance in desquamation (7).

There is a present uncertainty about the various mechanisms involved. One issue is clear, however, and this is that intracorneal cohesion must be high at the base of the stratum corneum, where strength is required to bond the structure together to provide a coherent water barrier and to provide some mechanical protection, and lower at the surface, where the horn cells drop off when stimulated by comparatively minor forces.

To measure intracorneal cohesion, the Cardiff group developed a device that has come to be known as the *cohesograph* (Figs. 1 and 2) (8). This instrument consists of a piston with a detachable cap that is set in a barrel containing a mechanism that can drive it back and forth and a force transducer that measures the force required to detach it from the skin surface. In operation the piston cap is stuck to the skin surface with a cyanoacrylate adhesive, and then the force required to distract it is measured using a force transducer.

Using this cohesograph we found that whenever the skin surface was broken up into scales, as in psoriasis or ichthyosis, there was an increase in the intracorneal force recorded (9). This was not unexpected, as indeed the presence of scaling signifies that there is failure of the usual release of corneocyte

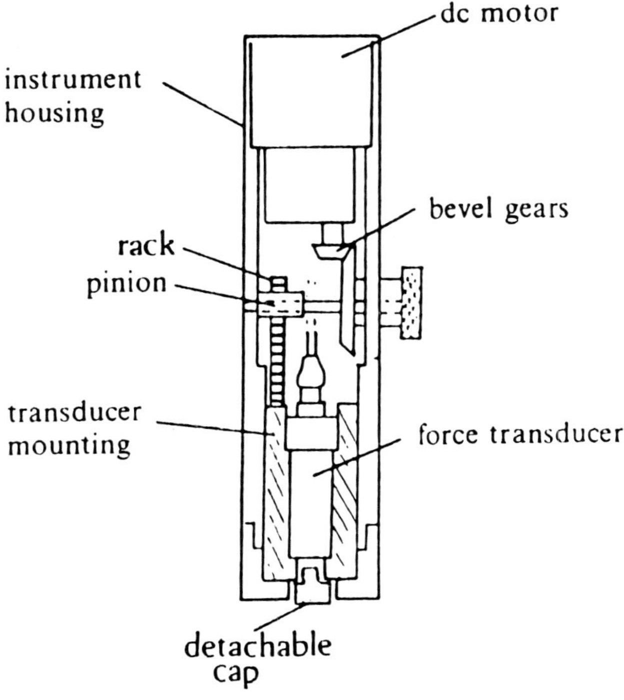

Figure 1 The cohesograph to measure intracorneal cohesion. The detachable cap is stuck to the skin surface by a cyanoacrylate glue. The force required to pull it from the skin surface is measured electronically.

bonds to allow single corneocytes to drop off at the surface and hence there is an increase in intracorneal cohesion.

The drop in binding forces within the stratum corneum was characterized using this device (10). Readings were taken from progressively adhesive tape-stripped adjoining sites on the flexor aspect of the forearms of volunteer subjects. The resulting relationship between the intracorneal binding forces recorded and the depth within the stratum corneum is portrayed in Figure 3. It can be observed that the binding forces gradually increase until, at a point deep within the horny layer, there is no further increase and a plateau is reached.

The intracorneal cohesion at the skin surface is influenced by the size of the corneocytes at that site. The smaller the value for mean corneocyte area,

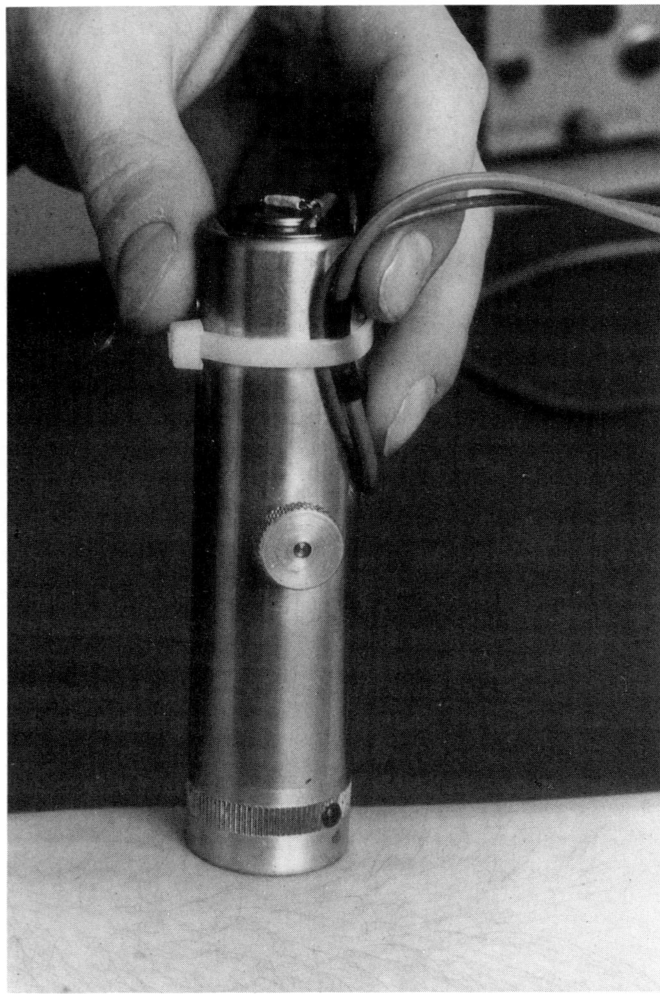

Figure 2   The cohesograph in use on the forearm of a normal subject.

the higher is the intracorneal cohesion (11). The explanation for this may well be that when there are smaller corneocytes there is comparatively more intercellular space per unit volume of horny layer—and obviously more intercellular junctions compared to an equal volume of stratum corneum containing larger corneocytes. It is well known that corneocytes increase in area

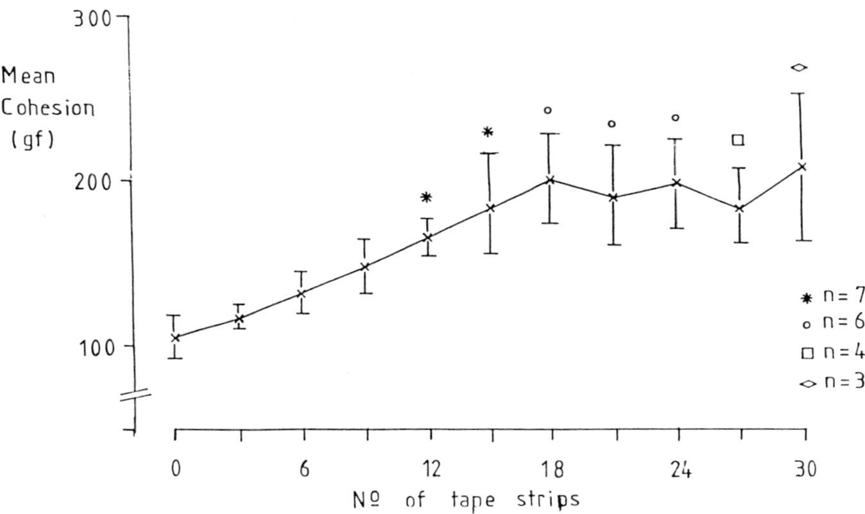

Figure 3   Relationship between stratum corneum cohesion as measured with the cohesograph and depth within the stratum corneum, performed in six normal individuals on adjoining areas of forearm skin that were progressively tape stripped.

with age (12–14), and it may be that this is the explanation for the drop in intracorneal cohesion with age (15).

III. RATE OF CORNEOCYTE LOSS

It is odd that there have been so few attempts at the direct measurement of the rate of corneocyte loss from the skin surface (desquamation). This is odd because desquamation is such a fundamentally important process. Epidermal population size depends not only on the rate of input into the system (epidermopoiesis) but is equally dependent on the rate at which cells are lost. It is not only the academic issue of understanding how the epidermis works and how it deviates in disease that make determination of the rate of desquamation important, however. Characterizing desquamation may also help in the evaluation of agents designed to treat scaling skin disorders. Part of the problem has been that convenient and reliable methods for the measurement of desquamation are unfortunately few and far between.

The easiest methods are those that rely on the clearance of some form of stratum corneum marker. Silver nitrate was among the first to be used (16). This soaks into and sticks to the first few layers of stratum corneum and is converted to visible silver by a solution of photographic developer. The density of the brown color observed at a time point after application is a function of the rate of desquamation. Unfortunately it is not possible to determine just how many cell layers become stained, so at best the method is an estimate.

Tetrachlorsalicylanilide (TCSA) is a fluorescing antimicrobial substance that penetrates the entire stratum corneum and becomes substantive after being in occlusive contact with the skin for 24 hs. The time between application and disappearance of the fluorescence is the turnover time (stratum corneum replacement or renewal time) (17). Dansyl chloride (DC) becomes fluorescent within the stratum corneum and is now used in preference to TCSA because it sensitizes the subjects tested much less frequently (18). The technique is an improvement on the silver nitrate method because DC penetrates the entire thickness of the horny layer, but the assumption that the stratum corneum has a particular thickness is still required to estimate the rate of cell loss in absolute terms. Baker and Blair (19) used TCSA to estimate the effect of age on desquamation and reported that there was a decreased replacement time for elderly individuals compared to young subjects. Interestingly, they found that the replacement time in elderly women was faster than that in elderly men. Roberts and Marks (20) investigated the effect of age on stratum corneum turnover using the dansyl chloride extinction time method. They found, as did Baker and Blair, a marked lengthening of the ''turnover time'' with increasing age.

The disadvantage of these extinction time methods is that in practice they are cumbersome. Subjects are required to attend daily so that the exact day on which the fluorescence is no longer visible can be accurately determined. The method is improved by measuring the degree of fluorescence present as a function of time. This was first accomplished photographically (21). Subsequently a fluorescence comparator was described (22), employing a gray wedge that is interposed between a standard fluorescing source and the viewing eyepiece to match the fluorescence with the ''unknown'' patch being studied. A further improvement eliminates the visual matching and employs a fluorimeter to measure the degree of fluorescence (23).

The lengthening of the turnover time implies a reduction in the rate of desquamation, but this decrease may not be as large as thought. The reason for this is the increase in size in corneocytes so that there are fewer corneocytes in an old individual's stratum corneum compared to a young person's stratum corneum per unit volume. It is clear that the issue needs to be reexamined using quantitative fluorescence techniques and careful measures of corneocyte size and stratum corneum thickness. There is, however, independent support for a ''slowing down'' of the rate of corneocyte shedding. When a standardized rotatory stimulus was applied using a device known as a desquamator, there was a trend to an age-related decrease in the number of corneocytes that could be released from the skin surface (24).

IV. EPIDERMAL CELL PRODUCTION

The epidermis shows a linear decrease in thickness with age, both in absolute terms and in cell number (11). The reduction in epidermal population size suggests that there may also be a decrease in the rate of production of epidermal cells, and the apparent lengthening of the stratum corneum renewal time seems to confirm this. In addition there is some evidence that the rate of reepithelialization of wounds decreases with age (25). These theoretical issues having been aired, it must be said that there are precious few experimental data reported on this issue. Once again there is the major problem of cumbersome, imprecise techniques. Using the tritiated thymidine autoradiographic labeling index method, Kligman (26) reported a reduced value for an elderly cohort compared to a younger group. In a study comparing the effects of aging on the tritiated thymidine autoradiographic labeling index at sun-exposed and nonexposed skin sites, we could not detect any decrease in the older subjects (Table 1) (27). We recently confirmed this ''negative'' finding using both tritiated thymidine and bromodeoxyuridine to label cells in DNA synthesis (Vijayasingam and Marks, unpublished data, 1991). The more sensitive but complicated technique of FACS analysis, in which dispersed cells are run through a fluorescence-activated cell sorter, was also performed and detected a small but significant age-related decrease in the proportion of cells in the DNA synthesis stage of the cell cycle (Fig. 4). The proportion of cells in DNA synthesis is of course only one parameter of epidermal growth and is anyway useful only if the time taken to complete this synthesis phase remains constant. Clearly it may be important to measure the lengths of the different phases of the epidermal cell cycle at different ages before concluding that there is an age effect on epidermopoiesis. Even this may not be sufficient

Table 1 Tritiated Thymidine Autoadiographic Labeling Indices (Mean ± Standard Deviation) for Sun-Exposed and Nonexposed Skin Sites in Different Age Groups

Age group, (years)	n	Exposed skin	Nonexposed skin
20–39	3	8.9 ± 2.2	4.5 ± 1.6
40–59	6	9.3 ± 1.8	5.6 ± 2.1
60–69	5	7.9 ± 2.8	3.7 ± 2.5
70$^+$	5	8.4 ± 2.4	4.9 ± 2.9

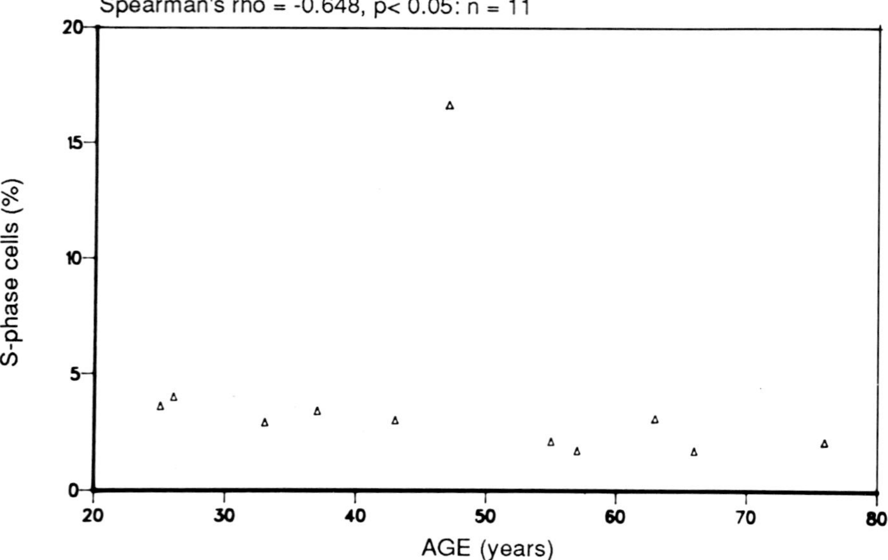

Figure 4 *S* phase analysis by fluorescein-activated cell sorting. It can be seen that the number of cells in *S* phase in the 11 individuals studied progressively decreased with age. The relationship is significant, but the decrease is comparatively small. No explanation was found to explain the anomalous result in 1 individual.

because two other imponderables influence the rate of production. The first is the proportion of stem cells to amplifying cells that are being evaluated with any of the techniques. The other issue concerns the fate of cells born into the system. It appears likely that a not inappreciable proportion may die prematurely in the process known as *apoptosis* (28).

From what has been said it is evident that although there are modest age-related alterations to the population dynamics of the epidermis, these are smaller than may be thought and the situation is not easy at present to characterize with precision. Basically inadequate methods are available for the study of all the parameters required for complete characterization.

REFERENCES

1. Zelickson AS. Ultrastrucure of normal and abnormal skin. London: Henry Kimpton, 1967.
2. Konohana A, Konohana I, Roberts GP, Marks R. Biological changes of bovine muzzle epidermis during differentiation. J Invest Dermatol 1987; 89(4):353–7.

3. Yardley HJ. Epidermal lipids. In: Goldsmith LA, ed. biochemistry and physiology of the skin, Vol. 1. New York: Oxford University Press, 1983; 363–81.

4. Williams ML, Elias PM. Stratum corneum lipids in disorders of cornification. Increased cholesterol sulfate content of stratum corneum in recessive X-linked ichthyosis. J Clin Invest 1981; 68:1404–10.

5. Lundström A. Cell cohesion and desquamation in plantar stratum corneum: the role of protein structures and their degradation. Thesis, University of Umeå, Sweden, 1989.

6. Dykes PJ, Williams DL, Marks R. Non identity of non-ionic detergent soluble (NIDS) protein and stratum corneum autoantigens. Arch Dermatol Res 1983; 275:239–41.

7. Dykes PJ, Williams DL, Marks R. Analysis of the non-ionic detergent soluble (NIDS) lipids of human stratum corneum. Br J Dermatol 1984; 110:283–92.

8. Nicholls S, Marks R. Novel techniques for the estimation of intracorneal cohesion in vivo. Br J Dermatol 1977; 96:596–602.

9. Marks R, Marks HV, Black D, Barton SP. Abnormalities of the stratum corneum in the ichthyotic disorders. Paediatric Dermatol News 1988; 7:22–31.

10. Marks R. Quantification of desquamation and stratum corneum cohesivity. In: Lévêque JL, ed. Cutaneous investigation in health and disease. New York: Marcel Dekker, 1988; 33–47.

11. Marks R, Barton SP. The significance of the size and shape of corneocytes. In: Marks R, Plewig G, eds. Stratum corneum. Heidelberg: Springer-Verlag, 1983; 161–70.

12. Grove G, Lavker RM, Hölzle E, Kligman AM. Use of non-intrusive tests to monitor age associated changes in human skin. J Soc Cosmet Chem 1981; 32:15–8.

13. Marks R. Measurement of biological ageing in human epidermis. Br J Dermatol 1981; 104:627–33.

14. Plewig G, Marples RR. Regional differences of cell sizes in human stratum corneum. Part II. Effects of age and sex. J Invest Dermatol 1970; 54(1):19–23.

15. Marks R, Lawson A, Nicholls S. Age-related changes in stratum corneum structure and function. In: Marks R, Plewig G, eds. Stratum corneum. Heidelberg: Springer-Verlag, 1983; 175–80.

16. Ascheim E. Experimental approach to the renewal of the skin surface. Nature 1965; 220:1242–3.

17. Baker H, Kligman AM. Technique for estimating turnover time of human stratum corneum. Arch Dermatol 1967; 95:408–11.

18. Jansen LH, Hojyo-Tomoko MT, Kligman AM. Improved fluorescence staining technique for estimating turnover of the human stratum corneum. Br J Dermatol 1974; 90:9–14.

19. Baker H, Blair CP. Cell replacement in the human stratum corneum in old age. Br J Dermatol 1968; 80:367–71.

20. Roberts D, Marks R. Determination of regional and age variations in the rate of desquamation. A comparison of four techniques. J Invest Dermatol 1979; 74:13–6.

21. Finlay AY, Marshall RJ, Marks R. A fluorescence photographic photometric technique to assess stratum corneum turnover rate and barrier function in vivo. Br J Dermatol 1982; 107:35–42.

22. Marks R, Black D, Hamami I, Caunt A, Marshall RJ. A simplified method for measurement of desquamation using dansyl chloride fluorescence. Br J Dermatol 1984; 111:265–70.

23. Takahashi M, Machida Y, Marks R. a new apparatus to measure rate of desquamation using dansyl chloride fluorescence. Arch Dermatol 1987; 279: 281–2.

24. Marks R. Measurement of biological ageing in human epidermis. Br J Dermatol 1981; 104:627–33.

25. Grove GL. Age related differences in healing of superficial skin wounds in humans. Arch Dermatol Res 1982; 272:381–5.

26. Kligman AM. Perspectives and problems in cutaneous gerontology. J Invest Dermatol 1979; 73:39–46.

27. Marks R, Berth-Jones J, Black DR, Gaskell SA. The effects of photoaging and intrinsic aging on epidermal structure and function. G Ital Chir Dermatol Oncol 1987; 2(3/4):252–63.

28. Marks R. The epidermal engine. A commentary on epidermopoiesis, desquamation and their interrelationships. J Cosmet Sci 1986; 8:135–44.

16

Age-Associated Changes in Integumental Reactivity

GARY L. GROVE

K.G.L.'s Skin Study Center
Broomall, Pennsylvania

I. INTRODUCTION

It is generally appreciated that a progressive decline in functional activity occurs in a variety of organ systems with advancing age. As a result of these physiologic changes, elderly adults may be less able to cope with adverse environmental conditions than they could when younger. Moreover, they tend to be more vulnerable to such external insults and less capable of repairing the ensuing damage. Since the skin serves as an interface of the organism with its environment, it is especially important to understand various age-associated changes in integumental reactivity because they can have dire clinical consequences. In this chapter, we briefly review our current understanding of this aspect of human cutaneous aging as measured by noninvasive techniques. For the most part we deal with visual observations made by expert graders and clinicians because the use of instrumental methods has unfortunately been extremely limited. On the other hand, it is becoming increasingly more appreciated that certain disagreeable sensations, such as pain and itching, are often not accompanied by visual signs and can only be evaluated by relying on subjective responses. For convenience we divide this review into two broad sections, one dealing with adverse reactions that produce visual changes, the other with those that do not but otherwise can be sensed by the subject.

II. CUTANEOUS REACTIONS THAT PRODUCE VISUAL SIGNS

A. Inflammatory Responses

The literature is contradictory regarding whether aged persons have diminished inflammatory responses to a variety of chemical and physical insults. Lorincz (1) remarked that the aged react more readily to formalin and adhesive tape. Nilzen and Voss-Lagerand (2) reported that patch test reactions to soaps and detergents increased with advancing age. In direct contrast, Bettley and Donoghue (3) found that patch test reactions to toilet soaps were less severe in the elderly. Carlizza and Bologna (4) demonstrated that there were fewer inflammatory cells in cantharidin blisters in older subjects. Moreover, Coenraads et al. (5) demonstrated that the number of positive reactions to croton oil decreased with advancing age but did not see any age-associated changes for either thymoquinone or crotonaldehyde.

In our own studies (6, 7), summarized in Figure 1, we found that under carefully controlled testing conditions the elderly respond far less sharply to croton oil, cationic and anionic surfactants, weak acids, and solvents, such as dimethylsulfoxide (DMSO) and kerosene. It seems that regardless of whether the end points are wheals, bullae, vesicles, pustules, or erythema, the reactions are less severe in the elderly. This can be explained in part by the attenuated microvasculature of the elderly.

Recent studies by Maibach's group (8) have confirmed and extended our initial reports of an age-associated decline in sodium lauryl sulfate (SLS) irritation. Although a limited number of individuals were followed, this study is of special interest because it used noninvasive instrumental methods to provide an objective measure of the differences in reactivity due not only to age but also to anatomic region. Visual scoring of erythema showed that the group of eight older (74.6 $\pm$ 1.9 years) females had a weaker irritation response compared to seven young (25.9 $\pm$ 1.4 years) adults whether compared on the basis of mean scores or number of responders. By comparing before and after measures of transepidermal water loss (TEWL) from these same test sites as obtained with the Servo Med Evaporimeter, they were able to demonstrate a fivefold increase in relative rates in young adults but only a threefold increase in elderly women. This age difference was especially striking in the thigh, where all of the young but none of the elderly showed an erythematous response. Despite this lack of visual redness, which might be interpreted as no response, the highest increase in TEWL among the elderly subjects occurred at this site.

Reduced inflammatory responses are not limited to chemical irritants. Gilchrest and her associates (9) irradiated buttock skin with 3 MED (minimal erythema doses) from a mercury vapor lamp. In comparison to young sub-

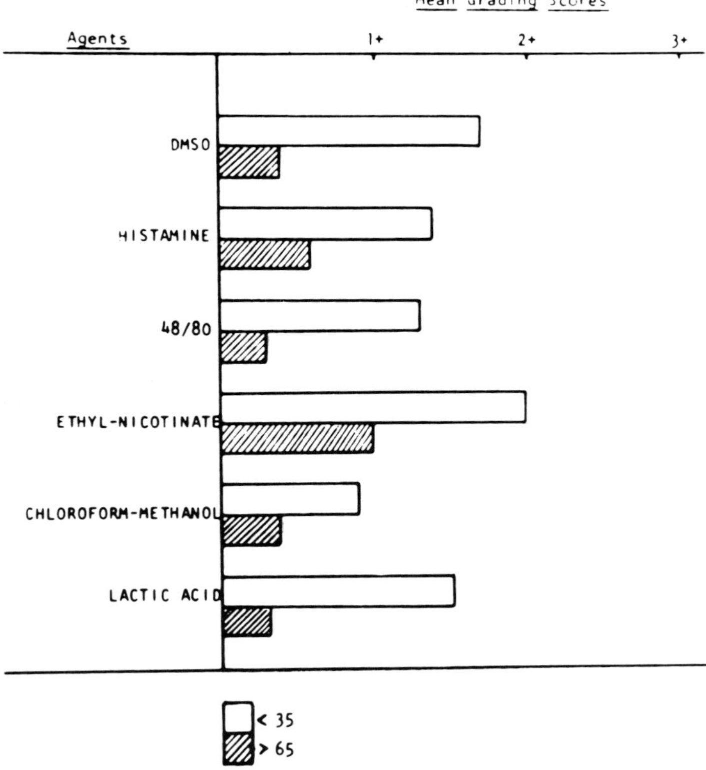

Figure 1 Comparison of the responses to croton oil, cationic and anionic surfactants, weak acids, and solvents, such as DMSO and kerosene, by young adults and older adults.

jects, individuals between 62 and 81 years of age showed diminished erythema, edema, sunburn cells, and histamine levels. Thus the total response was attenuated and evolved more slowly. This pattern is typical of the aged and in this case can be explained in part by there being fewer mast cells with perhaps a greater resistance to degranulation.

This failure of the skin to promptly mount an inflammatory response to a toxic stimulus means that they have a deficient ''early warning detection system.'' This is in contrast to a young individual, in whom redness most likely appears shortly after exposure to a noxious agent, signaling that something is amiss and leading the individual to discontinue use of the culprit product. Since pain perception is decreased as well, this means that the elderly can be continually exposed to harmful agents without experiencing any adverse reactions until considerable damage has been done.

B. Immunologic Impairments

Age-associated declines in both cell-mediated and humoral immunology have been well documented (10–13). Laboratory studies have demonstrated that intradermal reactions to ubiquitous antigens, such as tuberculin, *Candida*, and mumps, declines with age (14). It has also been found that the aged are also more resistant to contact sensitization with potent allergens, such as dinitrochlorobenzene (15,16).

Diminished immunologic reactivity also leads to waning responses in previously sensitized individuals (17). Because most people in the United States have become sensitized to poison ivy or oak plants, a number of investigators (18–20) have found *Rhus* dermatitis to be a convenient model for comparing the severity and time course of contact allergy in young and old persons. In the most comprehensive cross-sectional study, Lejman et al. (21) found that in the elderly an allergic response to an oleoresin patch test developed more slowly, the inflammatory response at peak was greatly diminished, and the dermatitis lasted longer. As shown in Figure 2, they found no clear correla-

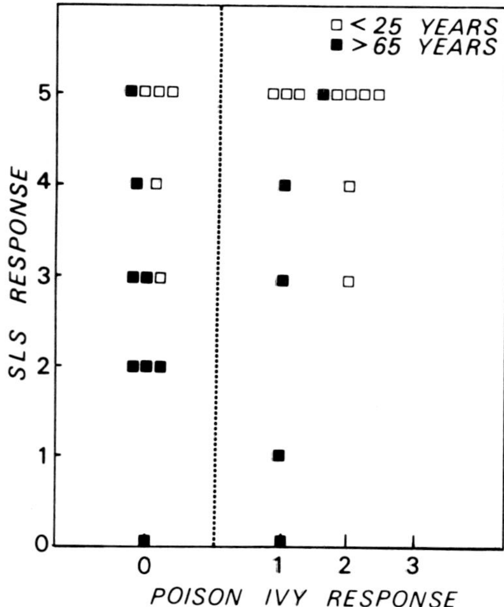

Figure 2 Scatter plot showing the ability to display an irritant response to SLS and an allergic response to *Rhus* oleoresin for both young adult and older adult cohorts.

tion between the intensities of concurrently provoked SLS and *Rhus* reactions in these same subjects. This means that the muted allergic response of the elderly cannot be wholly attributed to their decreased capacity to mount an inflammatory response.

III. RESPONSES THAT PRODUCE SUBJECTIVE SENSATIONS

A. Pain Perception

Laboratory tests employing various instruments to measure pain thresholds have shown that there is an age-associated loss of sensitivity, especially after age 50. For example, Sherman and Robillard (22) used the Hardy dolorimeter to compare pain perception on the foreheads of young and old persons. This device allows one to control the amount of radiant energy applied to the skin. The smallest amount of heat that causes a sharp, jabbing sensation is taken to be a measure of the pain threshold; the smallest stimulus that causes wincing is used to determine the pain reaction threshold. They found that both values were dramatically increased in the older group, indicating decreased sensitivity. Others (23,24) have shown similar age-associated results using "prick tests."

In more recent studies, Soschin and Kligman (25) compared the time required to perceive a burning sensation on the face of young and old persons after applying a 20:80 mixture of chloroform and methanol. A stopwatch was used to time how long it took for the subject to feel piercing burning. As described by Grove et al. (26), the subjects need not be trained to appreciate this end point as the onset; at least in young subjects, it is very sharp and soon deepens to intolerable pain if the provocative agent is not quickly removed. As shown in Figure 3, older persons consistently took longer to perceive this type of pain. In both groups, the shortest reaction times and greatest age differences were found in the nasolabial fold, a site extremely rich in pain receptors.

B. Stinging Sensations

Stinging seems to be a variant of pain that develops rapidly and fades quickly any time the appropriate sensory nerves are stimulated. As a result of an embarrassing experience with sunscreens containing Escolol 506, the amyl ester of *p*-aminobenzoic acid, Frosch and Kligman (27) were prompted to develop a practical test for uncovering new facial products that may have a potential for producing intolerable stinging. Such stinging sensations are completely subjective and typically not accompanied by visual clues. In further studies (26,28) involving such facial sting tests, we found that older subjects are not suitable for screening such culprit products for they are generally insensitive

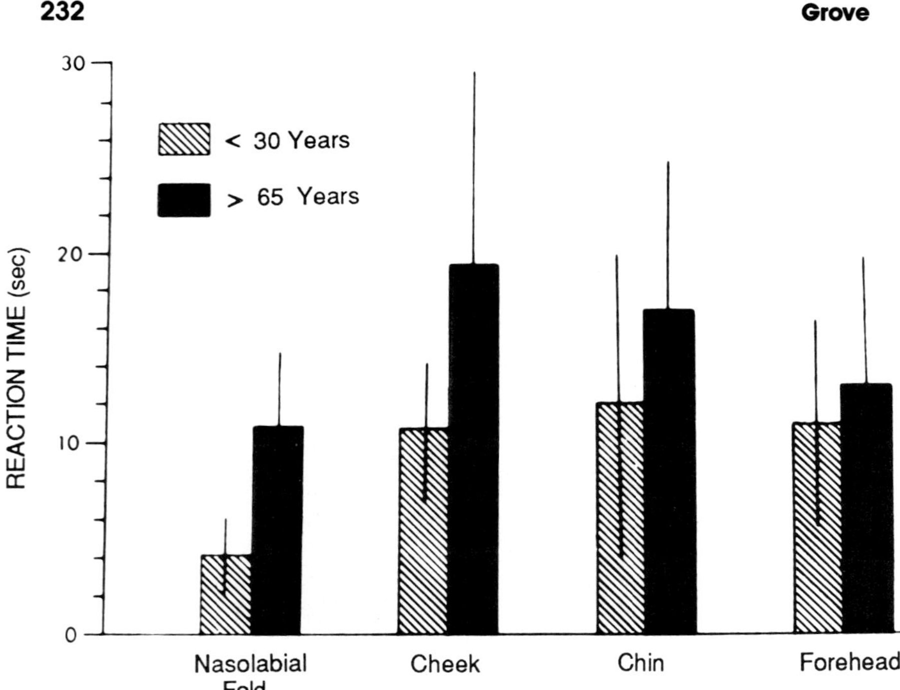

Figure 3 Comparison of the time required to perceive a burning sensation on the face of young adults and older adults after applying a 20:80 mixture of chloroform and methanol.

to various stinging agents. This seems to be especially true when the individual is heavily photodamaged. Indeed, most dermatologists (29) have come to recognize that topical retinoic acid at doses as high as 10% can be well tolerated by such individuals even though similar doses might well cause disagreeable stinging in younger patients. On the other hand, it should not be forgotten that this decreased ability to recognize pain can have dire consequences in that the elderly are thus less capable of sensing danger and reacting accordingly to topical insults. This is one reason thermal burns tend to be more serious and widespread in the aged (30).

C. Itching Response

The most recent laboratory study of the skin's response to poison ivy also revealed an important paradox in age-associated changes in cutaneous reactivity that needs to be considered. *Rhus* dermatitis is notoriously pruritic, and clinical observations by Lejman et al. (26) suggested that pruritus was more severe in the older group. They scratched more and often had fresh excoriations in the morning, with associated exudation and crusting in a linear "fingernail" pattern. Indeed it was thought that such scratching may be in part responsible for the longer duration of the dermatitis noted in the elderly.

There is no ready explanation for the greater itching of dermatitic skin in the elderly. As reviewed in more detail by Gilchrest (12) and Kligman (31), for some it is a minor annoyance but for others chronic pruritus leads to extensive, slowly healing excoriations or loss of sleep, resulting in impaired mental function and irritability. Since cutaneous inflammatory responses are muted, it is sometimes quite difficult to properly identify the causative problem.

Laboratory investigations of the itch response are quite limited. In attempting to develop a model for facial itching, we (26) tried various substances, such as proteolytic enzymes, mast cell degranulators, and vasoactive agents, but found they gave indifferent or inconsistent results. We had some success in a group of healthy, white, young adult females with a 4% histamine base. Since itching is graded solely by self-assessments by the subject, it is extremely important to check the reliability of the subject during a training session to ensure that she can distinguish itching from burning or stinging. If there are any doubts, the test must be repeated. After a 10 minute exposure period, a more objective measure of the instantaneous response can be obtained by observing the size of visible wheals and flares, at least in young subjects.

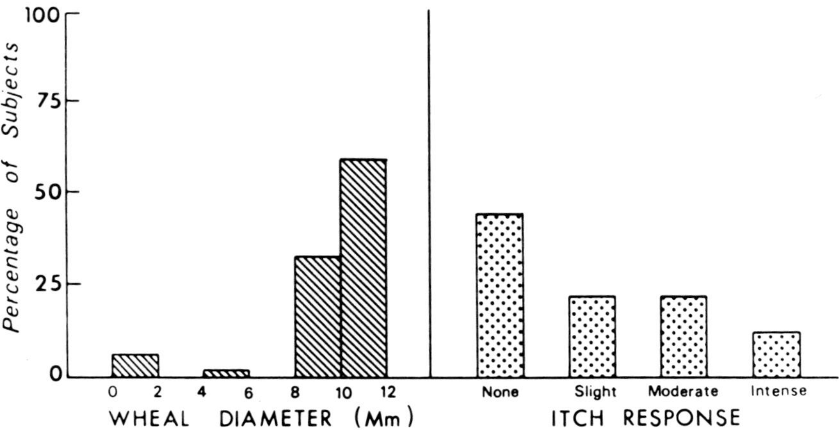

Figure 4 Comparison of whealing and itching responses produced at the same test site by topically applying 4% histamine base.

Figure 4 shows the distribution of the wheal size and intensity of itching response in a group of healthy, white, young adult females. As expected, measurable wheals developed in all subjects, with nearly 90% of the wheals greater than 8 mm in diameter. What is interesting is that nearly half these subjects failed to experience even the slightest pruritus. Large wheals were often unaccompanied by any signs of itching, and it is apparent that the two are not well correlated.

The relationship between itching and sting perception, if any, is extremely complicated (26). Figure 5 compares the cumulative lactic acid sting scores with the histamine itch scores of 32 healthy, white, young adults under age 30. These data show that almost all the subjects who were "stingers" (had sting scores > 3) were also at least moderate if not intense itchers. On the other hand, 50% of the moderate itchers (scores between 4 and 6) showed little or no stinging response. A clear-cut sex difference in both itching and stinging is apparent, with the clustering of most male values in the lower response levels for both tests. Whether this is a true physiologic difference or a reflection of differences in extent of cosmetic use needs to be examined.

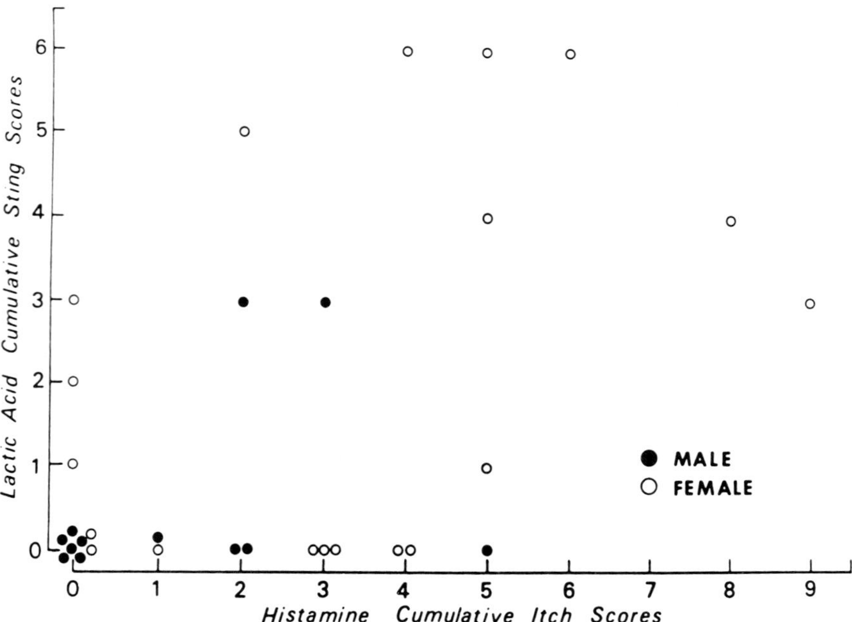

Figure 5   Scatter plot comparing the intensities of the stinging and itching responses of healthy, white, young adult subjects.

IV. SUMMARY

Although gerontologists have used a variety of objective methods to document various age-associated changes in all other organ systems, this approach has been little used to study cutaneous aging. For the most part what we know has been gained by having expert graders evaluate the severity of response induced after application of specific excitants by scoring such specific signs as erythema, vasodilation, wheals, and blisters. In general, it has been found that the elderly are less likely to produce such visual signs, and if they do they are generally lesser in magnitude. As a result, the elderly have been considered less reactive to such stimuli; however, it must be emphasized that this does not mean that the skin is not being adversely affected by such exposures. Indeed, instrumental measurements have clearly revealed in the elderly that transepidermal water loss rates can be dramatically increased as a result of disrupted barrier function due to detergent damage without visual signs of irritation. This age-associated decline in cutaneous displays of such adverse reactions has dire clinical consequences and greatly increases the risks for the elderly when exposed to noxious agents and physical trauma. The matter is further worsened since the elderly also apparently have decreased acuity for perceiving pain or stinging, which can also serve as early warning signals that the skin is being insulted. The only subjective sensation that seems to be enhanced in the elderly is that of itching, and this clearly is not a blessing as it can greatly lessen the quality of life.

REFERENCES

1. Lorincz AB. Physiology of aging skin. Ill Med J 1960; 117:59–62.
2. Nilzen A, Voss-Lagerand K. Epicutaneous tests with detergents and a number of other common allergens. Dermatologica 1962; 174:42–57.
3. Bettley FR, Donoghue E. The irritant effect of soap upon the normal skin. Br J Dermatol 1960; 72:67–76.
4. Carlizza l, Bologna E., Variazioni della reattivata, cutanea in rapporto con l'eta. Bull Soc Ital Biol Sper 1965; 41:344–8.
5. Coenraads PJ, Bleumink E Nofer JP. Susceptibility to primary irritants. Age dependence. Contact Dermatitis 1975; 1:377–81.
6. Grove GL, Lavker RM, Holzle E, Kligman AM. Use of nonintrusive tests to monitor age-associated changes in human skin. J Soc Cosmet Chem 1981; 32:15–26.
7. Grove GL. Physiologic changes in older skin. Clin Geriatr Med 1989; 5:115–25.
8. Cua AB, Wilhelm KP, Maibach HI. Cutaneous sodium lauryl sulfate irritation potential: age and regional variability. In Press.

9. Gilchrest BA, Stoff JS, Soter NA. Chronologic aging alters the response to UV-induced inflammation in human skin. J Invest Dermatol 1982; 79:11–6.

10. Kligman AM, Grove GL, Balin AK. Aging of human skin. In: Finch CE, Schneider EL, eds. The handbook of the biology of aging. New York: Van Nostrand-Reinhold, 1985; 820–41.

11. Weksler ME. Age-associated changes in the immune response. J Am Geriatr Soc 1982; 30:718–23.

12. Gilchrest BA. Skin and aging processes. Boca Raton, FL: CRC Press, 1984.

13. Lantis LR, Lantis SD. Allergic dermatoses in the older patient. Geriatrics 1974; 29:75–84.

14. Grossman J, Baum J, Gluckman J, Fosner J, Condemi J. The effect of aging and acute illness in delayed hypersensitivity. J Allergy Clin Immunol 1975; 55:268–75.

15. Robert-Thomson IC, Whittingham S, Youngchaiyud V, et al. Aging, immune response and mortality. Lancet 1974; 2:368–73.

16. Catalonia WJ, Taylor PT, Rabson AS, Chretein PB. A method of dinitrochlorobenzene sensitization: a clinicopathologic study. N Engl J Med 1972; 236:399–406.

17. Waldorf DS, Wilkens RR, Decker YL. Impaired delayed hypersensitivity in an aging population. JAMA 1968; 203:831–9.

18. Shelmire B. Contact dermatitis from weeds: patch testing with their oleoresins. JAMA 1939; 113:1085–93.

19. Kligman AM. Poison ivy (*Rhus*) dermatitis. Am Med Assoc Arch Dermatol 1958; 77:149–80.

20. Smith JG, Keim JM. Allergic contact sensitivity in the aged. J Gerontol 1961; 16:118–9.

21. Lejman E, Stoudemayer T, Grove G, Kligman AM. Age differences in poison ivy dermatitis. Contact Dermatitis 1984; 11:163–7.

22. Sherman ED, Robillard E. Sensitivity to pain in the aged. Can. Med Assoc J 1960; 83:944–7.

23. Procacci P, Bozza G, Buzzelli G, Cortz MD. The cutaneous pricking pain threshold in old age. Gerontal Clin 1970; 12:213–8.

24. Schluderman E, Zubeck JP. Effect of age on pain sensitivity. Percept Mot Skills 1952; 14:295–7.

25. Soschin D, Kligman AM. Adverse subjective responses. In: Kligman AM, Leyden JJ, eds. Safety and efficacy of topical drugs and cosmetics. New York: Grune and Stratton, 1982; 377–88.

26. Grove GL, Soschin D, Kligman AM. Adverse reactions to topical agents. In: Drill VA, Lazar P, eds. Cutaneous toxicity. New York: Raven Press, 1984; 203–11.

27. Frosch P, Kligman AM. A method for appraising the stinging capacity of topically applied substances. J Soc Cosmet Chem 1981; 28:197–209.

28. Grove GL, Soschin D, Kligman AM. Guidelines for performing facial sting tests. In: Proceedings of the 12th International Congress of the IFSCC, Paris, 1982; 249–55.

29. Leyden JJ 1992, personal communication.
30. Linn BS. Age differences in the severity and outcome of burns. J Am Geriatr Soc 1980; 28:118–30.
31. Kligman AM. Perspectives and problems in cutaneous gerontology. J Invest Dermatol 1979; 73:39–46.

17

Influence of Aging on the Barrier Function of Human Skin Evaluated by In Vivo Transepidermal Water Loss Measurements

KLAUS P. WILHELM

Medical University of Lübeck
Lübeck, Germany
and University of California–San Francisco, School of Medicine
San Francisco, California

HOWARD I. MAIBACH

University of California–San Francisco, School of Medicine
San Francisco, California

I. INTRODUCTION

Measurements of transepidermal water loss (TEWL) are used in many laboratories for characterization of skin barrier function in vivo, in clinical research, and as a supplementary tool to clinical examination for objective evaluation of certain diseases, including allergic and irritant contact dermatitis, psoriasis, atopy, and ichthyosis (1–6).

TEWL is higher in preterm infants than in term infants, although sweat glands are nonfunctioning (7–9). During the first 2–4 weeks of life the skin barrier gradually matures, and with increasing chronologic age, TEWL gradually becomes comparable to adult levels. At the other end of the age spectrum, that is, from adulthood through senescence, the age dependence of TEWL is controversial.

II. STRATUM CORNEUM AS A PHYSICAL BARRIER

The stratum corneum (SC), the outermost skin layer at the environment/individual interface, is the principal permeability barrier to transepidermal water loss and to percutaneous absorption of topically applied compounds

(10–12). SC is typically 6–20 μm thick, except in the palms and soles, where the thickness is approximately 400–600 μm (13,14).

As a part of the epidermis, SC is constantly renewed from the granular layer and the outermost corneocytes are gradually desquamated from the surface. The internal structure of SC is well organized and has often been schematically described as a brick wall model (12,15). Terminally differentiated, keratin-filled corneocytes of polyhedral shape, arranged as interdigitating vertical columns, represent the bricks; the intercellular lipoidal material in a multilamellar bilayer arrangement represents the mortar. Lipid metabolism within the SC has been documented, and TEWL seems to play a role in the regulation of lipid synthesis via regulation of 3-hydroxy-3-methylglutaryl-coenzyme A (HMG-CoA) reductase activity (16,17). Although today there is circumstantial evidence that SC is not homogeneous throughout its thickness (18,19), initial claims that the true barrier layer resides at the base of the SC (19–21) have been shown to be an inappropriate interpretation of experiments in which SC was removed, layer by layer, by adhesive tape stripping. More appropriate studies have shown the contrary, that the barrier properties are more evenly distributed across the entire thickness of the membrane (22,23).

III. TEWL MEASUREMENTS TO EXAMINE SKIN BARRIER PROPERTIES

Today measurement of TEWL is a generally accepted parameter for the evaluation of skin barrier function (7,24–27). The relationship between TEWL and percutaneous absorption has been clearly demonstrated in preterm infants (7) and with respect to anatomic variability (25).

Different methodologies have been used for assessing TEWL as reviewed by Wilson and Maibach (28) and by Grice (29). Today, the majority of clinical studies are performed with the open, unventilated chamber technique (Fig. 1) and instrumental calculation of the water evaporation gradient developing from the skin surface to atmospheric humidity (30). The instrument measures relative air humidity, water vapor partial pressure, and evaporation rate. The probe contains two sensors vertically placed at a known distance

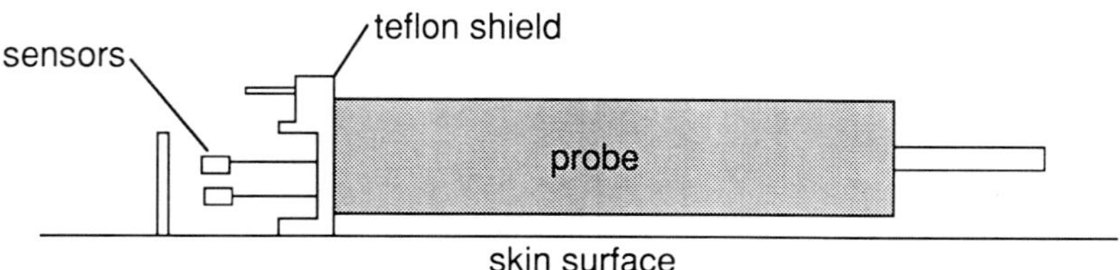

Figure 1 Measurement probe with the open, unventilated chamber.

from the skin surface. Each sensor is coupled to a fast thermistor, and both are enclosed in a cylindrically shaped Teflon capsule. For measurements the probe is held against the skin surface, orienting the sensors perpendicularly to the water vapor pressure gradient. To perform accurate and reliable measurements, several sources of variation should be taken into account as reviewed by Pinnagoda et al. (31). Most important are constant ambient temperature and relative humidity, minimizing air convection and recording skin temperature as the variable with the most significant influence on TEWL.

Skin temperature should always be reported since TEWL increases exponentially with skin temperature (32,33). Some investigators therefore prefer a correction of absolute TEWL to a standard skin temperature, conventionally 30°C (32,33), but others do not (31).

IV. TRANSEPIDERMAL WATER LOSS OF AGING SKIN

There is no doubt that the permeability barrier matures within the first 2–4 weeks of life, but no consensus has yet been established about the skin permeability barrier and baseline TEWL at the opposite end of the age spectrum, that is, from adulthood through senescence (Table 1). The majority of published studies, however, note a significant decrease in TEWL with age, especially after the age of 60–70 years. A study performed by Lévêque (34) on 145 healthy volunteers reports a significant decrease in TEWL on the forearm during the first 20 years of life and a second decrease after the age of 70 years compared with adulthood levels (Fig. 2). Wilhelm et al. (35) demonstrated that TEWL was significantly lower in an aged group (70.5 ± 13.8 years) than in young individuals (26.7 ± 2.8 years; Fig. 3). In the same study, however, no significant differences in skin capacitance as a measure of SC hydration were demonstrated (Fig. 4). In another study, Roskos and Guy (36) were not able to detect age-associated changes in TEWL. They then examined the water barrier in young and old individuals, again under "stressed" conditions, by first preventing TEWL for 24 h by occluding the skin and then monitoring the recovery of TEWL to baseline. The authors hypothesized that occlusion may enhance the signal-to-noise ratio associated with TEWL measurements. Indeed, with this stress test the authors demonstrated a relatively slower relaxation of TEWL in the aged group. Their results confirmed earlier work by Tagami et al. (37), who used conductance measurements in a water sorption-desorption test to distinguish between young and old skin. Whether this procedure of hydrating the SC first, either by occluding the skin or by applying water to it, and then measuring TEWL really reflects water permeability barrier properties remains open to discussion.

Table 1 Age Dependence of TEWL[a]

Group size	Result	Anatomic site	Author (ref.)
87	Lower water loss in individuals older than 70 years	—	Baker, 1971 (38)
39	No significant correlation between TEWL and age	Abdomen	Grice and Bettley, 1967 (58)
21	Significant negative correlation between TEWL and age	Onychial	Jemec et al., 1989 (59)
21	Lower TEWL in 66–81 year olds than in 19–26 year olds	Leg and forearm	Kligman, 1979 (39)
145	Decreased TEWL after 60 years of age	Forearm	Lévêque et al., 1984 (46)
33	No correlation with age (range 19–85 years)	Forearm	Roskos and Guy, 1989 (36)
23	No correlation with age	Upper arm	Rougier et al., 1988 (50)
22	TEWL decreased in aged group (19–22 versus 61–85 years)	Pretibial	Tagami, 1988 (37)
50	TEWL decreased in aged group	Upper arm	Thune et al. 1988 (40)
43	No correlation with age (range 20–48 years)	Forearm	Tupker et al., 1989 (24)
29	Significant decrease with age in most anatomic regions	11 Different regions	Wilhelm et al., 1991 (35)

[a]Summarized are the results of some recently published studies (without intention of completeness) on the effect of aging on in vivo TEWL measurements in humans.

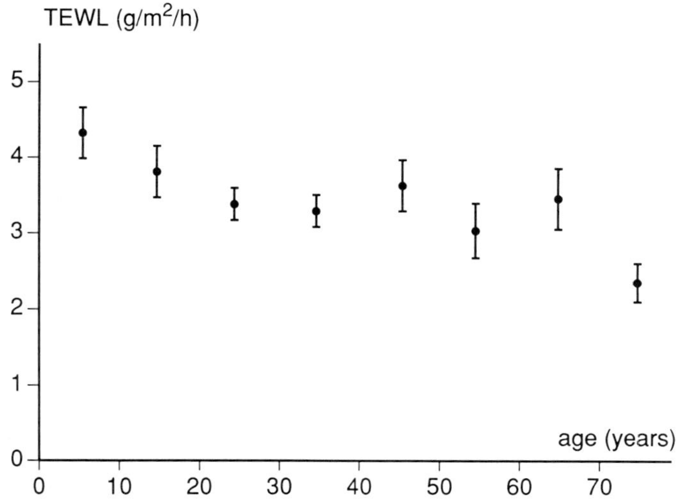

Figure 2 Baseline transepidermal water loss (TEWL) with increasing age ($n = 145$). (Modified from Ref. 34)

V. DISCUSSION

The clinical aspect of dry skin encountered in the majority of subjects age 65 or older has not been associated with a perturbed barrier to water permeability as evaluated by TEWL measurements (34,35). In contrast, the majority of studies demonstrated lower TEWL in individuals aged 60–70 and older (34,35,37–41). An explanation for reduced TEWL in the aged is not obvious. Skin physiology and biochemistry change in many regards with increasing age (42).

It is not expected that the barrier function is excluded from this modification. Reduced sweating associated with the aging process (43) may partially explain the observed decrease in TEWL, although no significant influence of sweating on baseline TEWL was demonstrated by Pinnagoda et al. (44). There is an inverse relationship between corneocyte size and TEWL (45). In skin senescence, however, there seems to be no clear correlation between these parameters (46). The relevance of the increased stratum corneum renewal time in aged skin is not known. Although the thickness of the SC is not altered by age, its renewal time is greatly prolonged; in young adults, SC transit time as estimated by the dansyl chloride staining method is about 20 days, whereas in older adults it is more than 30 days (47). Decreased density and efficiency of the skin microvasculature (48) resulting in decreased skin

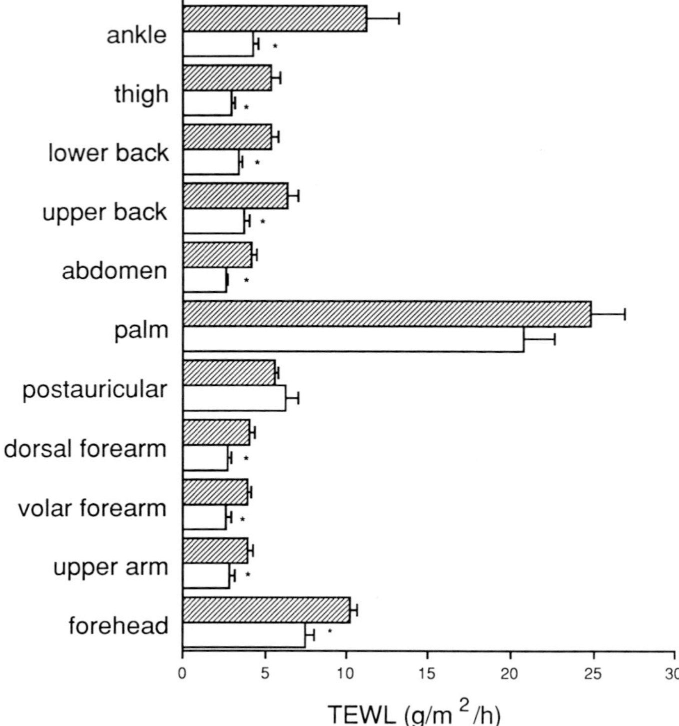

Figure 3 Age differences in TEWL rates at different anatomic locations: young group (hatched bars), aged group (open bars). Shown are mean ± Standard error of the mean (SEM; n = 14–15).
*Statistically significant difference between the age groups ($p \leq 0.05$). (Modified from Ref. 35)

temperature may explain the reduced TEWL in elderly individuals, although Wilhelm et al. (35) corrected their TEWL measurements to a standard skin reference temperature of 30°C and still noted lower TEWL values in the elderly.

A significant correlation between TEWL and the percutaneous absorption of diverse drugs has been demonstrated by several studies (25,49,50). It appears that the decreased TEWL in aged individuals also reflects a less permeable membrane to certain topically applied compounds (48,50–52). Rougier et al. (50) reported a decreased percutaneous absorption of 14-

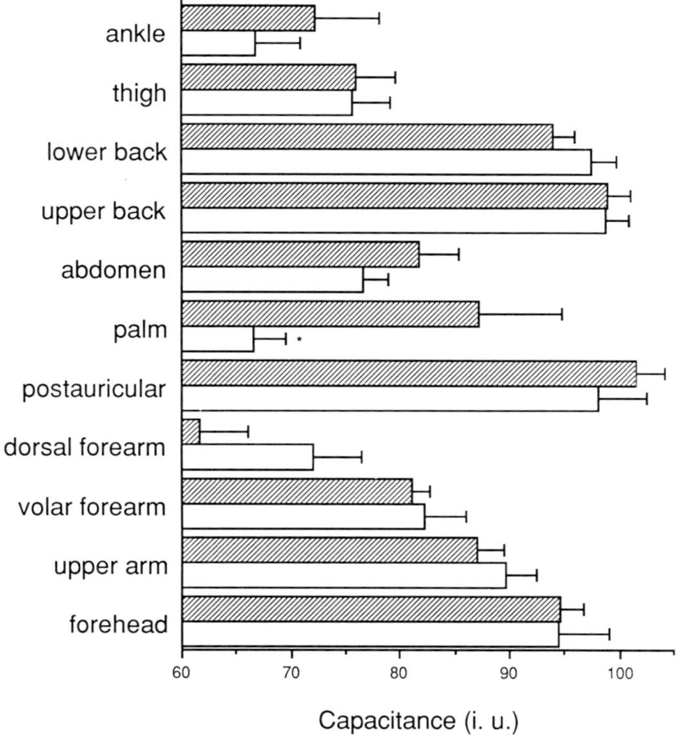

Figure 4　Age differences in stratum corneum hydration at different anatomic locations as evaluated by capacitance measurements: young group (hatched bars), aged group (open bars). i.u. = instrumental units (mean ± SEM; n = 14–15).
*Statistically significant difference between the age groups ($p \leq 0.05$). Since these age differences appear site specific, it is possible that the responsible mechanism(s) are local rather than systemic. (Modified from Ref. 35)

benzoic acid in old subjects (65–80 years). Roskos et al. (51) confirmed a decreased penetration for four of six radioisotope-labeled substances in old individuals. Only the percutaneous penetration of the two most lipophilic compounds considered was not significantly different in their experiments. This was in agreement with earlier studies by Christophers and Kligman (52) and Tagami (48), who concluded that the barrier function of human skin in vivo increases with increasing chronologic age. Furthermore, the recent study by Cua et al. confirmed a decreased irritant response after application of sodium lauryl sulfate in old individuals (41).

Since both TEWL measurements and percutaneous penetration experiments support a further increasing skin barrier function with increasing chronologic age, age-associated changes in the SC as the principle permeability barrier should be considered responsible.

The simplest way of modeling both the process of percutaneous absorption and TEWL is to assume that Fick's first law of diffusion is applicable, although the SC is not an inert membrane. The form of the equation often quoted is

$$\frac{dQ}{dt} = \frac{DK_pc}{h}$$

where: dQ/dt = rate of skin penetration (TEWL)

D = effective diffusion coefficient of drug (water) in stratum corneum

K_p = partition coefficient of drug (water) between membrane and solution

c = concentration gradient of drug (water)

h = effective thickness of skin barrier

For water diffusing through the SC in the opposite direction, dQ/dt is measurable at the skin surface as TEWL; all factors relevant to dQ/dt apply to TEWL. SC thickness is not altered by age (13,47) and may therefore not account for the increased in vivo barrier. One may also assume that c is constant, although epidermal atrophy and a reduced tissue hydration in the aged may decrease the concentration gradient for water (53).

Recent in vitro observations suggest that a lower lipid content leads to an increased penetration of tritiated water and of [14-C] salicylic acid (54). A lowered lipid content may reduce not only the diffusion coefficient but also K_p, as recently demonstrated by Surber et al. (55). They demonstrated that delipidization of isolated human SC significantly reduced K_p, especially for hydrophilic compounds. Interestingly, Roskos found an overall diminution of SC epidermal lipid content with increasing age in humans in vivo by means of attenuated total reflectance infrared spectroscopy (ATR-IR) (56).

No significant difference in SC water content between young and old individuals was demonstrated by capacitance or conductance measurements (35,37). Using more sensitive ATR-IR spectroscopy instrumentation, however, it has been demonstrated that the SC of the elderly is drier than the young adult equivalent (57). By using a water sorption-desorption test, Tagami confirmed a lower water-binding capacity of old SC (37). A reduced presence of water in the SC of old subjects (57) implies that the environment of aged skin is less attractive to hydrophilic molecules and to water, resulting in a decreased K_p and hence decreased dQ/dt.

VI. CONCLUSION

Today there is circumstantial evidence that aged individuals have reduced TEWL in vivo compared with midadulthood values. Several studies indicate that the permeability barrier in vivo in aged subjects is increased not only for water but also for topically applied compounds. Possible explanations for this phenomenon are discussed in this review. The exact mechanisms, however, are not yet known.

ACKNOWLEDGMENTS

The authors appreciate the collaboration with A.B. C'ua, who generated much of the experimental data considered for this chapter. Supported in part by the Deutsche Forschungsgemeinschaft (DFG Wi-879/3-1)

REFERENCES

1. Thune P. Evaluation of the hydration and the water-holding capacity in atopic skin and so-called dry skin. Acta Derm Venereol Suppl (Stockh) 1989; 144: 133–5.
2. Frost P, Weinstein GD, Bothwell JW, Wildnauer R. Ichthyosiform dermatoses. III. Studies of transepidermal water loss. Arch Dermatol 1968; 98:230–3.
3. Silverman RA, Lender J, Elmets CA. Effects of occlusive and semiocclusive dressings on the return of barrier function to transepidermal water loss in standardized human wounds. J Am Acad Dermatol 1989; 20:755–60.
4. Grice K, Sattar H, Baker H. The cutaneous barrier to salts and water in psoriasis and in normal skin. Br J Dermatol 1973; 88:459–63.
5. Serup J, Staberg B. Differentiation of allergic and irritant reactions by transepidermal water loss. Contact Dermatitis 1987; 16:129–32.
6. Van der Valk PJM, Nater JP, Bleumink E. Skin irritancy of surfactants as assessed by water vapor loss measurements. J Invest Dermatol 1984; 82:291–3.
7. Rutter N. The immature skin. Br Med Bull 1988; 44:957–70.
8. Hammerlund K, Sedin G, Stromberg B. Transepidermal water loss in newborn infants. Acta Paediatr Scand 1983; 72:721–8.
9. Wilson DR, Maibach HI. An in vivo comparison of skin barrier function. In: Maibach HI, Boisits EK, eds. Neonatal skin, structure and function. New York: Marcel Dekker, 1982; 101–10.
10. Blank IH, Scheuplein RJ. Transport into and within the skin. Br J Dermatol 1969; 81:4–10.

11. Scheuplein RJ. Percutaneous absorption after twenty-five years: or "old wine in new wineskins." J Invest Dermatol 1976; 67:31–8.

12. Elias PM. Epidermal lipids, membranes, and keratinization. Int J Dermatol 1981; 20:1–19.

13. Holbrook KA, Odland GF. Regional differences in the thickness (cell layers) of the human stratum corneum: an ultrastructural analysis. J Invest Dermatol 1974; 62:415–22.

14. Plewig G, Scheuber E, Reuter B, Waidelich W. Thickness of corneocytes. In: Marks R, Plewig G, eds. Stratum corneum. Berlin: Springer Verlag, 1983; 171–4.

15. Michaels AS, Chandrasekaran SK, Shaw JE. Drug permeation through human skin, theory and in vitro experimental measurement. AIChEJ 1975; 21:985–96.

16. Grubauer G, Elias PM, Feingold KR. Transepidermal water loss: the signal for recovery of barrier structure and function. J Lipid Res 1989; 30:323–33.

17. Proksch E, Elias PM, Feingold KR. Regulation of 3-hydroxy-3-methylglutaryl-coenzyme A reductase activity in murine epidermis. Modulation of enzyme content and activation state by barrier requirements. J Clin Invest 1990; 85:874–82.

18. Bommannan D, Potts RO, Guy RH. Examination of stratum corneum barrier function in vivo by infrared spectroscopy. J Invest Dermatol. 1990; 95:403–8.

19. Eriksson G, Lamke L. Regeneration of human epidermal surface and water barrier function after stripping. Acta Derm Venereol (Stockh) 1971; 51:169–78.

20. Bowser PA, White RJ. Isolation, barrier properties and lipid analysis of stratum compactum, a discrete region of the stratum corneum. Br J Dermatol 1985; 112:1–14.

21. Blank IH. Further observations on factors which influence the water content of the stratum corneum. J Invest Dermatol 1953; 21:259–71.

22. Blank IH, Gould E. Location and reformation of the epithelial barrier to water vapor. Arch Dermatol 1962; 78:702–14.

23. Blank H, Gould E. Study of mechanisms which impede the penetration of synthetic anionic surfactants into skin. J Invest Dermatol 1962; 37:311–5.

24. Tupker RA, Coenraads PJ, Pinnagoda J, Nater JP. Baseline transepidermal water loss (TEWL) as a prediction of susceptibility to sodium lauryl sulphate. Contact Dermatitis 1989; 20:265–9.

25. Lotte C, Rougier A, Wilson DR, Maibach HI. In vivo relationship between transepidermal water loss and percutaneous penetration of some organic compounds in man: effect of anatomic site. Arch Dermatol Res 1987; 279:351–6.

26. Onken HD, Moyer CA. The water barrier in human epidermis. Arch Dermatol 1963; 87:90–6.

27. Murahata RI, Crowe DM, Roheim JR. The use of transepidermal water loss to measure and predict the irritation response to surfactants. Int J Cosmet Sci 1986; 8:225–31.

28. Wilson DR, Maibach HI. Transepidermal water loss: a review. In: Lévêque J-L, ed. Cutaneous investigation in health and disease. Noninvasive methods and instrumentation. New York: M Dekker 1989; 113–34.

29. Grice KA. Transepidermal water loss. In: Jarret A, ed. The physiology and pathophysiology of the skin. Vol. 6, London, Academic Press, 1980; 2115–27.
30. Nilsson GE. Measurement of water exchange through skin. Med Biol Eng Comput 1977; 15:209–18.
31. Pinnagoda J, Tupker RA, Agner T, Serup J. Guidelines for transepidermal water loss (TEWL) measurement. Contact Dermatitis 1990; 22:164–78.
32. Mathias CGT, Wilson DM, Maibach HI. Transepidermal water loss as a function of skin surface temperature. J Invest Dermatol 1981; 77:219–20.
33. Grice K, Sattar H, Sharratt M, Baker H. Skin temperature and transepidermal water loss. J Invest Dermatol 1978; 57:108–10.
34. Lévêque J-L. Measurement of transepidermal water loss. In: Lévêque J-L, ed Cutaneous investigation in health and disease. Noninvasive methods and instrumentation. New York: M. Dekker 1989; 135–52.
35. Wilhelm KP, Cua AB, Maibach HI. Skin Aging. Effect on transepidermal water loss, stratum corneum hydration, skin surface pH, and casual sebum content. Arch Dermatol 1991; 127; 1806–9.
36. Roskos KV, Guy RH. Assessment of skin barrier function using transepidermal water loss—effect of age. Pharm Res 1989; 6:949–53.
37. Tagami H. Aging and the hydration state of the skin. In: Kligman A M, Takase Y, eds. Cutaneous aging, Tokyo: University of Tokyo Press, 1988; 99–109.
38. Baker H. Deperdition d'eau par voie trans-epidermique. Ann Dermatol Syphiligr 1971; 98:289–96.
39. Kligman AM. Perspectives and problems in cutaneous gerontology. J Invest Dermatol 1979; 73:39–46.
40. Thune P, Nilsen T, Gustavson T, Lövig Dahl H. The water barrier function of the skin in relation to the water content of stratum corneum, pH and skin lipids. Acta Derm Venereol (Stockh) 1988; 68:277–83.
41. Cua AB, Wilhelm KP, Maibach HI. Cutaneous sodium lauryl sulfate irritation potential: age and regional variability. Br J Dermatol 1990; 123:607–13.
42. Gilchrest BA. Skin aging and photoaging: an overview. J Am Acad Dermatol 1989; 21:610–3.
43. Sato K, Timm DE. Effect of aging on pharmacological sweating in man. In: Kligman A M, Takase Y, eds. Cutaneous aging, Tokyo: University of Tokyo Press, 1988; 111–26.
44. Pinnagoda J, Tupker RA, Coenraads PJ, Nater J P. Transepidermal water loss with and without sweat gland inactivation. Contact Dermatitis 1989; 21:16–22.
45. Marks R, Nicholls S, King CS. Studies on isolated corneocytes. Int J Cosmet Sci 1981; 3:251–8.
46. Lévêque J-L, Corcuff P, de Rigal J, Agache P. In vivo studies of the evolution of physical properties of the human skin with age. Int J Dermatol 1984; 23:322–9.
47. Grove GL, Kligman AM. Age-associated changes in human epidermal cell renewal. J Gerontol 1983; 38:137–42.
48. Tagami H. Functional characteristics of aged skin. 1. Percutaneous absorption. Acta Dermatol (Kyoto) 1971/1972; 66/67:19–21.

49. Dupuis D, Rougier A, Lotte C, Wilson DR, Maibach HI. In vivo relationship between percutaneous absorption and transepidermal water loss according to anatomic site in man. J Soc Cosmet Chem 1986; 37:351–7.

50. Rougier A, Lotte C, Corcuff P, Maibach HI. Relationship between skin permeability and corneocyte size according to anatomic site, age, and sex in man. J Soc Cosmet Chem 1988; 39:15–26.

51. Roskos KV, Maibach HI, Guy RH. The effect of aging on percutaneous absorption in man. J Pharmacokinet Biopharm 1989; 17:617–30.

52. Christophers E, Kligman AM. Percutaneous absorption in aged skin. In: Montagna W, ed. Advances in biology if skin, Vol, 6 Aging. Oxford: Pergamon Press, 1965; 163–75.

53. Miyake I. Histological aging of facial skin. In: Kligman AM, Takase Y, eds. Cutanous aging, Tokyo: University of Tokyo Press, 1988; 571–88.

54. Elias PM, Cooper ER, Korc A, Brown BE. Percutaneous transport in relation to stratum corneum structure and lipid composition. J Invest Dermatol 1981; 76:297–301.

55. Surber C, Wilhelm KP, Hori M, Maibach HI, Guy RH. Optimization of topical therapy: partitioning of drugs into stratum corneum. Pharm Res, 1990; 7:1320–4.

56. Roskos KV. The effect of skin aging on the percutaneous penetration of chemicals through human skin. Dissertation, University of California–San Francisco, 1989.

57. Potts RO, Buras EM. In vivo changes in the dynamic viscosity of human stratum corneum as a function of age and ambient moisture. J Soc Cosmet Chem 1985; 36:169–76.

58. Grice KA, Bettley FR. Skin water loss and accidental hypothermia in psoriasis, ichthyosis and erythrodermia. Br Med J 1967; 4:195–201.

59. Jemec G, Agner T, Serup J. Transonychial water loss. Relation to sex, age and nailplate thickness. Br J Dermatol 1989; 121:443–6.

18

Variations in Skin Surface Lipids During Life

D. SAINT-LÉGER

L'Oréal, Clichy, France

PIERRE G. AGACHE

University Hospital, Besançon, France

> We grow old too soon, and smart too late!
> —*Pennsylvania Dutch proverb*

I. INTRODUCTION

Although this old proverb may philosophically hold true, it cannot apply to skin. As summarized in a recent volume (1), skin slowly ages and is "smart" enough to maintain most of its properties until the final act.

In contrast to other organs, whose functional properties decline linearly with age (2), the aging process of the skin integrates those of its various compartments (epidermis, and dermis) and appendages (sebaceous glands, hair follicles, sweat glands, and so on). This raises difficulty in making a global description of the skin aging process since this assembly of highly differentiated tissues may show different responses to the same stimuli. This even holds true in comparable structural elements: the 5α-reductase pathway is a major culprit of hair loss in male pattern alopecia, although it greatly stimulates beard and pubic hair growth (3).

The skin surface lipids (SSL) in the human illustrate these comments with regard to their dual origins: the sebaceous cells (sebocytes), producing sebum, and epidermal cells, producing epidermal lipids, are structural elements located mostly within the intercellular spaces of corneocytes (4).

251

Since the sebaceous gland is not uniformly distributed in the human body, the lipidic mixture (sebum and epidermal lipids) that is spread over the skin surface is obviously of a ''mosaïc'' pattern. This is the reason the choice of a given region of the human skin surface, as a model, has great importance. The scalp and forehead, where the lipids are 95–97% of sebum origin (5), are regions of choice for studying both quantitative and qualitative variations with age. Inversely, the lower leg, where sebaceous glands are sparse, is privileged when the subject of research is epidermal lipids or stratum corneum lipids.

Can all these lipids adequately reflect the aging process of the skin? Can they be reliable markers? The present review aims to address such questions.

II. SEBACEOUS FUNCTION AND AGING

A. Quantitative Aspect

It is well established that sebaceous function is primarily governed by androgenic stimulation (6,7), mostly through the synthesis of dihydrotestosterone (DHT) from testosterone through the action of 5α-reductase within the cytoplasm of the sebocyte.

In 1980, Agache et al. (8) found that in newborns, however, sebum levels were high during the first week of life and declined thereafter, suggesting that sebaceous function was strongly stimulated before birth.

The most common way of assessing sebaceous function in vivo is to determine through various noninvasive techniques (9–11) the sebum production (SP) or sebum excretion rate (SER), that is, the amount of sebum recovered some hours following prior defatting of the forehead. In this way it is clear that from the first week of life until age 8–10, the levels of sebum found on the forehead and the scalp are extremely low (8,12).

It has been shown that sebaceous function strongly increases long before puberty, implying an initial stimulus through androgens of adrenal origin. In this regard, ''sebaceous puberty'' precedes sexual puberty. Once the latter occurs, the SP becomes higher and is accompanied in many adolescents by the formation of acneic lesions, illustrating the close link between sebum and acne (13).

In a study of individuals ranging from puberty to old age (age 15–65), Nazzaro-Porro et al. (14) (Fig. 1) and Pochi et al. (12) showed that aging exerts a weak influence on SP accumulated over a 24 h period.

However, females, with lower levels compared to males, show a rather constant decline from the forties, illustrating the impact of menopause on sebaceous function. This is likely related to the decrease in androgen produc-

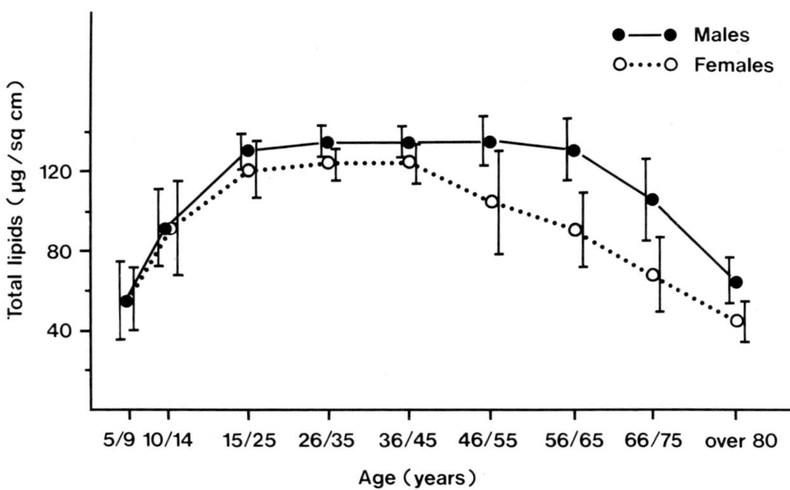

Figure 1 Variations in sebum production with age in men and women. (From Ref 14, used with kind permission.)

tion rather than a decline of the capacity of sebocytes to respond to androgenic stimulation. The SP of postmenopausal women increased following treatment with fluoxymesterone (12). However, despite a low SP in the elderly, the sebaceous glands appear paradoxically enlarged, since it is generally agreed that high SP positively correlate with the size of the sebaceous glands.

However, Plewig et al. (15,16) showed that in aged people the approximately twofold enlargement of the sebaceous gland is related to an increase in sebocyte size but the gland output is actually reduced. The enlarged gland would arise from a greater reduction in sebocyte maturation or transit time within the gland rather than from cell production.

Using both the Lipometre (10) and the Sebutape techniques (11), our group and that of Grove in Philadelphia (17) found the same pattern of age-related changes in SP as that found by Nazzaro-Porro (Fig. 1).

These comparable findings logically allow us to conclude that sebaceous function remains rather constant over most of the life span and that the late drop in SP reflects merely the decrease in the production of androgens. Such a clear-cut conclusion may not necessarily be valid.

In 1982, Downing et al. (18) introduced a new technique for collecting sebum on the forehead, using successive applications of bentonite gel over a long period (12 h), depleting skin surface sebum and part of that present within the follicular reservoir. A further 3 h contact with a fresh benzonite gel yields a "sustainable excretion rate" of a much lower value (5–10 times) than that obtained by other methodologies.

Using this technique, Jacobsen et al. (19) recorded the variations in this sebum production rate with age. Taking the wax ester (WE) fraction—a purely sebaceous marker—as an index of the SP, these authors found a regular (log arithmic) decrease in the wax ester secretion with age from 15 to over 90 (Figs. 2 and 3). The best-fit equation of the correlation indicated that these regular decreases were about 23 and 32% per decade in men and women, respectively.

Since the WE fraction is of constant concentration within the bulk of sebum (26%), these results imply that the human sebaceous gland, as other tissues, continuously ages, in contrast to the findings previously mentioned. According to these authors, the most likely explanation of such a regular decline is a drop in the responsiveness of the gland to androgens. Such a paradox in these two series of studies remains unexplained. The first dealt mostly with the excretion phase of sebum (i.e., the ability of the pilosebaceous duct reservoir to excrete sebum), whereas the second very likely depicted changes in the low secretionsynthesis phase of the gland with age.

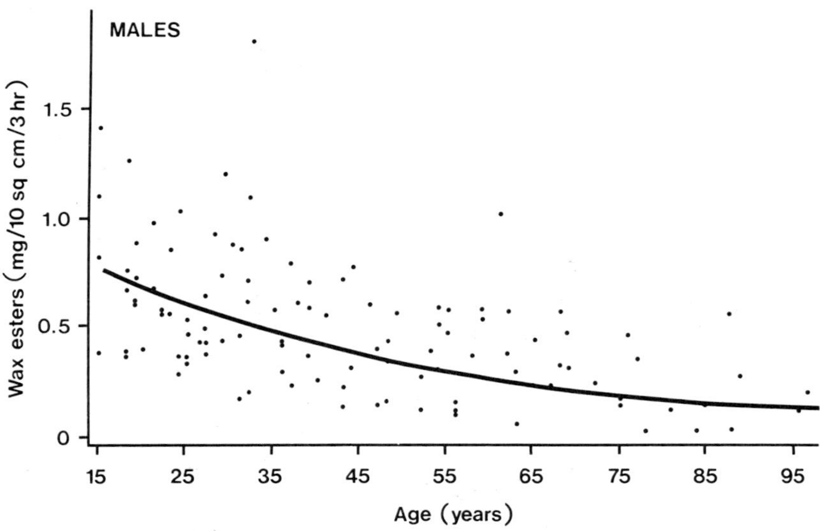

Figure 2 Variations in the wax ester secretion with age, in men. (From Ref. 17, used with kind permission.)

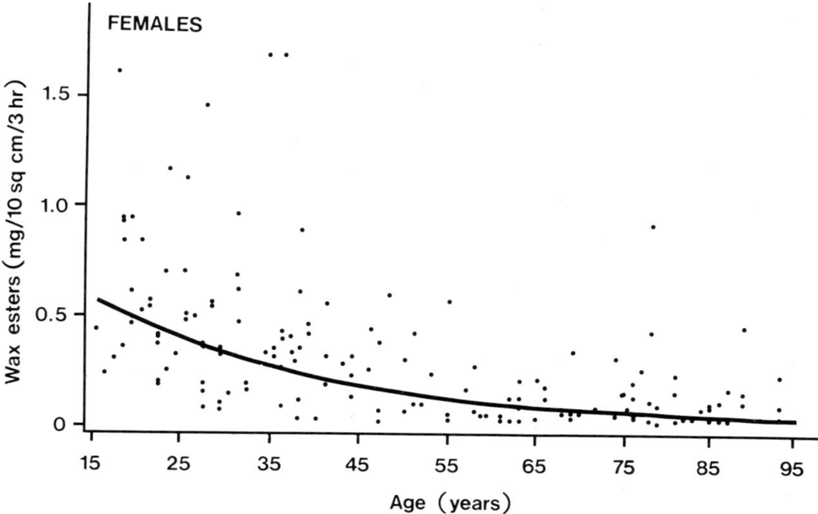

Figure 3 Variations in wax ester secretion with age in women. (From Ref. 17, used with kind permission.)

B. Qualitative Changes

In 1958, an elegant study carried out by Kellum (20) on dissected human sebaceous glands showed that native sebum was comprised of about 15% squalene, 60% triglycerides (TG), and 25% wax esters. The TG and WE comprise an unusual variety of unique and complex fatty acids (even and odd carbon chains, unusual location of unsaturation, iso and anteiso, and others), as shown by the pioneering studies of Nicolaides (21). The biochemical explanation of the synthesis of such fatty acids is that the human sebaceous gland is able to utilize many other precursors in the fatty acid synthesis pathway than the classic acetylcoenzyme A.

The holocrine process of sebaceous gland physiology implies that the sebocytes, when terminally active, disintegrate and liberate the bulk of sebum in the infundibulum of the pilosebaceous duct. It is now well established that the resident flora progressively hydrolyze the triglyceride fraction, explaining the presence of complex free fatty acids (FFA) at the surface of the skin (22).

The WE fraction, which is not hydrolyzed by bacterial and fungal lipases, therefore remains constant. This is mostly the reason many authors focused their attention on the profile of the fatty acids comprising the WE fraction. As stated earlier, the WE fraction is of a purely sebaceous origin, whereas the

TG fraction arises from both sebaceous gland and epidermis (see later) and is not suspected to be metabolized by exogenous events.

With regard to the aging process, the profile of these FFA, analyzed by gas chromatography–mass spectrometry (GC/MS), varies with age and sex. In 1979, Nazzaro-Porro et al. (14), showed that the surface lipids of very old individuals were similar to those of prepubertal children, whereas pubertal subjects show significant changes in this profile in 11–16 year children compared to the 6–9 year group (23). Analyzing the profiles of the FFA included in the WE fraction led Yamamoto et al. (24) to record a significant correlation between the C16:1 straight and C16:1 iso-branched chains (the former increasing from infancy) and age.

A possible daily or weekly variation in the FFA profile, which would yield misleading results, is unlikely, since it has been shown (25) that over a 2 month period the FFA profile for a given subject remains rather constant.

Significant differences were observed from subject to subject, however, implying the existence of a personal "chemical signature" of sebum, which in turn varies with age. Such a signature is very likely under genetic control, as shown by Stewart et al. (26). This clever study showed very small differences in the FFA from WE in 13 identical twins by assessing intrapair comparisons in the proportions of iso-even fatty acids. However, interpair differences were found to be as large as in the nontwin population. This observation is of importance because it implies that follow-up of these subtle qualitative variations in the biosynthesis of lipids with age must be recorded on an individual basis. This unfortunately raises obvious technical difficulties for assessing a global and statistical impact of aging on sebaceous physiology.

III. EPIDERMAL (STRATUM CORNEUM) LIPIDS AND AGING

Epidermal lipids are structural elements of the keratinocytes consisting of a complex mixture of sterol esters (SE) triglycerides, free fatty acids, free sterols (FS), and more polar lipids, such as ceramides and cholesteryl sulfate. Along with keratinization, their profiles show considerable variations within the depth of the epidermal layers (27). For example, no phospholipids can be recovered from the stratum corneum, although phospholipids are enriched at the basal layers. Epidermal lipids are very likely located within the intercellular spaces between corneocytes, showing a typical multilamellar organization (28). Their role in the process of desquamation remains unclear. However, recent findings suggest they play an important role in maintenance of the skin barrier in the hydration state (29, 30), a role mostly attributed to the ceramide fraction.

Assessing the impact of aging in vivo in the human on epidermal lipids requires the fulfillment of two conditions:

1. The site of sampling should be a region where the sebaceous glands are sparse or absent.
2. The technique of sampling should be noninvasive, allowing numerous analyses from large groups of subjects.

Technically speaking, the first and simplest approach concerns the analysis of profiles of the classes of stratum corneum lipids (SCL), between the first three to five layers of the stratum corneum, which are very accessible by superficial noninvasive techniques (e.g., direct solvent extraction and cyanoacrylate sampling). With regard to the first condition, the forearm and the lower leg are appropriate. This is the approach with which our group initially described the variations in the SCL profile with age, sampled on the lower leg through a direct solvent extraction technique (31). Although the total amount of collected SCL did not vary with age, the profile showed an increase in SCL polarity, mostly in the ceramide fraction (Fig. 4).

When this study was carried out, ceramide standards as described by Long et al. (32) were not available, and these were therefore analyzed by thin-layer chromatography. An increase in the index of sterol esterification was also observed (Fig. 5), suggesting that sterol is increasingly in a free form with age.

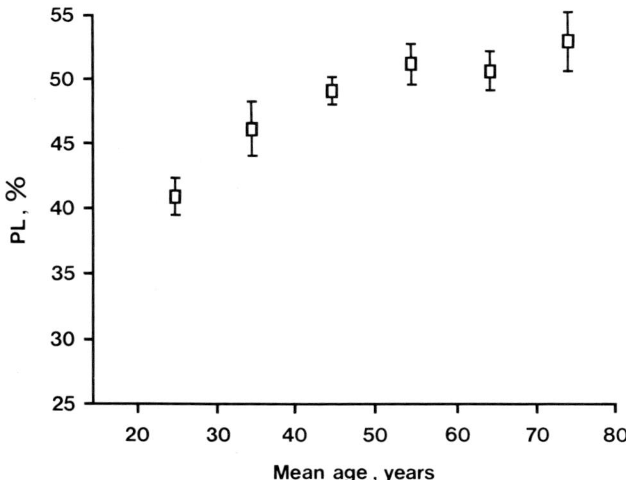

Figure 4 Increase in the percentage of polar stratum corneum lipids (ceramides + cholesteryl sulfate) with age.

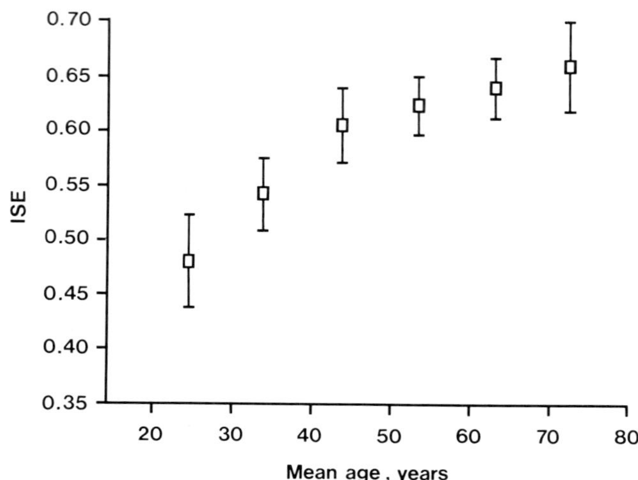

Figure 5 Changes in the index of sterol esterification (ISE) with age. The ISE is defined as the ratio of free sterols (%) to free sterols (%) + esterifed sterols (%).

The general pattern of SCL shows a large variation from the twenties to the fifties, plateauing from this age (Fig. 6). We interpreted such a plateau as the impact of menopause since our subjects were predominantly females. We need not consider the influence of skin xerosis (a common affliction on the lower leg) on such a profile, since a further study (33) found a rather stable SCL pattern in premenopausal, age-matched women who showed various grades of severity of skin xerosis.

However, a recent study carried out by Imokawa et al. (34), analyzing 65 cyanoacrylate strippings of the forearm, showed a statistical decrease in the total ceramide content per milligram stratum corneum with age. According to these authors, such a finding would explain, though a progressive alteration of keratinization, the variations in the maintenance of SC hydration that accompany the aging process as well as dryness of the skin. This latter is a common sign of the impact of aging on epidermal physiology.

IV. CONCLUSION

All these conflicting results lead us to admit that, at the present time, much more work must be carried out to address the issue of the actual influence of aging on both sebaceous and epidermal lipids to make clear-cut conclusions. For example, as far as epidermal lipids are concerned, it remains possible that, compared to sebaceous production, their profile may vary from subject

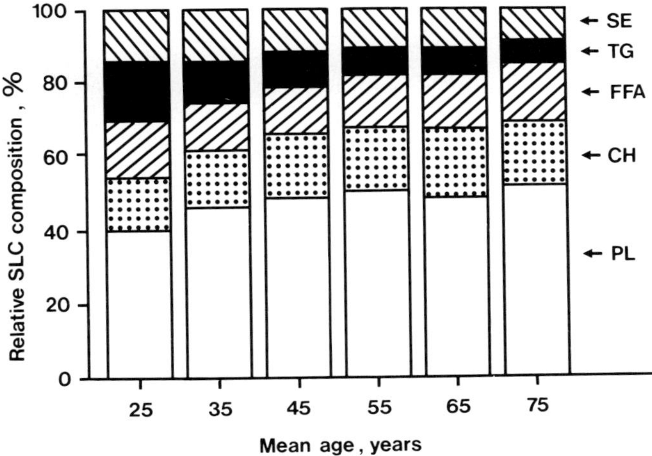

Figure 6 Variations in the relative composition of SCL with age, illustrating the increase in the overall polarity of SCL.

to subject, under genetic control. Taken as a whole, both sebaceous and epidermal tissues show complex and subtle modifications with age, although exogenous events (e.g., sun exposure and flora) may exert additional influence.

Such multifactorial causes obviously call for numerous additional studies. These necessarily require more sophisticated protocols with regard to the genetic control of the unusual biochemical pathways leading to the synthesis of sebaceous and epidermal lipids. It is likely that it will be in such difficult approaches that their precise role(s) in skin physiology will be more adequately defined.

ACKNOWLEDGMENT

The authors express their deep gratitude to Mrs. Marie-Marguerite Sarrot for her kind and skillful help in the preparation of the manuscript.

REFERENCES

1. Balin KK, Kligman AM. Aging and the skin. New York: Raven Press, 1989.
2. Shock NW. Discussion on mortality and measurement. In: Strehler BL, Ebert JD, Glass HB, Schock NW, eds. The biology of aging: a symposium. American Institute of Biological Sciences, 1960; 22–3.
3. Lucky AW. The paradox of androgens and balding: where are we now? New York: J Invest Dermatol 1988; 91(2):99–100.

4. Lampe MA. Burlingame LAL, Whitney J. Human stratum corneum lipids: characterization and regional variations. J Lipid Res 1983; 24:120–30.

5. Greene RS, Downing DT, Pochi PE, Strauss JS. Anatomical variation in the amount and composition of human skin surface lipids. J Invest Dermatol 1970; 54:240–7.

6. Strauss JS, Kligman AM, Pochi PE. The effect of androgens and oestrogens on the human sebaceous gland. J Invest Dermatol 1962; 39:139–55.

7. Simpson NB, Cunliffe WJ, Hodgins MB. The relationship between the in vitro activity of 3-hydroxysteroid dehydrogenase 4, 5 isomerase in human sebaceous glands and their secretory activities in vivo. J Invest Dermatol 1983; 81(2): 139–44.

8. Agache P, Blanc D, Barrand C, Laurent R. Sebum levels during the first year of life. Br J Dermatol 1980; 103:643–9.

9. Strauss JS, Pochi PE. The quantitative gavimetric determination of sebum production. J Invest Dermatol 1980; 103:643–9.

10. Saint-Léger D, Berrebi C, Duboz C, Agache P. The lipometre: an easy tool for rapid quantitation of skin surface lipids in man. Arch Dermatol Res 1979; 265(1):79–99.

11. Nordstrom KM, Schmus HG, McGinley KJ, Leyden JJ. Measurement of sebum output using a lipid absorbent tape. J Invest Dermatol 1986; 87:260–4.

12. Pochi PE, Strauss JS, Downing DT. Age related changes in sebaceous gland activity. J Invest Dermatol 1979; 73:108–11.

13. Cotterill JA, Cunliffe WJ, eds. The acnes, clinical features, pathogenesis and treatment. Philadelphia: W. B. Saunders, 1975; 176.

14. Nazzaro-Porro M, Passi S, Boniforti L, Belsito F. Effects of aging on fatty acids in skin surface lipids. J Invest Dermatol 1979; 73:112–7.

15. Plewig G, Klingman AM, Proliferative activity of the sebaceous glands in the aged. J Invest Dermatol 1975; 70:314–7.

16. Luderschmidt C, Plewig G. Circumscribed sebaceous gland hyperplasia. Autoradiographic and histoplanimetric studies. J Invest Dermatol 1978; 70:207–9.

17. Saint-Léger D, Grove G. Unpublished results, 1984.

18. Downing DT, Stranieri AM, Strauss JS. The effect of accumulated lipids on measurements of sebum secretion in human skin. J Invest Dermatol 1982; 79:216–20.

19. Jacobsen E, Billings JK, Frantz RA, Kinney CK, Stewart ME, Downing DT. Age related changes in sebaceous wax ester secretion rates in men and women. J Invest Dermatol 1985; 85:483–5.

20. Kellum RE. Human sebaceous gland lipids. Analysis by thin layer chromatography. Arch Dermatol 1958; 95:218–20.

21. Nicolaides N. Skin lipids: their biochemical uniqueness. Sciences 1974; 186(4158):19–26.

22. Pablo G, Hammons A, Bradley S, Fulton JE. Characteristics of the extracellular lipases from *Corynebacterium acnes* and *Staphylococcus epidermidis*. J Invest Dermatol 1974; 63(2):231–8.

23. Sansone Bazzano G, Cummings B, Seeler AK, Reisner RM. Differences in the lipid constituents of sebum from pre-pubertal and pubertal subjects. Br J Dermatol 1980; 103:131–7.

24. Yamamoto A, Srizawa S, Masaaki I, Sato Y. Effect of aging on sebaceous gland activity and on the fatty acid composition of wax esters. J Invest Dermatol 1987; 89(5):507–12.

25. Green SC, Stewart ME, Downing DT. Variation in sebum fatty acid composition among adult humans. J Invest Dermatol 1984; 83:114–7.

26. Stewart ME McDonnell MW, Downing DT. Possible genetic control of the proportions of branched-chain fatty acids in human sebaceous wax esters. J Invest Dermatol 1986; 86(6):706–8.

27. Lampe MA, Williams ML, Elias PM. Human epidermal lipids: characterization and modulations during differentiation. J Lipid Res 1983; 24(2):131–40.

28. Elias PM, Brown BE, Fritsch P, Goerke J, Gray GM, White R. Localization and composition of lipids in neonatal mouse stratum granulosum and stratum corneum. J Invest Dermatol 1979; 73:339–48.

29. Imokawa G, Hattori M. A possible function of structural lipids in the water-holding properties of the stratum corneum. J Invest Dermatol 1985; 83:282–4.

30. Imokawa G, Akasaki S, Hattori M, Yoshizvka N. Selective recovery of deranged water holding properties by stratum corneum lipids. J Invest Dermatol 1986; 87:758–61.

31 Saint-Léger D, Francois AM, Lévêque JL, Stoudemayer TJ, Grove GL, Kligman AM. Age associated changes in stratum corneum lipids and their relation to dryness. Dermatologica 1988; 177:159–64.

32. Long SA, Wertz PW, Strauss JS, Downing DT. Human stratum corneum polar lipids and desquamation. Arch Dermatol Res 1985; 277:284–7.

33. Saint-Léger D, Francois AM, Lévêque JL, Stoudemayer TJ, Kligman AM, Grove GL. Stratum corneum lipids in skin xerosis. Dermatologica 1989; 178:151–5.

34. Imokawa G, Akihito A, Jin K, Higaki Y, Kawashima M, Hidano A. Decreased level of ceramides in stratum corneum of atopic dermatitis: an etiologic factor in atopic dry skin. J Invest Dermatol 1991; 96(4):523–6.

19

Objective Assessment of Skin Xerosis in the Aged

OLIVIER de LACHARRIÈRE

L'Oréal
Aulnay-sous-Bois, France

I. INTRODUCTION

By analogy with the appearance of "dry mud" and because of the particular aspects of xerotic skin, it is wrongly referred to as "dry skin." Dry skin is not representative of all the clinical aspects of xerosis (from the Greek *Xeros*, dry, rough). Thus, before considering skin xerosis in the aged, we must first define what we mean when we use this term.

The diagnosis of xerosis is based on a clinical description of the skin surface, which depends mainly on the status of the stratum corneum. According to Franchimont and Pierard (1), we propose to describe the clinical status of the skin surface using three basic parameters, each defined by pairs of antonyms: (1) desiccated or moisturized, (2) rough or smooth, and (3) asteatotic or seborrheic. *Skin xerosis* can thus be described as a nonexhaustive association of desiccation, roughness, and asteatosis. Variations in the intensity of these conditions enable the entire diversity of the clinical aspects of skin xerosis to be described. In the elderly, skin xerosis is very common and takes on a particular clinical form called senile xerosis.

II. CLINICAL ASPECTS OF SENILE XEROSIS

The incidence of xerosis increases with age. Clinically examining the feet of 1366 elderly people, Kligman (2) found that 80% had severe xerosis. Similarly, in a systematic examination of 68 noninstitutionalized elderly subjects, Beauregard and Gilchrest (3) found that 85% had xerosis.

Xerosis of the aged appears in the postmenopausal period in women and at around 60 years of age in men. In both sexes, the clinical features of senile xerosis are frank after 70 years of age. The semiologic signs vary in intensity according to the different areas of the body. A papery, dull, mat appearance, due to desiccation, is present over the entire surface of the body. Roughness and desquamation are less frequently observed and are localized predominantly on the lower legs but may occur on the arms and trunk. Asteatosis is often found on the face of women, but less commonly in men.

There are several clinical patterns of senile xerosis. Besides the rough and desquamative forms, the condition is often limited to desiccation alone, and this is usually associated with smoothness of the skin surface.

Senile xerosis can be associated with pathologic conditions, particularly on the limbs and the trunk, where affected skin can be fissured and pruritic, with consequent eczematization. In such cases, scaling and fissuring of the skin can create a "puzzlelike" or "pavementlike" appearance known as *eczema craquelé* (4).

Although senile pruritus is frequently associated with senile xerosis, the opposite is not true.

III. PATHOPHYSIOLOGIC CONSIDERATIONS IN SENILE XEROSIS

The clinical features of senile xerosis give rise to a variety of questions about its pathophysiology.

1) The dryness itself (see Table 1):
   a. Is the water content of the stratum corneum (SC) altered?
   b. Is physiologic water input into the stratum corneum altered?
   c. Is the water output by the SC altered?

Table 1 Main Elements Involved in the Water Content of the Stratum Corneum

Input elements	Water from viable epidermis
	Water from eccrine sweat
Output mechanisms	Water-holding capacity of stratum corneum (natural moisturizing factors)
	Barrier effect of stratum corneum (intercellular lipids)

2)   The roughness:
    a. Is skin microrelief altered?
    b. Is the cohesion of corneocytes altered?
3)   The asteatosis: Is sebum secretion altered?

If such alterations exist, are they involved with the mechanisms of senile xerosis? A further question is whether the pathophysiologic patterns of senile xerosis are similar to those observed in other forms of skin xerosis, such as atopic dermatitis. Objective methods, particularly noninvasive methods, are of real interest in answering these questions.

IV. OBJECTIVE METHODS FOR EVALUATING SKIN XEROSIS IN THE ELDERLY

A. Assessment of Hydration of Stratum Corneum

1. Assessment of Water Content of Stratum Corneum

Hydration of the stratum corneum can be measured directly in vivo by means of spectroscopy, although infrared and photoacoustic spectroscopy do not give absolute values of water content. Potts et al. (5) proposed a technique for direct quantitative measurements, but no data are yet available for senile xerosis.

Among the indirect methods, impedance measurement (6,7) is the most relevant for evaluating the hydration state of the skin surface. Skin conductance decreases with age (Fig. 1) (8,9).

The hydration status of SC induces deep changes in its plasticity and biomechanical properties. The measurement of such parameters is therefore another indirect approach to determining the water content of the SC

The torsional technique developed by de Rigal and Lévêque shows that some of the parameters recorded with this technique are related to the elasticity of the stratum corneum (10). Intrinsic extensibility U_E^* at low torque is the most relevant parameter, and it decreases from the age of 70 years (11).

By measuring the propagation and attenuation of shear waves in the skin (range of frequencies 8–1016 Hz) (12), Potts et al. (13) showed that the water content of the skin decreases with age; their experimental results suggest that the site of altered water content is the stratum corneum. All these in vivo measurements suggest that the water content of the stratum corneum decreases slightly with age. In vitro experiments have similarly shown a decrease in the amount of water bound within the SC in senile xerosis: 31.7 versus 38.2 mg per 100 ml in dry normal SC from glabrous skin (14). No experimental data are available for free water.

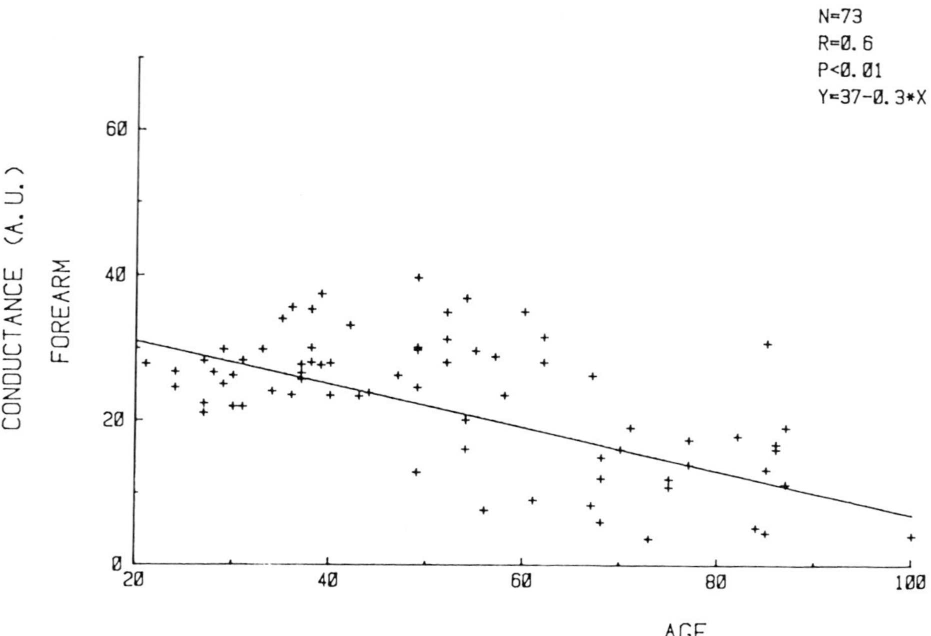

Figure 1 Conductance versus age (forearm, ventral side). (From Lévêque, Ref. 9, with permission.)

It is important to remember that aging does not modify the thickness of the stratum corneum; as a result, the changes observed could be linked to alterations in physiologic water input and/or output mechanisms.

2. Assessment of Physiologic Water Input Mechanisms in the Stratum Corneum

Physiologic water input in the SC involves two sources: the viable epidermis and the eccrine sweat glands. No data are available on the changes in the water content of the viable epidermis with age. It is known that the water content in the dermis increases with age (15) and that the ration between free and bound water probably changes. Whatever the case, it is not yet possible to assess physiologic water input from the viable epidermis.

Sweat secretion also decreases with age. This is probably related to a fall in the capacity of each gland to produce sweat, since sweat gland density is unchanged (16,17). Although in vivo measurements of eccrine sweat gland secretion are possible with L-lactate biosensors (18), no data are yet available in the literature on age-induced variations.

3. Assessment of Water Output Mechanisms in the Stratum Corneum

Water output by the stratum corneum is regulated by its permeability barrier and its water-holding capacity.

a. Barrier Property of the Stratum Corneum.   The effect of age on the cutaneous barrier is extensively reviewed by Wilhelm and Maibach in Chapter 17. We simply recall the following points:

> The barrier effect of the stratum corneum can be assessed in vivo by measurement of transepidermal water loss (TEWL). Using an Evaporimeter, the TEWL values are lowered in elderly subjects (19,20).
> The intercellular lipids of the stratum corneum play a critical role in the barrier function (21).

b. Water Holding Property.   It is believed that the water-holding property of the stratum corneum is linked to

> Water-soluble substances (24), called natural moisturizing factors (NMF), which originate in keratinocytes (histidine-rich protein, profilaggrine) and eccrine sweat. The composition of NMF is shown in table 2.
> Intercellular lipids, mainly ceramides (25,26).

1. Analysis of Natural Moisturizing Factors.   Noninvasive collection of corneocytes by stripping (27) or by skin scraping (28) permits the chemical analysis of samples of stratum corneum. Horii et al. (27) reported quantitative information. They found a decrease in free amino acid content in the SC (extractable amino acids) on the legs and volar forearm in senile xerosis. Furthermore, these authors found that "the amino acid content of SC showed a gradual increase in the aged skin with the number of strippings and reached

Table 2   Natural Moisturizing Factor Composition (%)

Free amino acids		40
Pyrrolidone carboxylic acid		12
Lactates		12
Urea		7
Mineral salts		18
Chloride	6	
Sodium	5	
Potassium	4	
Calcium, magnesium	3	
Other compounds		
(organic acids, sugars, citrate, peptides)		11

Source: From References 22 and 23.

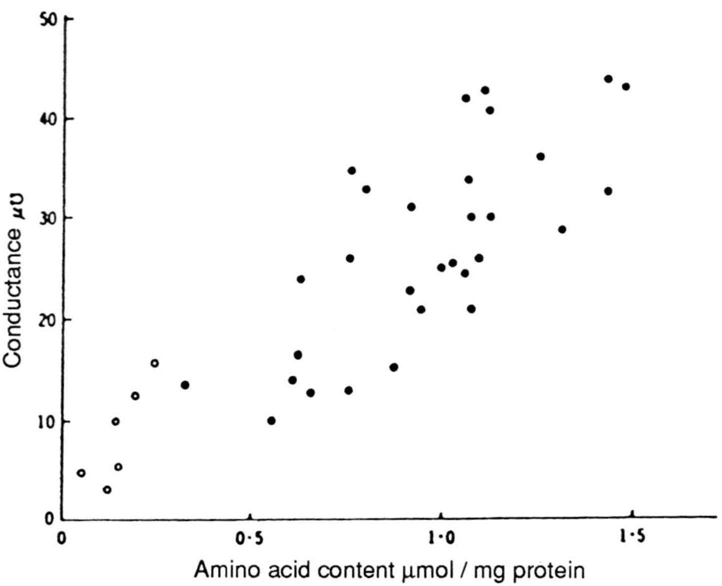

Figure 2 Relationship between amino acid content of the stratum corneum and skin surface conductance in patients with senile xerosis and those with ichthyosis vulgaris (r = 0.81). (From Hoorii et al., Ref. 27, with permission.)

a plateau after the fifth stripping.'' The intensity of senile xerosis (assessed by clinical examination and conductance measurements) correlates directly with amino acid content (Fig. 2). However, clinical improvements following topical therapy are not associated with significant changes in the amino acid content.

Jacobson et al. (28) published qualitative data. They compared the amino acid composition on the legs of young people (less than 30 years) and old people (more than 60 years) with and without "dry skin." They noted a decrease in the amino acid content and changes in composition that varied according to age and the presence or absence of dry skin. However, the clinical basis for the diagnosis of dry skin was not given and no physical measurements for the objective assessment of water content were done, making it difficult to compare these results with others.

2. Analysis of Stratum Corneum Lipids. Stratum corneum lipids (SCL) play a role in both water retention and the permeability barrier function of the SC (21,29–31). It has been shown that ceramides, the major component of SCL, are important to both functions (26,32). Noninvasive collection of SC by means of a turbine device and direct lipid extraction (33) or by stripping with cyanoacrylate glue and secondary lipid extraction (34) has been used, but the results are controversial.

Saint-Léger et al. found no statistical correlation between the total amount of SCL collected and age or skin dryness (33). In an another study (34), however, they found a significant association between dry skin scores and both the decrease in neutral lipids (sterol esters, wax esters, and triglycerides) and the increase in free fatty acids. They discussed the relationship of these modifications to the decline in the activity of the sebaceous glands, but the absence of squalene—a sebaceous marker—suggests a weak contribution of sebaceous lipids to SCL in this case. Imokawa et al. (35) reported that the total amount of SCL per mg stratum corneum declines with age; the ceramide content of the SC was significantly lower with age. By analogy with results for uninvolved skin of patients with atopic dermatitis and associated xerosis, these authors find it conceivable that the decrease in ceramide content is associated with the dry appearance of xerotic skin.

The different modes of SCL collection must be taken into account in interpreting these opposing results. In any event, it is not yet possible to reach a conclusion about changes in SCL with age.

3. Assessment of the Water-Holding Capacity of the Stratum Corneum.

Overall water-holding capacity can be assessed by the water sorption-desorption test developed by Tagami et al. (36). Comparing dry skin in old people, normal skin in young people, and uninvolved dry skin in patients with atopic dermatitis, the measurements on the upper arm reported by Thune (37) gave conflicting data: the hydration state (assessed by conductance measurement) was better in old people, and the water-holding capacity was higher. There is no clear explanation for these surprising results.

B. Assessment of Skin Roughness

1. Skin Microrelief and Roughness

An extensive review of skin microrelief changes with age is presented by Corcuff and Lévêque in Chapter 13. As we have seen, roughness can be a component of xerosis. Therefore, profilometry measurements of skin microrelief can provide interesting information. There is full agreement that the depth of furrows increases with age (19,38–40), doubling on the volar forearm and increasing by one-half on the outer legs (39). In contrast, the mean line density decreases with age (19). From a clinical point of view these results are somewhat surprising, since roughness is undoubtedly greater on the leg than on the volar forearm. This suggests that the depth and density of furrows are not correlated with clinical skin roughness.

2. Corneocyte Cohesion and Roughness

The cohesiveness of the stratum corneum and the way in which it changes with age are developed by Marks in Chapter 15. The cyanoacrylate strip biopsy technique (41–43) is of value in the assessment of senile xerosis. Using this method, Pierard-Franchimont and Pierard (43,44) showed that the cleavage plane of the horny layer is marked by an irregularity. "Corneocytes are torn away as single cells or in sheets," suggesting a change in corneocyte cohesion in the outer part of the SC, a phenomenon that is probably involved in clinical roughness.

C. Assessment of Sebum Secretion

Changes in sebum secretion with age are reviewed by Saint-Léger and Agache in Chapter 18. We simply recall here that the sebum secretion rate declines with age. The intuitive belief that low-level secretion of sebum (composed of nonpolar lipids) is linked to skin xerosis has not been confirmed. Investigating a possible link between dry skin and sebum secretion in 76 old people, Downing et al. (45) found no correlation in either sex.

V. CONCLUSION

As previously mentioned, the term "dry" is misleading in the description of skin xerosis. The absence of a consensus for the definitions of skin xerosis and senile xerosis should be borne in mind. The clinical pattern we considered for our purpose is, in our opinion, the closest to the clinical presentations encountered.

In this review devoted to senile xerosis, we considered the main features, independently of variations according to body area and sun-exposed or unexposed zones.

Although no direct measurements of the water content of the SC in senile xerosis have been possible, indirect methods indicate that there is a slight decrease. Even if such indirect assessments reflect a true physiologic change, it is not known which fraction of water is concerned (free or bound). Some experimental results indicate that several factors probably play a role in modification of the water content of the SC with age, as well as input (mainly sweat secretion?) and output mechanisms (mainly water-holding capacity). However, there is a marked lack of data in this field. Skin roughness changes in senile xerosis, based on clinical assessments, are difficult to understand, although there may be a link with the depth of skin furrows. In this field, anomalies in the desquamation of the SC must be further evaluated using objective noninvasive methods. Sebum secretion is not correlated with xerosis.

Senile xerosis, a condition with both dermatologic and cosmetologic implications, has not yet yielded all its secrets.

REFERENCES

1. Franchimont C, Pierard GE, Kératinisation, xéroses et peau séche. In: Robert P, ed. Dermatopharmacologie clinique. Quebec: Edisem; Paris: Maloine, 1985; 215–21.
2. Kligman AM, Perspectives and problems in cutaneous gerontology. J Invest Dermatol 1979; 73:39–46.
3. Beauregard S, Gilchrest BA. A survey of skin problems and skin care regimens in the elderly. Arch Dermatol 1987; 123:1638–43.
4. Kaplan LA. Xerosis. In: Newcomer VD, Young EM, eds. Geriatric dermatology. New York: Igaku-Shoin, 1989; 309–14.
5. Potts RO, Guzek DB, Harris RR, McKie JE. A noninvasive, in vivo technique to quantitatively measure water concentration of the stratum corneum using attenuated total-reflectance infrared spectroscopy. Arch Dermatol Res 1985; 277:489–495.
6. Lévêque J-L, de Rigal J. Impedance methods for studying skin moisturization. J Soc Cosmet Chem 1983; 34:419–428.
7. Tagami H, Ohi M, Iwatsuki K, Kanamaru Y, Yamada M, Ichijo B. Evaluation of the skin surface hydration in vivo by electrical measurement. J Invest Dermatol 1980; 75:500–7.
8. Tagami H. Impedance measurement for evaluation of the hydration state of the skin surface. In: Lévêque J-L, ed. Cutaneous investigation in health and disease—noninvasive methods and instrumentation. (New York: Marcel Dekker, Basel) 1989; 79–111.
9. Lévêque J-L. Méthodes expérimentales d'étude du vieillissement cutané chez l'homme in vivo. Ann Dermatol Venereol 1987; 114:1279–83.
10. De Rigal J, Lévêque J-L. In vivo measurement of the stratum corneum elasticity. Bioeng Skin 1985; 1:13–23.
11. Escoffier C, de Rigal J, Rochefort A, Vasselet R, Lévêque J-L, Agache PG. Age-related mechanical properties of human skin: an in vivo study. J Invest Dermatol 1989; 93:353–7.
12. Potts RO, Chrisman DA, Buras EM. The dynamic mechanical properties of human skin in vivo. J Biomech 1983; 16:365–72.
13. Potts RO, Buras EM, Chrisman DA. Changes with age in the moisture content of human skin. J Invest Dermatol 1984; 82:97–100.
14. Takenouchi M, Suzuki H, Tagami H. Hydration characteristics of pathologic stratum corneum—evaluation of bound water. J Invest Dermatol 1986; 87: 574–6.
15. Pearce RH, Grimmer BJ. Age and the chemical constitution of normal human dermis. J Invest Dermatol 1972; 58:347–61.
16. Anderson RK, Kenney WL. The effect of age on heat-activated sweat gland density and flow during exercice in dry heat. J Appl Physiol 1987; 63:1089–94.

17. Kenney WL, Anderson RK. Responses of older and younger women to exercise in dry and humid heat without fluid replacement. Med Sci Sports Exerc 1988; 20:155–60.

18. Bernard D, Bazin R, Kermici M, Prunieras M. Utilisation d'une électrode à enzyme pour la mesure in vivo du L-Lactate cutané. English/French Symposium on Skin Ageing—causes and prevention: April 25–27, 1990, Blois, France.

19. Lévêque J-L, Corcuff P, de Rigal J, Agache P. In vivo studies of the evolution of physical properties of human skin with age. Int J Dermatol 1984; 23:322–9.

20. Tagami H. Aging and the hydratation state of the skin. In: Kligman AM, Takase Y, eds. Cutaneous aging. Tokyo: University of Tokyo Press, 1988; 99.

21. Imokawa G, Akasaki S, Hattori M, Yoshizuka N. Selective recovery of deranged water-holding properties by stratum corneum lipids. J Invest Dermatol 1986; 87:758–61.

22. Jacobi O. Water and water-vapor absorption of the stratum corneum of the living human skin. J Appl Physiol 1958; 12:403–7.

23. Spier HW, Pasher G. Quantitative untersuchungen über die freien aminosäuren der hautoberfläche. Zur frage ihrer genese. Klin Wochschr 1953; 31:997–1000.

24. Middleton JD. The mechanism of water binding in stratum corneum. Br J Dermatol 1968; 80:437–50.

25. Elias PE. Epidermal lipids, barrier function and desquamation. J Invest Dermatol 1983; 80:44s–9s.

26. Downing DT, Wertz PW, Stewart ME. The role of sebum and epidermal lipids in the cosmetic properties of skin. Int J Cosmet Soc 1986; 8:115–23.

27. Hoorii I, Nakayala Y, Obata M, Tagami H. Stratum corneum hydration and amino acid content in xerotic skin. Br J Dermatol 1989; 121:587–92.

28. Jacobson TM, Yüksel U, Geesin JC, Gordon JS, Lane AT, Gracy RW. Effects of aging and xerosis on the amino acid composition of human skin. J Invest Dermatol 1990; 95:296–300.

29. Imokawa G, Hattori M. A possible function of structural lipids in the water-holding properties of the stratum corneum. J Invest Dermatol 1985; 83:282–4.

30. Elias PM. Epidermal lipids, barrier function and desquamation. J Invest Dermatol 1983; 80:44s–9s.

31. Lévêque J-L, Escoubez M, Rasseneur L. Water-keratin interaction in human stratum corneum. Bioeng Skin 1987; 3:227–42.

32. Kawashima M, Morita K, Higaki Y, Hidano A, Abe A, Imokawa G. Quantitative analysis of ceramides in the stratum corneum of aged skin and atopic dermatitis (abstract). J Invest Dermatol 1990; 94:541.

33. Saint-Léger D, François AM, Lévêque J-L, Stoudemayer TJ, Grove GL, Kligman AM. Aged-associated changes in stratum corneum lipids and their relation to dryness. Dermatologica 1988; 177:159–64.

34. Saint-Léger D, François AM, Lévêque J-L, Stoudemayer TJ, Kligman AM, Grove G. Stratum corneum lipids in skin xerosis. Dermatologica 1989; 178:151–5.

35. Imokawa G, Abe A, Jin K, Higaki Y, Kawashima M, Hidano A. Decreased level of ceramides in stratum corneum of atopic dermatitis: an etiologic factor in atopic dry skin? J Invest Dermatol 1991; 96:523–6.

36. Tagami H, Kanamaru Y, Inoue K, et al. Water sorption-desorption test of the skin in vivo for functional assessment of the stratum corneum. J Invest Dermatol 1982; 78:425–8.

37. Thune P. Evaluation of the hydration and the water-holding capacity in atopic skin and so-called dry skin. Acta Derm Venereol Suppl (Stockh) 1989; 144: 133–5.

38. Corcuff P, de Rigal J, Lévêque J-L, Makki S, Agache P. Skin relief and aging. J Cosmet Chem 1983; 34:177–90.

39. Mignot J, Zahouani H, Rondot D, Nardin P. Morphological study of human skin relief. Bioeng Skin 1987; 3:177–96.

40. Agache PG, Mignot J, Makki S. Microtopography of the skin and aging. In: eds. Cutaneous aging. Kligman AM, Takase Y, Tokyo: University of Tokyo Press, 1988; 475–99.

41. Lachapelle JM, Gouverneur JC, Boulet M, Tennstedt D. A modified technique (using polyester tape) of skin surface biopsy. Br J Dermatol 1977; 97:49–52.

42. Marks R, Dawber RPR. Skin surface biopsy: an improved technique for the examination of the horny layer. Br J Dermatol 1971; 84:117–23.

43. Pierard-Franchimont C, Pierard GE. Lex xéroses: structure de le peau rêche. Int J Cosmet Soc 1984; 6:47–54.

44. Franchimont C. The stratum corneum xerotic from aging and photochemotherapy (PUVA). A Study by scanning electron microscopy. Am J Dermatopathol 1980; 2:295–304.

45. Downing DT, Wertz PW, Stewart ME. The role of sebum and epidermal lipids in the cosmetic properties of skin. Int J Cosmet Soc 1986; 8:115–23.

20

Psychologic Aspects of Skin Disorders in the Elderly

ALBERT M. KLIGMAN

University of Pennsylvania
Philadelphia, Pennsylvania

I. INTRODUCTION

Skin problems in aged persons must be viewed differently from the diseases that receive much attention from geriatricians, for example, arthritis, malignancy, and cardiovascular disorders. Skin disorders generally do not end life, nor are they disabling or immobilizing. No one dies of old skin. As structurally degraded as it might become, skin never wears out. We are well packaged in our integuments and protected from external assaults to the very end. Of course, old age brings with it physiologic deficits in skin as in all organs. For example, there occurs a marked deletion of superficial blood vessels. As a result the skin is less able to mount a vigorous inflammatory reaction against chemicals and microorganisms (1). With modest care, however, decreased responses are neither troublesome nor dangerous. Indeed, one might view this diminished reactivity as a biological blessing; inflammatory signs (redness, swelling, and pain) become muted, and predictably, some stubborn, chronic dermatoses tend to regress or disappear in old age, namely atopic dermatitis and psoriasis.

Malignancies of the skin are exceedingly common, with an annual prevalence rate almost equal to that of all others combined. In this case also, however, except for the relatively uncommon malignant melanoma, the major tumors (basal and squamous cell cancers) are rather benign. They usually do not metastasize and are generally not killers, although they may be locally quite destructive. Fear of skin cancer cannot be placed high on the list of diseases that frighten the elderly.

The worst disorders, decubitus ulcers for example, are really secondary to other medical problems that result in immobility. If this perspective is accurate, should problems associated with aging skin be of much concern to caretakers of the elderly or to the aged themselves? The skin troubles of old people are generally unrecognized, and standards of care are very low. This negligence can be attributed to ignorance rather than callousness. Skin specialists who have looked into the extent of the severity of skin problems among the aged know that these are often the bane of existence (2). These disorders do not end life, but they can certainly ruin and spoil it. Dry, scaly, rough skin, an unwanted possession of *all* people over 70, feels uncomfortable, is itchy and disquieting, and disturbs sleep. Reflexive scratching worsens the disturbance, increasing irritability and restlessness. Moisturizers, not tranquilizers, are the proper response. Many other superficial conditions can be cited that comprise what older people themselves call their "skin miseries." Itching, in fact, is far less tolerable than pain and, unfortunately, less controllable by drugs. Pain alone rarely drives sufferers to suicide, in contrast to the desperation of patients with generalized pruritus.

Gerontologists are not aware that the pattern of aging changes in skin is different from that in other organs. Covered areas of skin, such as the inner arm or buttock, endure the passage of time beautifully, showing very little change until after about age 50. Physiologic functions, like the reproductive activity of epidermal cells, then begin to decline gradually and usually not noticeably (3). Even after 60, except for looseness and some loss of elasticity, the skin remains smooth and unblemished. By the late sixties, the slope steepens and the changes become more evident. Still, it is only in the exposed sun-damaged areas that diverse lesions make their appearance.

This discussion is a prelude to the theme I develop here. It is not frank disease or functional deficits that are the chief sources of the skin sufferings of the aged. It is psychology, not pathology, that is the focus of interest here. It will come as a surprise to many geriatricians that the major complaints relate to the social and psychologic consequences of "badly" aged skin, which no longer looks and feels good. These are largely subjective matters, relating to the psychosocial, not the biologic, functions of skin. When the skin becomes uncomfortable as a biologic garment, distress signals are sent to the higher centers of the brain, inciting irritable moods and behaviors. Moreover, as the skin becomes increasingly unhandsome, it repels physical contact by self and by others. Having skin that no one "loves to touch," including the possessor, is a serious matter (4). The need to be touched, fondled, caressed, rubbed, and massaged does not end in infancy. Studies of animals and humans deprived of touching after being born show they do not develop normally, physically or mentally (5). We can only guess what happens when an old person becomes nontactile, literally forced out of contact and deprived of the pleasurable sensations nice skin long provided. The skin's role as an organ of expression has been keenly recognized by poets and peasants less so than by physicians. We all know that deep emotions can turn on feeling-specific displays, including blanching, blushing, reddening, sweating, and bristling.

The sociologic aspects of skin, what might be called "social skin," need much greater emphasis. The skin is an organ of communication; it sends varied messages (6). Depending on care and adornment, it can communicate status, age, health, sex, wealth, and so on. In all societies skin has never been left alone but has been the object of systematic transformations.

II. SKIN PROBLEMS OF THE AGED

After adolescence, the percentage of people with skin disorders steadily increases. Moreover, each person has an increased number of skin conditions (7). Most people over 65 have 2–3 conditions that warrant medical attention. Indeed, the diversity of problems is noteworthy; 10% of those over 70 may have 10–15 skin complaints simultaneously.

The most common complaints do not affect the general health; they are mainly nuisances, troublesome because of discomfort and high visibility. High on the list are dry skin, fungus infections of the feet, seborrheic dermatitis, and a host of facial alterations that comprise the well-known unattractive portrait of old age, namely, wrinkles, sags, bags, blotches and splotches, fleshy nevi, pigmented lentigines, dilated sprays of vessels, seborrheic keratoses, actinic keratoses, and yellow, leathery, loose skin (7). It cannot be too strongly stated that virtually all these facial lesions are preventable; they do not represent intrinsic aging but are better described as *photoaging*, imposed largely by needless exposure to sun and the elements (8). Still, this assorted collection of disfigurements does not raise health issues. Their importance lies in debauched, deteriorated appearance and the resultant psychologic effects. It is difficult to feel good when one looks bad. It is a meritorious maxim that says that "looking better is feeling better." We do, all of us, take things at face value. Every blemish, every imperfection affronts us, damaging our self-image, which in turn lowers our self-esteem (9).

Prophylaxis against these delayed cutaneous distresses is easy and highly effective. One does not have to seek the shade or wear wide hats, grotesque pastes, or imprisoning clothing. Modern sunscreens are exceptionally efficacious and come in multiple forms to suit every need and style (10). Some form invisible films that resist swimming and perspiration. Whether a solution, cream, ointment, or spray is chosen, it is best to screen out as much of the harmful rays as possible; thus, the proper choice is the high-potency, sun protection factor (SPF) 15 sunscreen available in any supermarket.

III. SOCIAL REACTIONS TO SKIN DISEASE

One can better understand the heavy psychologic penalties imposed by skin disorders by examining the problem in historical context.

The records show that in all societies at all times, persons with skin diseases have suffered severe discrimination (11). They are viewed as lepers (biblical leprosy embraced a half-dozen disorders) and are repulsed and reviled. People with heart disease or cancer elicit sympathy, not the disgust and fear that sick skin produces. Thus, it is scarcely surprising that patients with skin disorders typically have fears and anxieties far out of proportion to the severity of the illness. This is not an inappropriate, neurotic reaction. The patient with an eruption can directly *see* how the disease affects others. Why are skin afflictions such a special curse, different from all other diseases?

For one thing, in ancient times skin sores were recognized, often correctly, as contagious. Indeed, today in crowded inner cities, skin infections are still common and highly transmissible. Yet the contagiousness of skin lesions, including leprosy, the most loathsome of diseases, has been enormously exaggerated. Following the historical thread, we can trace the pervasive notion that skin disease reflects not only physical dirtiness but spiritual filth and decadence as well. (12) This idea cuts across all cultures, although possibly most clearly enunciated in the Old Testament, in which skin disorders are regarded as punishment for sins. Thus, transgressors were visibly marked with disease, notifying everyone of their sinful nature. Consistently, clearing of the eruption was taken as a sign of expiation, the sinner having suffered enough to be redeemed. This association of skin disease with evil within persists to this very day. When asked what they think caused their chronic, unexplained skin disease, many patients attribute it to wrongdoing, not necessarily old-fashioned sins but more modern versions: poor diet, drinking, sexual irregularities, hostile actions, and others (13). In short, skin lesions represent blameworthiness.

IV. PSYCHOLOGIC EFFECT OF BLEMISHES

Inflammatory skin disease, with its spilling of internal contents onto the surface, alarms the ordinary observer. The blistered, oozing, smelly, crusted skin is as offensive as someone vomiting or having diarrhea in public. Leaking from either end of the gastrointestinal tract or through the skin is vile and despicable.

The skin stigmata of the aged face, however, are not inflammatory spillages or smelly, dirty rashes. They are mainly discolorations, creases, and growths, better described as disfigurements. They are alterations of the surface that mainly affect esthetic appearance. It turns out, however, that these defacements evoke strongly negative reactions in the observer. Photoaged skin, in short, is repugnant, generating aversive behaviors (14).

Insight into this negativism can be gained by examining patients whose disorders consist solely of discolorations. For example, studies of patients with no pigment (vitiligo and albinism) and those with purple-red discolorations (port-wine stains) make it clear that the afflicted suffer a great deal of psychic pain (15, 16). In some societies, such persons have often been banished, literally a death sentence. There is a good deal of truth in the saying that beauty is skin deep. We love to look at smooth, unblemished skin (associated with youth and health), and conversely we turn away from blemished skin (associated with old age and ill health).

The core of the problem is that disfigurements are unattractive, displeasing, and disturbing, especially in the elderly. The changes are, of course, ugly. Much more than esthetics is involved in the aversive behavior of the young to the elderly, however. My speculation is that the facial portrait of the aged person disturbs us because it reminds us of our own coming physical decrepitude and eventual death. The prospect of looking old, even more than being old, is frightening and unnerving. Much better to keep the elderly out of sight in nursing homes and retirement communities.

In this sense, the first wrinkle is an unnerving event. A face full of wrinkles is an emotional disaster. I suggest that the aged might be treated more kindly if their integuments were better preserved in old age.

V. APPEARANCE, HEALTH, AND LONGEVITY IN THE AGED

In our laboratory we presented photographs of aging females to a neutral panel of men and women who were asked to rate 48 stimulus persons on a seven-point, bipolar scale (17). From these 16 females were selected who were the most physically attractive and an equal number from the bottom of the unattractive group. These two polar groups were then intensively interviewed with regard to psychologic differences. Not surprisingly, the attractive groups perceived themselves far more positively by a number of important dimensions.

They thought they were in better health and had a better overall feeling of well-being. They were emotionally more cheerful and better adjusted, which enabled them to have a more positive outlook on life. The latter finding is extremely important in view of the high frequency of depression in the aged. The attractive aged were also more satisfied with their lives, more socially engaged, and more realistic. All this says, unequivocally, that the positive attributes associated with beauty in youth and adult life extend as well as to the aged.

These findings complement those of Connor et al., who found that the attractive elderly are perceived more favorably by others (18). Evidence is accumulating that the benefits of being attractive are more medically significant later in life. The physically attractive may not only have greater satisfactions, they may actually be healthier and live longer. More than 1000 elderly males have been participating in a longitudinal study requiring annual checkups during which a battery of 24 age-related variables has been administered (19). In addition to assessment of lung, heart, kidney, hearing, eye, functions, and so on, the participants were divided into an upper and lower 15% based on whether they looked younger or older to physicians than their chronologic age. The similarly aged men who looked good, that is, young, were then contrasted physiologically with those who looked bad, that is, old. In 15 of 24 tests, the old-looking group was indeed biologically older. Moreover, the young-looking group actually lived longer. It is extraordinary that physical appearance predicts physical health so well. There may be some truth in packaging!

It requires no imaginative effort to account for the evident advantages the attractive elderly seem to enjoy. The dynamics are not very different than for the young. Those who are good-looking in old age were assuredly comely when younger. The beautiful people receive automatic approval and endorsement, reinforcing a sense of high worth, self-regard, and confidence (20). Persons who feel good about themselves are likely to behave more generously and agreeably to others, which of course elicits favorable responses contributing to well-being. Conversely, the unattractive, who are treated less favorably, are likely to have less esteem, fewer social opportunities, and, in the face of late life's increasing uncertainties, fewer resources to deal with stress. Indeed, the unattractive may surrender to their fate when needed social support is not forthcoming.

It should be emphasized that being physically unattractive poses real risks of becoming emotionally ill (14). The elderly themselves turn away from persons whose faces are badly wrinkled and blotched, studded with growths and with hanging, flabby skin. Emotionally disturbed persons in institutions are far worse off if they happen to be unattractive. Again, even in this setting, beauty counts heavily.

VI. APPEARANCE MODIFICATION IN THE ELDERLY

An enormous range of services are available to overcome the sizable handicaps that accrue from loss of good looks in the elderly, whether or not the deterioration is self-induced, as in the case of photoaging.

Tumors and excrescences can be destroyed or removed in a dozen different speedy, inexpensive ways with splendid cosmetic results. Soft tissue defects, such as wrinkles and scars, can be inflated with silicone or collagen. Pigmented lesions can be bleached out with liquid nitrogen. Saggy, baggy skin can be corrected by face-lifting, and blotchy, yellow skin can be completely resurfaced by phenol peels. In short, of the many types of skin lesions in the exposed body areas, practically all can be corrected or ameliorated by a range of surgical procedures. The technical services are widely available, and the required skills are, for the most part, not hard to master.

The greater problem is educational—to convince the elderly that the eradication of appearance-detracting lesions is worthwhile, not simply for vanity's sake, but for the sake of physical and mental health. We need to enlighten the elderly that negative appearance predisposes to negative reactions in every encounter, while shopping, partying, socializing, or whatever. Caring for appearance establishes positive behavior patterns that enhance good health and caring for self and others.

The "psychology of cosmetic therapy" is a new, rapidly burgeoning field that is receiving increasing attention from dermatologists, psychologists, social scientists, surgeons, cosmeticians, and estheticians. The nonsurgical aspects of cosmetic therapy have barely reached the consciousness of professionals. An astounding array of products are available for highlighting good facial features and subduing bad ones.

In an earlier study we were surprised to find that the physically unattractive aged did not differ materially in their usage or attitudes toward cosmetics (17). The unattractive did not achieve their undesirable visage by being ignorant of or neglectful of daily cosmetics. It was apparent that the elderly, whether attractive or not, were much in need of instruction regarding the proper use of cosmetics, their purposes and benefits. Questioning revealed that the elderly had a good deal of anxiety about cosmetics, especially concerning the possibility of being judged frivolous and ludicrous—trying to recapture youth by cosmetic cunning. The fact is that elderly women do not know how to use cosmetics effectively.

The makeover is an art form insufficiently known to health care professionals and older persons in general. Administered by a professional, it takes 30–45 minutes and results in a dramatic enhancement of appearance. The materials are familiar—lipstick, powders, rouge, eye shadow, and foundation—expertly exploited. Hair styling and coloring add to the esthetic impact. The result is a stunning and pleasing transformation that has immediate social consequences.

We compared the effect of makeovers on physically attractive older women with unattractive women of the same age. The psychologic and social benefits were instantly obvious to both groups (21). There was an immediate psychologic boost. The women felt more optimistic and became more outgoing, more social, and more confident. Naturally, self-esteem was enriched. Interestingly, the unattractive experienced greater benefits, perhaps because of starting at a lower level, which of course would intensify the contrast. Moreover, the skills involved in the makeover can be taught to become part of the individual's daily cosmetic practice.

This study showed us that cosmetic therapy could help the elderly adopt more positive attitudes and improve their self-regard and confidence. A better appearance may result indirectly in more favorable attitudes and actions toward the elderly. Moreover, cosmetic therapy can help to close the wide gap that currently separates the badly aged from those whom time has treated more gently.

We also see a place for cosmetic therapy as a supportive measure in general geriatric practice. With aging come more chronic disorders, and these have greater negative impacts on well-being and mental health. Depression and worry are constant companions of the chronic diseases that burden the elderly. Any tactic that aids coping and improves life's little pleasures should be incorporated into medical management.

VII. SUMMARY

The aged have many skin problems. However, these are not like the "high-visibility" diseases that are the subject of geriatric texts. Skin diseases are not disabling, do not hamper self-care, and are not killers. Nonetheless, they are important for reasons of which geriatricians are mainly unaware. Simply stated, they spoil the quality of life. An aged, degraded skin is uncomfortable to live in. It is often dry, scaly, and itchy. It does not fit very well and is not pleasant to feel or to touch. Even worse, a garment disfigured and reformed by time is exceedingly unattractive and leads to averse reactions by others. The unhandsome aged have trouble maintaining self-esteem when they recollect the smooth, unmarked, turgid skin—the clothing of their youth. They are repellent to themselves and to others. All this conduces toward lessening contact between the aged and potential providers of support, including health care providers.

Enhancement of appearance provides a psychologic boost that may feed back to positive thoughts and actions. ''Looking good is feeling better'' is a sound maxim for improving health.

Cosmetic therapy is a neglected aspect of geriatric care. Instruction in the selection, use, and value of cosmetics should start at an early age. In old age, the benefits of appearance enhancement should not be denied or ignored. The elderly are largely incompetent in the effective use of cosmetics to subdue the visible ravages of age. Dermatologists, too, need education and enlightenment. For example, instead of merely treating the lesion or disease, it is equally important to keep the blemishes out of sight, to maintain an appearance that provokes neither stares nor separateness. Masking and camouflaging cosmetics are available in marvelous colors and textures to conceal almost every disfigurement.

Psychiatrists dealing with the varied mental illnesses of the aged, including irreversible brain disease, should begin to explore cosmetic therapy as a therapeutic adjunct.

REFERENCES

1. Kligman AM. Perspectives and problems in cutaneous gerontology. J Invest Dermatol 1979; 73:39–46.
2. Tindall JP, Smith JG. Skin lesions of the Aged. JAMA 1963; 186:1039–42.
3. Grove GL, Kligman AM. Age-associated changes in human epidermal cell renewal. J Gerontol 1983; 38:137–42.
4. Graham JA, Jouhar AJ. The importance of cosmetics in the psychology of appearance. Int J Dermatol 1983; 22:153–6.
5. Kastenbaum R. On the significance of skin in human aging and survival. Psychobiological observations. Columbia Point Campus. University of Massachusetts, 1974.
6. Adams GR. Physical attractiveness research: toward a developmental social psychology of beauty. Hum Dev 1977; 20:217–39.
7. Johnson MLT, Robert J. Relevance of dermatologic disease among persons 1–74 years of age. Vital and Health Statistics of the National Center for Health Statistics, No. 4, Bethesda, MD: U.S. Department of Health, Education and Welfare, January 26, 1977.
8. Kligman AM. Early destruction effect of sunlight in human skin. JAMA 1969; 210:2377–80.
9. Shuster S, Fisher GH, Harris E, Bennell D. The effect of skin disease on self-image. Br J Dermatol 1978; 99:18–24.
10. Kaidbey KH, Kligman AM. Laboratory methods for appraising the efficacy of sunscreens. J Soc Cosmet Chem 1978; 29:525–36.
11. Mathis EW, Kahn A. Physical attractiveness, happiness, neuroticism and self-esteem. J Psychol 1975; 90:27–30.

12. Hughes GR. The cosmetic arts in ancient Egypt. J Soc Cosmet Chem 1959; 10:159–63.
13. Parrish JA, Gilchrest BA, Fitzpatrick TB. Between you and me. Boston: Little Brown, 1980.
14. Farina A, Fischer E, Sherman S, Smith WT, Groh T, Merman P. Physical attractiveness and mental illness. J Abnorm Psychol 1977; 86:510–7.
15. Porter J, Beuf A, Nordlund J, Lerner AB. Personal responses of patients and vitiligo. Arch Dermatol 1978; 114:1384–5.
16. Kalick SM, Goldwyn RM, Noe JM. Social issues and body image concerns of port wine stain patients. Lasers Surg Med 1981; 1:205–13.
17. Graham J, Kligman AM. Physical attractiveness, cosmetic use and self-perception in the elderly. Int. Jour. Cosm. Sci. 7:85–97, 1985.
18. Connor CL, Walsh RP, Litzelman DK, Alvarez MG. Evaluation of job applicants: the effects of age versus success. J Gerontol 1978; 33:246–52.
19. Borkan GA, Norris AH. Assessment of biologic age using a profile of physical parameters. J Gerontol 1980; 35:177–84.
20. Dion K, Berscheid E, Walster E. What is beautiful is good. J Pers Soc Psychol 1972; 24:285–90.
21. Graham JA, Kligman AM. Cosmetic therapy for the elderly. J Soc Cosmet Chem 1984; 35:133–45.

21

Efficacy of Topical Treatment of Aging Skin

JEAN-LUC LÉVÊQUE

L'Oréal
Aulnay-sous-Bois, France

ROLAND BAZIN

L'Oréal
Chevilly-Larue, France

I. INTRODUCTION

Noninvasive methods aimed at giving an objective estimation of skin changes during the aging process can also be sued to evaluate the efficacy of a given treatment. As we see later, numerous cosmetic products provide a clear benefit. In addition, the results of such noninvasive techniques generally correlate well with clinical assessments and the subjective appreciation by the person concerned, although there are some exceptions that can usually be explained in rational terms (1).

The treatment of aged-related pathologies is not discussed in this chapter, and neither is the important role of makeup products in covering the symptoms of skin aging. Although some noninvasive methods can provide valuable information in this setting, ''psychosensory'' methods and simple enquiries based on rating scales with parametric or nonparametric criteria are generally more suitable for evaluating both ''efficacy'' and ease of use, since the main aim of such products is to change the esthetic aspect. The psychosocial impact of makeup preparations is important, as shown in several concrete experiments (this aspect was dealt with in Chap. 20).

Age-related modifications of the skin can be classified into the following three categories, for which various types of product exist:

1. Problems of dry skin and skin firmness
2. Problems of wrinkles and skin texture
3. Problems of skin color and pigmentation

These three categories are first dealt with in the light of published data on cosmetic products and then with regard to the effect of all-*trans*-retinoic acid (RA).

II. EFFECT OF COSMETICS

A. Dry Skin

After the sixth or seventh decade of life, most elderly people suffer from skin dryness over almost the entire body surface (see Chap. 19). In addition to the discomfort and esthetic aspect, dry skin is usually associated with pruritus, which can be painful.

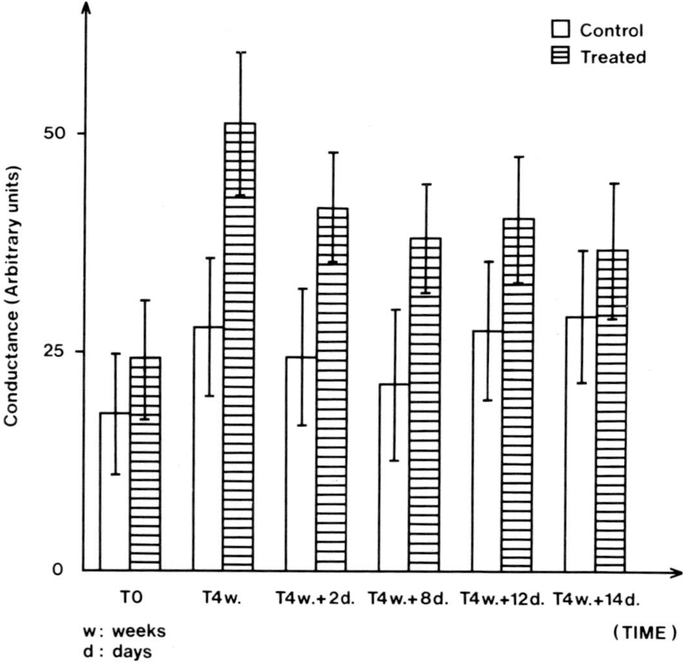

Figure 1 Effects of cosmetic treatment on the electrical conductance of the skin of the forearm. The conductance of the treated forearm was still significantly higher than that of the control forearm 12 days after a 4 week treatment period. (Courtesy of R. Bazin, L'Oréal.)

Several moisturizing products are highly effective in improving and sometimes eliminating these problems, and several examples have been published in the clinical and instrumental literature (2) . The instrumental technique most commonly used (being the simplest) is measurement of cutaneous electrical conductance, although the exact nature of the phenomenon measured is not entirely clear (3).

Figure 1 shows the type of result one might expect to obtain during repeated treatment over a 4 week period. The data are from a study of 25 volunteers; one arm was treated; the other served as a control. That the effect persisted for 2 weeks after the end of the treatment period shows that the observed improvement was not only due to the presence of the product on the skin, but that there was a certain modification of the stratum corneum (SC) in its full thickness.

Another way of checking the efficacy of cosmetic products is to measure the viscoelastic properties of the SC in vivo. This is now possible using an apparatus known as the Twistometer. Figure 2 shows an example of the results obtained after repeated treatment for 24 days relative to the untreated contralateral arm in terms of elastic recovery (UR/UE) (4). This parameter decreases linearly with age (5) and is a component of skin "firmness."

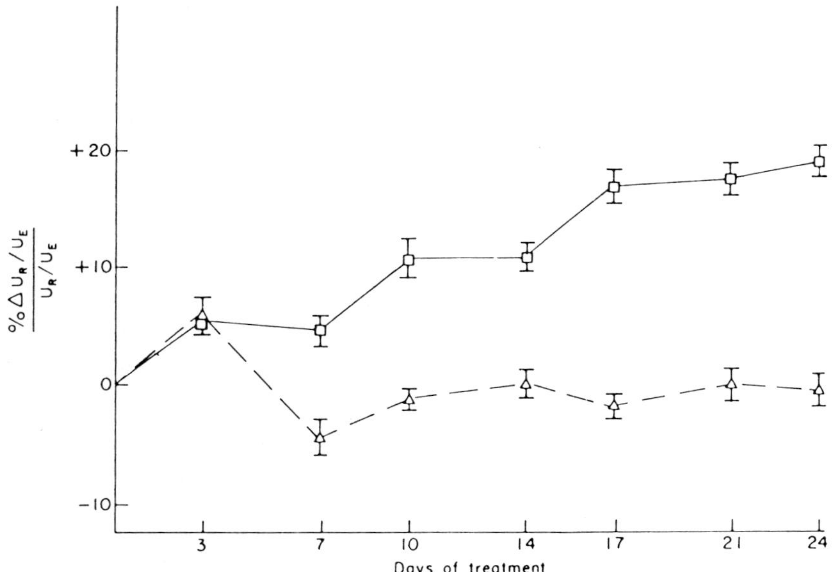

Figure 2 Effect of a cosmetic treatment on the elasticity of the skin (U_R/U_E). (Courtesy of Aubert et al., Ref. 4.)

The various techniques (conductance and measurement of mechanical parameters) do not all provide exactly the same type of information, and their joint use can help to optimize the efficacy of cosmetic preparations with respect to hydration (6). In general, there is an excellent correlation between the results of these methods and clinical evaluation by the specialist, although it is clear that the opinion of the volunteers is also necessary to predict the user's response (1). This triple experimental approach has enabled cosmetic products for dry skin to be developed, with proven efficacy before marketing.

B. Pigmentation and Microcirculation

Quantitative results concerning the efficacy of cosmetic products on these two parameters are far less abundant, even though a number of techniques exist (laser Doppler and photoplethysmography for microcirculation and portable colorimetry for skin color).

Figure 3 shows an example of the results one can obtain for comparison of various cosmetic products designed to treat dark skin spots (senile lentigo of the hands and face). Five groups of 25 elderly subjects applied a cream to one hand twice daily for 2 months; the other hand served as an untreated control. Color measurements *(L, a,* and b) were made at the beginning and end of the

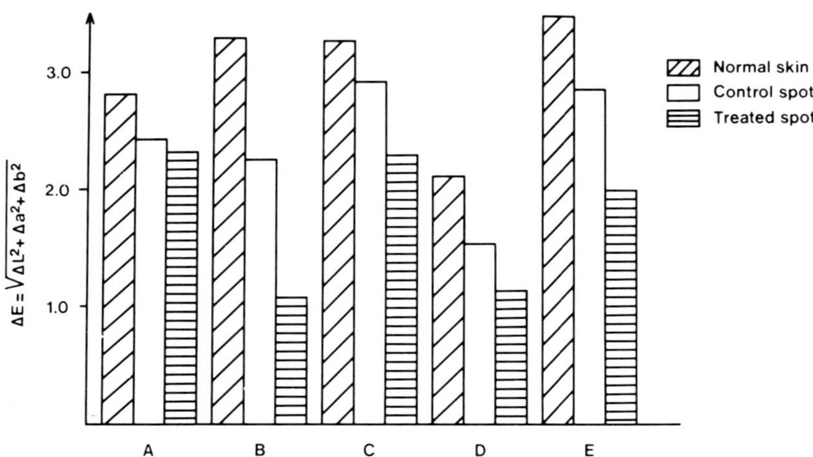

Figure 3 Comparative efficacy of five different cosmetic products on the depigmentation of actinic lentigo plaques on the hands of 125 volunteers. The intensity of the color $\Delta E = (\Delta L^2 + \Delta a^2 + \Delta b^2)^{1/2}$ was measured with a Minolta chromameter. The results for products B, D, and E are statistically significant. (Courtesy of C. Montastier, L'Oreal.)

treatment period. The statistical analysis, which took into account changes on the untreated hand, showed that products B, D, and E very significantly lightened the spots.

Certain cosmetic products can also improve skin complexion. Figure 4 shows typical results obtained after 6 months of treatment with such a preparation. The significant increase in parameter $a*$ reflects a certain degree of pinking.

More generally, the techniques used in the development of products active on the complexion are usually based on "psychosensory" methods and, thus, on questionnaires. Although they have become highly scientific and objective, these methods are not considered noninvasive and are therefore not discussed in this short review.

C. Antiwrinkle Products

There are at least two published studies concerning the efficacy of cosmetic preparations aimed at treating wrinkles. Using a profilometric method, Meybeck and Chanteloube (11) compared the effect of 14 different cosmetic products on the crow's-feet in a panel of 10–53 women.

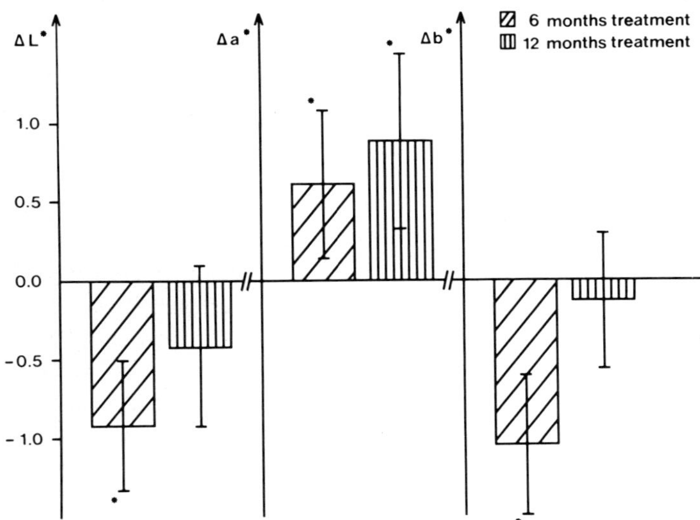

Figure 4 Effect of chronic application of a cosmetic product on the chromametric parameters of the cheek ($n = 32$). The asterisks correspond to statistically significant differences. (Courtesy of R. Bazin, L'Oreal.)

After 4 or 5 weeks of treatment, the improvement in the roughness parameters *Ra* and *Rz* ranged from 0 to 15% and was significant for the most active products (11). Similar results were obtained by Corcuff et al. (12), who used two different methods (profilometry and image analysis) to analyze the efficacy of a product applied for 4 weeks to the crow's-foot in 140 subjects. The profilometric method showed a reduction in mean line depth of 23% and in mean line density of 27%. Image analysis confirmed these results, although the reductions were slightly smaller (16% for both parameters). Although the data were highly significant ($p < 0.001$), a more detailed analysis showed that, despite an overall improvement in the number and depth of the lines, only the effect on deep lines was in fact significant because of a redistribution.

Given the kinetics of the treatment-related changes (4–6 weeks), they may well be accounted for by phenomena occurring in the epidermis. Figure 5 shows changes in crow's-foot wrinkles during long-term treatment with a cosmetic product.

III. EFFECT OF TOPICAL TRETINOIN TREATMENT

Over the past 5 years, there have been numerous reports concerning the efficacy of RA on the actinic aging of the human skin. Most have been descriptions of clinical effects or discussions of the biologic mechanism of action. With regard to publications concerning the clinical benefit of RA treatment, few have involved the use of noninvasive methods. The following concerns only those employing such methods.

A. Treatment of Dry Skin

Marks et al. observed a large increase in conductance after 7 days of treatment, but a similar effect was observed with the vehicle alone and no statistical difference could be shown because of the small number of subjects (7). Renal transplant recipients receiving oral steroid therapy showed an increase in skin conductance of about 20% after 180 days of treatment with 0.05% RA relative to the area treated with the excipient (8). There was also a 10% increase in skin elasticity. Using an indentation method, Berardesca et al. found a significant increase in skin elasticity in 18 subjects treated with 0.05% RA for 4 months (9), although no such improvement was found in other types of experiment based on longitudinal extension of the skin. For example, Marks et al. found no significant change in extensibility after 8 weeks of treatment with 0.05% RA (10).

In any event, the relatively small effects obtained with RA should be seen in the light of increases in the thickness of the various skin layers. Table 1 shows the data available in the relevant literature. RA-induced skin thickening is most marked at the level of the epidermis (about 30 μm) and is therefore best evaluated by means of histologic studies, even though at least three experiments based on ultrasound echography have been reported in which significant differences were obtained. Finally, it should be noted that transepidermal water loss increases after 3 months of treatment with 0.05% RA (13), although smaller values have been obtained by de Lacharriére et al. (14) after a 12 month treatment period. We consider that these data objectively illustrate the great improvement in skin smoothness and softness evidenced in the various clinical studies.

B. Pigmentation and Microcirculation

The main clinical effect of long-term treatment with RA-based creams on skin prematurely aged by exposure to sunlight is a clear improvement in color. This is particularly the case on the face, with marked lightening and evening of the color due to the removal of brown-pigmented spots; in addition, there is a slight but esthetically positive pinking. These phenomena are mainly due to three distinct properties of RA: a depigmenting action, a ''keratolytic'' effect (causing exfoliation of superficial corneocytes), and an angiogenic effect.

Published results on pigmentation have been derived only from clinical studies, which all tended to show a reduction in pigmentation leading to a lightening and evening of skin color.

With regard to the angiogenic effect, there have been at least two published studies based on noninvasive methods. Grove et al. showed in 1988 that the concentration of moving blood cells was enhanced in tretinoin-treated arms relative to contralateral controls (15). This study involved measurement of the microcirculatory response of the skin to a vasodilator, Trafuril®.

The effect of RA on the microcirculation has also been measured directly in terms of blood flow by means of the laser Doppler technique. After 8 weeks of treatment with a cream containing 0.05% RA, Marks et al. found a clear increase in blood flow, with values rising from 0.18 ± 0.19 to 0.35 ± 0.57 V (16). According to Marks, the effect was nonspecific, however, since treatment with a cream containing a simple abrasive gave similar results.

As in treatment with cosmetic products, data concerning skin complexion are somewhat disappointing in the light of most clinical results. This is probably because skin complexion is a far more complex notion than skin

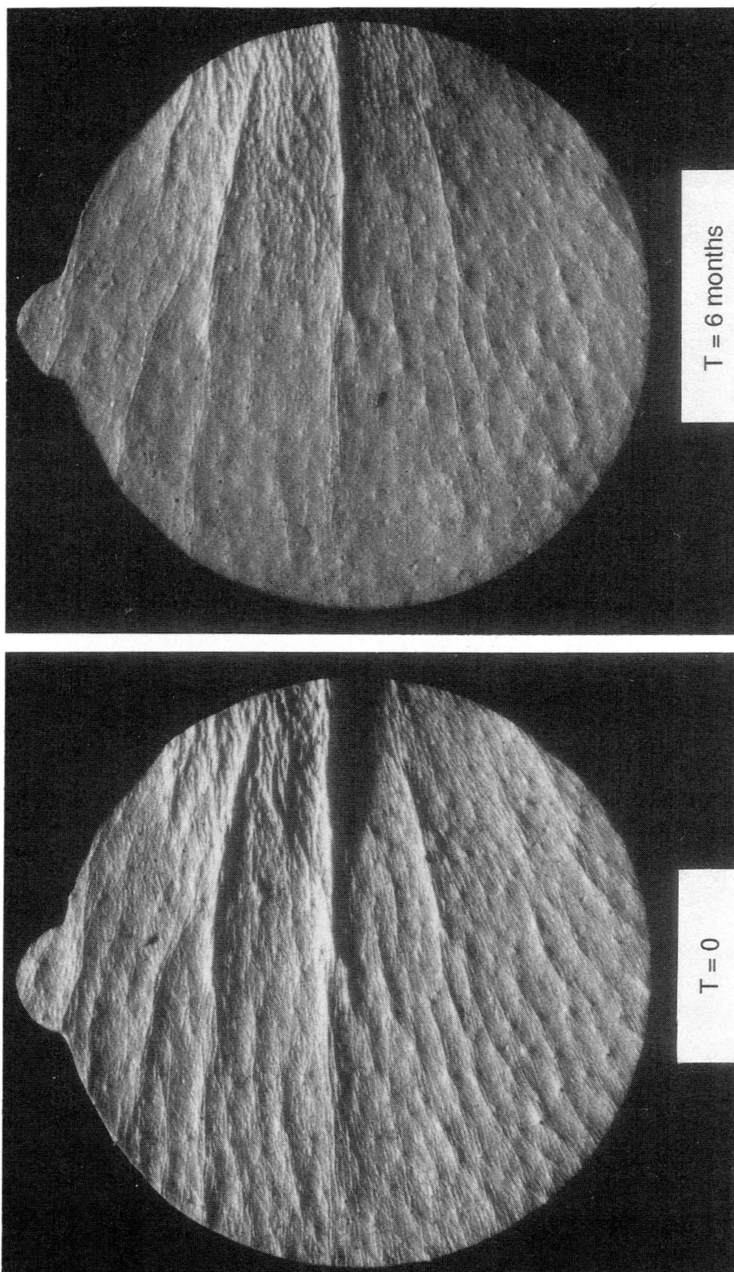
T = 6 months
T = 0

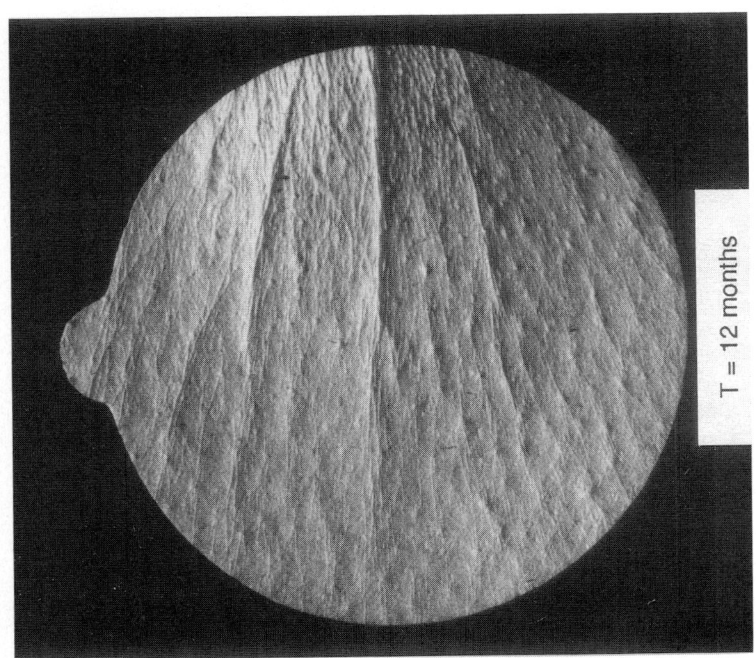

Figure 5 Effect of chronic treatment with an antiwrinkle cosmetic. This result is not representative of the overall group of volunteers. (Courtesy of R. Bazin, L'Oreal.)

Table 1 Literature Survey on the Effect of Retinoic Acid on Skin Thickness

Treatment	Technique	Site	Tissue	Thickness variation (%)	Reference
0.05%, 4 months	Ultrasound	Forearm	Total skin	NS	Berardesca et al. (9)
0.05%, 6 months	Ultrasound	Forearm	Total skin	4 ($p < 0.05$)	De Lacharrière et al. (8)
0.05%, 3 months	Histology	Forearm	Epidermis	40 significant	Kligman et al.(13)
0.05%, 8 weeks	Ultrasound	Forearm	Total skin	14 ($p < 0.05$)	Marks et al. (10)
0.05–0.1%, 22 months	Histology	Forearm	Epidermis	~50 (significant)	Ellis et al. (19)
0.05%, 12 weeks	Ultrasound	Forearm	Total skin	12 ($p = 0.005$)	Lever et al. (20)
	Histology	Forearm	Epidermis	28 ($p = 0.019$)	
0.025%, 21 days	Histology	Forearm	Epidermis	30 significant	Marks et al. (7)
	Ultrasound	Forearm	Total skin	NS	
0.1%, 16 weeks	Histology	Forearm	Epidermis	270 ($p = 0.02$)	Weiss et al. (21)
			Granular layer	110 $p < 0.01$	
			Dermis	50 NS	
0.01%, 24 weeks	Histology	Crow's-feet	Epidermis	26 <0.001	Weinstein et al. (22)
0.05%,24 weeks	Histology	Crow's-feet	Epidermis	33 < 0.001	
0.001%, 24 weeks	Histology	Crow's-feet	Epidermis	NS	Bhawan et al. (23)
0.01%, 24 weeks				17	
0.05%, 24 weeks				18	

surface color, which can be measured simply using commercially available equipment.

C. Problems Concerning Wrinkles

The data in the literature appear to agree that long-term treatment of wrinkles with RA leads to a decrease in depth and number of thin lines. In general, this is supported by clinical data, which are often confirmed by the volunteers' personal appreciation. It should be mentioned that the relevant publications can include highly spectacular photographs, which are probably not representative of the average case.

There are, however, a number of published results obtained using noninvasive methods. Using a profilometric technique to study replicas of crow's feet, Caputo et al. reported decreases in Rt, Ra, and Rz of 10, 15, and 16% following 6 months of treatment with a cream containing 0.05% RA (the concentration being progressively increased) (17). For their part, Grove et al. developed a special method called optical profilometry (18) and studied the effect of a cream containing 0.05% RA on volunteers after 24 weeks of treatment. The areas examined were crow's feet and the cheek. The results differed according to whether the profilometric measurement was made vertically or horizontally. The parameters Ra and Rz (the mean roughness and the mean of the maxima for each line, respectively), fell by 10–20% on the cheek (according to the measurement axis) and from 0 to 10% on crow's feet; both results were statistically significant. The values obtained on the contralateral sites (treated with the excipient alone) varied between 10 and −5%.

These improvements may appear slight compared to the clinical data, but it should be borne in mind that they are mean values taking into account both large wrinkles (little affected by the treatment) and small lines.

IV. Conclusion

Noninvasive methods have developed rapidly over the last two decades, and most cutaneous parameters can now be measured directly. Such techniques are not used by all the teams working in this area, however, and this is probably one of the reasons that objective data on the efficacy of drugs and cosmetics are still so few and far between. However, it is now clear that products are available that improve the state of the elderly skin, even though the ideal preparation, that is, one that would eliminate all wrinkles and lines, does not exist. Work triggered by studies of the effects of topical RA relative to its excipient (which may itself be an excellent cosmetic) has enabled a number of dermatologists to agree on the relative efficacy of a number of cosmetic preparations (Fig. 5).

The wide variability in the responses of a given population to a given treatment remains a major problem. All those involved in such studies know that spectacular results can be obtained in some subjects, despite only moderate efficacy in the overall group (Fig. 6).

Finally, with regard to noninvasive methods, it should be emphasized that the efficacy data obtained in experiments with RA are less impressive than those derived from subjective clinical observations. This is partly because clinical studies generally concern the face and noninvasive methods concern the forearm. The differences between these two sites, together with the sometimes significant effect of the excipient (used as a control), suggest that comparative studies of new active agents should involve the two sides of the face.

Given the small number of published studies of the efficacy of topical treatments for aged skin based on noninvasive methods, it appears difficult to compare the efficacy of RA-based treatments with that of cosmetic preparations. On the one hand, the nature of the products used is different; on the other hand, the conditions of application, the frequency, and the compliance are also different. RA-based preparations are drug products aimed at treating a particular form of aging (actinic aging). They are relatively irritant and

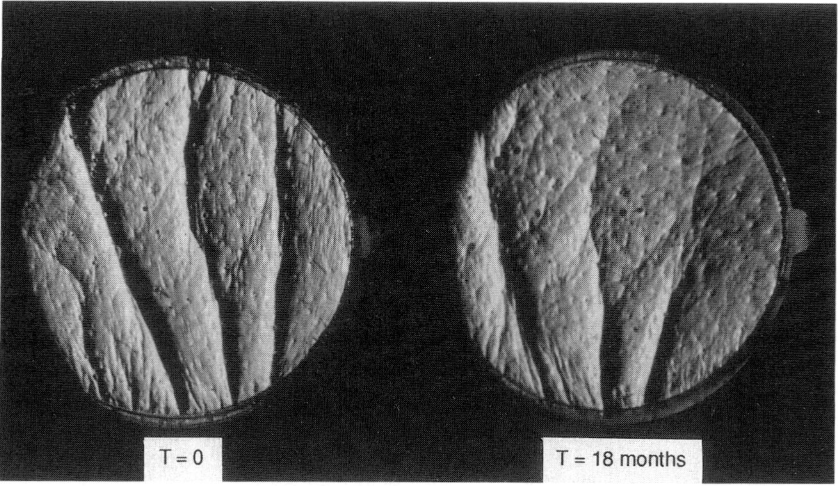

Figure 6 Effect of chronic treatment (18 months) with a retinoic acid preparation (0.05%) on the crow's-foot of a volunteer. Again, the result is not representative of the overall group of volunteers.

should be applied under medical control; they induce a clear cosmetic benefit, but this is slow to appear. The effects in terms of hydration, wrinkles, and pigmentation are generally best evaluated globally following at least 6 months of treatment.

Many cosmetic preparations are designed and formulated for specific problems in given areas of skin and for different skin types. Their efficacy and claimed effects vary, but most are well tolerated. The results of noninvasive methods now suggest that, for a given problem (dry skin or wrinkles or pigmentation), certain preparations have objective efficacy close to that of retinoic acid-based products.

REFERENCES

1. Grove G. Design of studies to measure skin care product performance. Bioeng Skin 1987; 3:359–73.
2. Prall JK, Theiler RF, Bowser PA, Walsh M. The effectiveness of cosmetic products in alleviating a range of skin dryness conditions as determined by clinical and instrumental techniques. Int J Cosmet Sci 1986; 8:159–74.
3. Lévêque JL, de Rigal J. Impedance methods for studying skin moisturization. J Soc Cosmet Chem 1983; 34:419–26.
4. Aubert L, Anthoine P, de Rigal J, Lévêque JL. An in vivo assessment of the biomechanical properties of human skin modifications under the influence of cosmetic products. Int J Cosmet Sci 1985; 7:51–9.
5. Escoffier C, De Rigal J, Rochefort A, Vasselet R, Lévêque JL, Agache P. Age related mechanical properties of human skin: an in vivo study. J Invest Dermatol 1989; 93:353–7.
6. Lévêque JL, Aubert A. Methodes d'étude du pouvoir hydratant des cosmétiques. J Med Esth et 1987; 54:117–22.
7. Marks R, Black D, Pearse AD, Hill S. Techniques for assessing the activity of topically applied retinoids. J Am Acad Dermatol 1986; 4:810–6.
8. De Lacharrière O, Escoffier C, Gracia AM, et al. Reversal effects of topical retinoic acid on the skin of kidney transplant recipients under sytemic corticotherapy. J Invest Dermatol 1990; 95:516–22.
9. Berardesca E, Gabba P, Farinelli N, Borroni G, Rabbiosi G. In vivo tretinoin-induced changes in skin mechanical properties. Br J Dermatol 1990; 122:525–9.
10. Marks R, Hill S, Barton SP. The effects of an abrasive agent on normal skin and photoaged skin in comparison with topical tretinoin. Br J Dermatol 1990; 123:457–66.
11. Meybeck A, Chanteloube F. Cosmetic wrinkle smoothing. In: Morganti P, Montagna W, eds. (A new look at old skin.) Int. Ediemme, 1986; 243–59.
12. Corcuff P, Chatenay F, Brun A. Evaluation of anti-wrinkle effects on humans. Int J Cosmet Sci 1985; 7:117–26.

13. Kligman AM, Grove GL, Hirose R, Leyden JJ. Topical tretinoin for photoaged skin. J Am Acad Dermatol 1986; 15:836–58.

14. De Lacharriére O, Escoffier C, Teillac D, et al. Reversal effects of systemic corticotherapy by topical tretinoin in grafted kidney patients. In Reichert U, Shroot B, edrs. Pharmacology of retinoids in the skin, vol. 3. Basel: Karger 1989; 259–62.

15. Grove GL, Grove MJ, Zerweck CR, Leyden JJ. Determination of topical tretinoin effects on cutaneous microcirculation in photoaged skin by laser Doppler velocimetry. J Cut Aging Cosmet Dermatol 1988; 1:27–32.

16. Marks R. Methods for the assessment of the effects of topical retinoic acid in photoaging and actinic keratoses. J Int Med Res 1990; 18:29–34.

17. Caputo R, Monti M, Motta S, et al. The treatment of visible signs of senescence; the Italian experience. Br J Dermatol 1990; 35:97–103.

18. Grove GL, Grove MJ, Leyden JJ, et al. Skin replica analysis of photodamaged skin after therapy with tretinoin emollient cream. J Am Acad Dermatol 1991; 25:231–7.

19. Ellis CN, Weiss JS, Hamilton TA, Headington JT, Zelickson AS, Vorhees JJ. Sustained improvement with prolonged topical tretinoin for photoaged skin. J Am Acad Dermatol 1990; 23:629–37.

20. Lever L, Kumar P, Marks R. Topical retinoic acid for treatment of solar damage. Br J Dermatol 1990; 122:91–8.

21. Weiss JS, Ellis C, Headington JT, Tincoff T, Hamilton TA, Vorhees JJ. Topical tretinoin improves photoaged skin. JAMA 1988; 259:527–32.

22. Weinstein GD, Nigra TP, Pochi PE, et al. Topical tretinoin for treatment of photodamaged skin. Arch Dermatol 1991; 127:659–65.

23. Bhawan J, Gonzalez-Serva A, Nehal K, et al. Effects of tretinoin on photoaged skin. Arch Dermatol 1991; 127:666–72.

Index

About the Editors

Jean-Luc Lévêque is Director of the Biophysics Department in the Basic Research Laboratories of L'Oréal in Aulnay-sous-Bois, France, where he has served since 1969. His research interests include the measurement of the skin's biophysical properties, and in particular the effects of age, sun, cosmetics, and drugs on the skin. The editor of *Cutaneous Investigation in Health and Disease: Noninvasive Methods and Instrumentation* (Marcel Dekker, Inc.), the author or coauthor of more than 100 professional papers, and the holder of several patents, he is a member of the International Society for Bioengineering and the Skin, the American Academy of Dermatology, the French Society of Cosmetic Chemists, and the French Society for Dermatological Research. Dr. Lévêque received the Doctorat es Sciences degree in physics from the University of Grenoble, France.

Pierre Agache is Professor of Dermatology and Venerology at the University of Besançon, France, and Head of the Dermatology Department at the University Hospital Center, Besançon. The author of numerous professional papers, he is a former President of the French Society of Dermatology and Venereology and a member of the French College of Vascular Pathology, the International Society for Bioengineering and the Skin, the European Society for Dermatological Research, and the British Association of Dermatologists, among other organizations. Dr. Agache received the M.D. degree (1958) from the University of Lille I, Villeneuve d'Ascq, France.